FETAL ALCOHOL
ABUSE SYNDROME

FETAL ALCOHOL ABUSE SYNDROME

Ernest L. Abel

Wayne State University School of Medicine
Detroit, Michigan

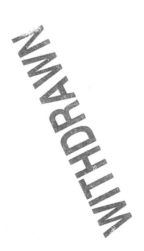

PLENUM PRESS • NEW YORK AND LONDON

Library of Congress Cataloging-in-Publication Data

Abel, Ernest L., 1943-
    Fetal alcohol abuse syndrome / Ernest L. Abel.
        p.   cm.
    Includes bibliographical references and index.
    ISBN 0-306-45666-4
    1. Fetal alcohol syndrome.   I. Title.
    [DNLM: 1. Fetal Alcohol Syndrome.   WQ 211 A139fb 1998]
    RG629.F45A317   1998
    618.3'268--dc21
    DNLM/DLC
    for Library of Congress   98-26505
                                                                    CIP

ISBN 0-306-45666-4

© 1998 Plenum Press, New York
A Division of Plenum Publishing Corporation
233 Spring Street, New York, N.Y. 10013

http://www.plenum.com

Printed in the United States of America

Preface

My initial purpose in writing this book was to offer readers an update of my book *Fetal Alcohol Syndrome and Fetal Alcohol Effects* (Plenum, 1984), which contained a broad overview of the history (actually the absence of any history) of the awareness of alcohol's teratogenic potential; a review of alcohol's pharmacology, especially with respect to pregnancy; a survey of the physical and behavioral effects of prenatal alcohol exposure; and an overview of the mechanisms suspected of being responsible for those effects.

I have omitted most of the previously examined historical and pharmacological information because not much of what was previously discussed needed revision. On the other hand, because much more has been learned about the consequences of prenatal alcohol exposure and its potential mechanisms of action, I have considerably expanded my discussion of these topics. In doing so, I have attempted to include as much new material as possible without (I hope) being overly pedantic and thereby losing the proverbial forest for the trees.

No book is ever entirely neutral in the topics it discusses, the issues it raises, or in its conclusions. In sifting through hundreds and oftentimes thousands of articles, writers have to choose which facts to emphasize and which to ignore. Every idea cannot be chronicled and every article cannot (and should not) be cited. In going about the business of picking and choosing, however, a writer has an obligation to present the arguments for and against a particular conclusion. Readers may disagree with the topics I have chosen or my conclusions, but at least they have been presented with the facts and the reasoning behind them.

That said, it is now time to express my sincerest appreciation to my colleagues who read and provided detailed comments and criticisms on various chapters in the book. In many cases, those comments allowed me to fine tune issues that were otherwise unfocused or revise weak and abstruse arguments. Those to whom I owe a special debt of appreciation for their corrections and viewpoints, many of which often differ from my own, are Robert Berman, Michael Church, Claire Coles, Stan Fisher, Zehava Gottesfeld, John Hannigan, Chris Loock, and Michael Kruger. I would also like to express my appreciation to Rebecca Goodemoot and Myra Meredith for their secretarial assistance, and Marlene Visconti for editorial comments.

Contents

Introduction

When I decided to write the present book, I promised my editor that I would have
it to him within a year. I underestimated my commitment. Instead of one year, it
has taken me three, mainly because I was unable to reconcile the many contradictions and the new ideas that now characterize this literature. A mere listing of the
references I had cited in my earlier drafts ran to over 100 pages!

As I continued trying to make sense of all this information, it seemed to me
that what was needed was less of a cataloging of effects and ideas and more of a
reconciliation and interpretation of these facts. Let me explain.

While my purpose remains that of informing readers about the latest findings
concerning the impact of FAS on the individual and society, our understanding of
these issues has broadened. At the same time, our knowledge base has become
confusing with respect to the effects of "moderate" drinking and the related issue
of "safe levels of drinking." A new diagnostic paradigm—implying that some
children previously identified as having fetal alcohol syndrome may have been
misdiagnosed and vice-versa—has been proposed. Questions have been raised as
to whether the related diagnosis of "fetal alcohol effect" should be jettisoned, and
so on.

Bothered by the many contradictions raised by these and related issues, I
began searching for a clarifying principle to bring some coherence to these issues.
In doing so, I was reminded of the Greek poet Archilochus's maxim: "The fox
knows many things, the hedgehog knows but one big thing."

Several years ago, Sir Isaiah Berlin (1957), one of this century's most
eminent philosophers, called on Archilochus to explain the two basic ways people
go about trying to make sense of their worlds:

> There exists a great chasm between those, on the one side (the hedgehogs), who relate
> everything to single central vision ... a single universal organizing principle in terms of
> which alone all that they are and say has significance—and, on the other side (the

foxes), those who pursue many ends, often unrelated and often contradictory, connected, if at all, only in some de facto way.

When it comes to the growing list of birth effects attributed to prenatal alcohol exposure, especially to what has in the past been called "fetal alcohol syndrome," I confess to being both a hedgehog and a fox. (This, of course, makes me a fox despite my avowed duality.)

My "hedgehoginess" comes from my first organizing principle, which I argue throughout this book, that all of the effects attributed to maternal drinking during pregnancy are due to binge drinking—and especially alcohol abuse—during pregnancy. In this regard, I am but following the argument made by many others in the alcoholism field, most forcefully by Knupfer (1987a), who succinctly stated her view as follows:

> A great deal of time and money is currently spent interviewing light drinkers and abstainers, while those who drink enough to be of interest are lumped together in a vast, heterogenous category of "heavier" drinkers. A more detailed study of heavier drinkers would enable us, for one thing, to arrive at a better idea of what we are talking about when we speak of "problem drinkers."

Knupfer also commented that researchers vary considerably in how they define "heavy" drinking, an issue also explored in the present book. I prefer to label the kind of drinking Knupfer says leads to "problem drinking," and what I propose leads to alcohol-related birth effects, as *heavy* drinking rather than *binge* drinking or *alcohol abuse*. By heavy drinking, I mean drinking that results in a blood alcohol level of 0.15 g% or above at least once a week but, in fact, is usually much higher. Alcohol abuse refers to drinking this amount more than once a week. All the effects experimentally attributed to *moderate, social, occasional,* or whatever other term is used to reflect the kind of behavior the overwhelming majority of drinkers engage in during pregnancy, I contend are due to the artifice of "lumping" the children of alcohol abusers in with the children of these latter drinkers. Although this conclusion will undoubtedly raise hackles on the part of those who for some time have been arguing that their research puts them totally at odds with any such conclusion, I ask forbearance until they have considered my arguments.

My "foxiness" comes from the fact that although alcohol abuse during pregnancy is the "necessary" cause of birth effects, it alone is not sufficient to cause these effects. Just as relatively few alcoholics develop liver cirrhosis, relatively few alcoholics have children with fetal alcohol syndrome. Knupfer (1987a) likewise has asked "why, among really heavy drinkers—those, for example who drink enough to get inebriated several times a week—some seem not to experience or cause any trouble and have no regrets about their way of life." These being the case, foxiness demands we expand our search for the causes of this disorder rather than remain narrowly focused on *the* cause.

In keeping with the hedgehoginess side of my character, I have, as Professor Berlin so adroitly put it, "related everything to (my) single central vision" and have built my presentation around the "universal organizing principle" that the main cause of alcohol-related birth effects, such as "fetal alcohol syndrome," is related to the kind of heavy drinking associated with alcohol abuse. Accordingly, Chapter 1 argues the merits of replacing the current term *fetal alcohol syndrome* with the more descriptively appropriate *fetal alcohol abuse syndrome*.

In calling this birth effect caused by alcohol abuse "fetal alcohol abuse syndrome," rather than "fetal alcohol syndrome," I am not simply suggesting a difference without a distinction. Because words represent articulated thought–if all one has to go by is a name—then that name (and the thought behind it) ought to be more explicit, especially when that thought directs clinical practice. Because "fetal alcohol syndrome" conveys a message about alcohol and not alcohol abuse, one of my reasons for "revisiting" the concept behind fetal alcohol syndrome is to argue it ought to be renamed, and that the implications of such a name change must be considered. I believe that the arguments presented in Chapter 1 are persuasive, and in anticipation of those arguments, when the acronym FAS is encountered, it should be regarded as standing for "fetal alcohol abuse syndrome" unless the context demands otherwise.

Chapter 2 proceeds to an examination of the criteria by which FAS has been diagnosed in the past and then considers the new diagnostic paradigm developed by the Institute of Medicine (IOM). Although FAS refers to a pattern of anomalies that occur in children born to alcoholics, until recently, maternal alcohol abuse was not considered in the formal criteria used in diagnosing the syndrome. In part, this was an attempt to keep the diagnosis objective—the idea being that if a diagnostician knew a mother were an alcohol abuser, that information would bias his or her diagnosis in favor of FAS even before that woman's child was seen. However, the features associated with FAS, and especially "alcohol abuse-related birth effects" (which I will discuss momentarily), are often difficult to discern and come down to an educated opinion. The more information a diagnostician has about a mother's drinking behavior during pregnancy, the more confidence he or she can put in that opinion. Because diagnosis is at the heart of FAS treatment, research, and prevention, clinicians and biomedical researchers have to agree on the criteria for a particular disorder. The various paradigms currently used for identifying individuals with FAS in detail, including an in-depth examination of the newly revised set of criteria recently proposed by the Institute of Medicine, are examined in Chapter 2.

Closely related to the diagnostic conundrum is the equally enigmatic problem of identifying individuals with partial expression of the syndrome, a condition that, until recently, has been referred to as *fetal alcohol effects* or alcohol-related birth defects. Like FAS, these two terms are also undergoing revision, albeit in this case, some clinicians have recommended the former be dropped from the clinical lexicon entirely. The rationales for discarding and retaining these concepts in conjunction with the more global issue of diagnosis are discussed in Chapter 2. The discussion about terminology segues into the next 8 chapters that survey the profusion of effects currently attributed to prenatal alcohol exposure, which I collectively refer to throughout this book as *alcohol-abuse-related birth effects* (*ARBEs*). In addition to reviewing much of this vast literature, the knotty questions mentioned earlier regarding the extent to which these effects occur as partial expressions of the syndrome or alternatively as the consequences of lower levels of alcohol exposure, are examined.

Following this detailed examination of ARBEs, Chapter 11, "The American Paradox," introduces the foxiness aspect of these disorders by comparing the incidence of FAS in different countries with that in different parts of the United States. On the basis of this comparison, risk factors are identified that increase/decrease vulnerability for the disorder.

Chapter 12, "Permissive and Provocative Factors in FAS," develops the theme of alcohol as a necessary but not sufficient cause of FAS/ARBEs. Researchers have known this for some time but until recently have been reluctant to articulate this fact. The Institute of Medicine's (IOM) recent report on FAS, however, clearly stated:

> While alcohol is the necessary teratogen, it alone may not be sufficient to produce FAS in humans or birth defects in animals. As with most teratogens, not every fetus exposed to significant amounts of alcohol is affected. The outcomes might be modulated by numerous biologic and environmental factors. (IOM, 1996, p. 20)

Although epidemiological studies have provided us with considerable information about these environmental conditions, in many instances these studies have stopped short of explaining how these conditions attenuate or exacerbate them.

Chapter 12 examines the most important of these environmental factors and explains how they may "modulate" the outcome of in utero alcohol exposure. In doing so, it takes as its starting point associations known to affect the outcome of in utero alcohol exposure and relates them to changes in the biological milieu that increase or decrease vulnerability to alcohol's toxic effects. Unless these associations can be related to the broader context of biological "mechanisms of action," epidemiological research aimed at uncovering such associations will appear to have no apparent purpose beyond that of accumulating data simply for the sake of data accumulation.

Chapter 13 turns to a discussion of potential mechanisms through which alcohol causes ARBEs and relies on examples from the previous chapter to illustrate those mechanisms that I argue have the best heuristic potential for generating new ideas with respect to treatment and prevention.

Chapter 14 provides a broad overview of the earlier chapters and offers "conclusions and implications" about issues mentioned in those chapters.

CHAPTER 1

Why Fetal Alcohol Abuse Syndrome?

About three days after a human egg is fertilized, it passes through the fallopian tunnel and reaches the uterus, where it spends about four days floating in the uterus's fluids, after which it begins to implant itself into the uterine wall. By the 12th day, it is completely embedded. Prior to implantation, the embryo draws on its own reserves and those present in the fluids of the fallopian tube and uterus for sustenance. Other substances, like alcohol, may be present in these fluids, but there is little evidence these foreign substances adversely influence embryonic development.

After implantation, the embryo begins receiving nutrients—and alcohol if it is present—from the maternal circulation. Various organs of the body begin forming and become functional, following a cascade of cellular events involving their genesis, proliferation, adhesion, migration, differentiation, growth, connections with one another, death, and reconnections among the survivors.

Structural organization occurs during discrete "critical periods" of development called *organogenesis*. In humans, with their 260–280-day gestation period, organogenesis lasts from about gestation day 20 to day 55. In the rat, which has a 21-day gestation period, it starts on day 9 and ends on day 17.

The principle of *critical periods* is the cornerstone of teratology (the science of "birth defects"). The essence of this principle is that an agent can only cause a malformation if encountered during organogenesis, when cell groups and tissues are forming into organs. Although every other principle in teratology is shared by other disciplines (like pharmacology or toxicology), this principle applies only to teratology. It explains why developing organisms have unique responses to foreign substances, responses that are never observed in adults. If an agent such as alcohol, for example, is found to cause a structural abnormality, exposure could only have occurred during organogenesis.

The most dramatic example of this critical periods principle is the thalidomide

5

tragedy of the 1960s. Only mothers who took the drug after being 34-days pregnant and before they were 50-days pregnant gave birth to children with missing limbs or damaged organs. Children exposed on gestation days 34–37 were born with duplicated thumbs; those exposed on gestation days 38–43 had abnormal ears, kidney defects, shortened arms, and urogenital and respiratory defects. Those exposed after organogenesis had no abnormal limbs or organs.

Malformations, however, are not the only response to foreign substances. If exposure occurs during the latter phases of gestation, these substances can kill cells, interfere with cellular growth, and/or interfere with growth of specific cells, so that fine-tuning events whereby organs develop their functional capacity are compromised. The discipline devoted to these kinds of functional birth defects is called *behavioral teratology*, to distinguish it from the more traditional teratology, which focuses on structural damage.

Behavioral and cognitive dysfunction are among the most common consequences of exposure to substances such as alcohol because the actions of these substances are not confined to any critical period. The brain continues to fine-tune itself throughout gestation and beyond. When finally developed, the brain's 1,400 cubic centimeters contains several hundred different cell types, each with their own distinctive morphological, physiological and biochemical characteristics— about 15 billion nerve cells in all. Because all of these cells come into existence during the first 12 weeks of life, the developing brain must produce about 150,000 of them a minute! If this first "growth spurt" is interfered with, it may result in malformations, microcephaly, or in a normal-sized brain with decreased cells in a particular area, such as the corpus callosum or cerebellum. A second growth spurt begins in the final two months before birth. Because all of the brain's neurons have been formed during organogenesis, this latter growth period reflects increases in the size of individual neurons and changes in their shapes, for example, sprouting of axons and dendrites or myelination of axons. Final maturation does not end until the second year of life. These latter cellular refinements underlie the brain's unique functional abilities. If exposure to toxic levels of alcohol occurs during this second growth spurt, children may develop behavioral and cognitive disorders even though their brains are normal in size.

A pregnant woman who drinks every day and exposes her unborn child to toxic doses of alcohol during periods of cell proliferation and growth creates the potential for a syndrome related to such exposure to occur in her unborn child. In this context, the term *syndrome*, refers to a pattern of similarly occurring anomalies in most patients. In this regard, it is not very different from the way in which the term disease is often understood.

In contrast to the woman who consumes toxic amounts of alcohol throughout pregnancy, a woman who consumes toxic amounts in sporadic binges will expose her child during fewer days of pregnancy, and, therefore, her child is more likely to exhibit individual anomalies than a syndrome. Based on the principle of critical periods, it follows that malformations involving the face or bodily organs can arise if toxic exposures occur during the first trimester of pregnancy, when the proliferative stage of cell development occurs. Exposure during the last trimester cannot give rise to malformations because the proliferative stage is over. However, exposure during this last period could result in decreased overall growth or decreased growth of specific organs. There is no "safe time" for toxic levels of exposure during pregnancy because dynamic changes occur throughout gestation.

What's in a Name?

When Drs. Ken Jones and David Smith, the dysmorphologists (physicians specially trained in the identification of birth defects), christened the pattern of anomalies they observed in children born to alcoholic women *fetal alcohol syndrome (FAS)* (Jones & Smith, 1973, p. 999), their label did more to bring this birth defect to international attention than anything else they could have called it. Their term, however, is misleading because it implies that any amount of drinking is toxic. Instead, as they clearly stated, the pattern of anomalies comprising the syndrome only occur in children born to alcohol-abusing mothers:

> Eight unrelated children of three different ethnic groups, all raised in the fetal environment provided by an *alcoholic* mother, had a similar pattern of craniofacial, limb, and cardiovascular defects with prenatal-onset growth deficiency and developmental delay (Jones & Smith), 1973, p. 1270; italics added).

Because it was not alcohol per se but its abuse that led to the pattern of anomalies, *fetal alcohol abuse syndrome* would have been then, and still is, sui generis, more apt than fetal alcohol syndrome.

Making this distinction is not merely persiflage. In Michigan, one third of the more than 500 obstetricians, pediatricians, and general practitioners who responded to a 1996 questionnaire about fetal alcohol syndrome stated that the syndrome could result from consumption of as little as one drink a day (Abel & Kruger, 1998), despite the fact there isn't a single instance in the hundreds of case reports and clinical studies in which the syndrome has been found in which the mother was not an alcoholic. Dr. Hans-Ludwig Spohr, whose clinical experience with this disorder spans several decades, commented that whereas clinicians were once skeptical a condition such as fetal alcohol syndrome even existed, this skepticism has given way to glib diagnoses: "When FAS was first detected, paediatricians didn't believe it was a specific syndrome. Now they start to make a diagnosis by association.... They see a 'funny-looking' child, they have heard about FAS, and *if somebody says the mother is drinking, they make the diagnosis*" (Spohr, 1984, p. 153; italics added). Dr. Jo Nanson had a similar experience working with aboriginal children in Canada. If one of these children has an unusual appearance, she said, and "*a mother who drank at all during pregnancy*, (she) receives a very glib diagnosis of fetal alcohol syndrome by primary care physicians" (Nanson, personal communication, 1995; italics added). Needless to say, the result of these glib diagnoses is that these children could very well receive inappropriate treatment or no treatment at all.

The simple fact is that the term fetal alcohol syndrome has created such a false impression that large numbers of clinicians now believe even minimal amounts of alcohol consumption during pregnancy can produce the syndrome. Because no cases of this syndrome have ever been found outside the context of alcohol abuse, renaming it fetal alcohol abuse syndrome should, at the very least, preclude the kind of glib diagnosis Spohr and Nanson alluded to and the kind of error the survey of physicians uncovered. More importantly, it should also keep many children from being misdiagnosed and receiving treatment, if any, for a condition they do not have.

The mistaken impression that minimal amounts of alcohol can cause individual anomalies is also rampant. Individual anomalies resulting from alcohol toxicity in utero were initially called "possible fetal alcohol effects." The "possible" was subsequently dropped and, like fetal alcohol syndrome, the term *fetal alcohol effect* (*FAE*) took on a life of its own (Aase, 1994).

In some instances, fetal alcohol effect began and continued to be used to imply an attenuated severity of FAS (Aase, 1994). A related term, *alcohol-related birth defect* (*ARBD*), also began to be used to denote a less severe form of FAS (Aase, 1994). However, people with FAEs or ARBDs did not differ from those with FAS when individual anomalies were compared (Streissguth, LaDue, & Randelsk, 1987). In other words, the damage to a particular area of the body is the same whether it occurs as a singular anomaly or as a component of a pattern of anomalies. The incorrect use of these terms to designate less severe forms of FAS, along with their indiscriminate use as in clinical diagnoses, has prompted three leading dysmorphologists to recommend that FAE and ARBD no longer be applied to individual patients (Aase, Jones, & Clarren, 1995).

This recommendation does not mean FAEs or ARBDs do not exist, or that the concept of individual anomalies has no validity. If children or animals prenatally exposed to toxic amounts of alcohol as a group have a higher prevalence of anomalies than a comparable group of children or animals not so exposed, it is reasonable to refer to these differences as fetal alcohol effects or alcohol-related birth defects (Aase et al., 1995), If, however, as I will argue momentarily, it is alcohol abuse rather than simply alcohol that is responsible for these abnormalities, then it is even more reasonable to refer to them as *fetal alcohol abuse effects.*

A More Realistic Relationship

If all that were at stake in revisiting alcohol's prenatal effects were a name change, there would be little reason to go beyond conceding that fetal alcohol syndrome does not encapsulate the true etiology of the disorder. However (as Chapters 3–10 indicate), in the last ten years, a hodgepodge of studies have appeared which are seemingly in conflict with one another as to alcohol's involvement in spontaneous abortion, low birth weight, cognitive dysfunction, and so on. Although the role of alcohol abuse in producing such effects is recognized, the role of relatively low levels of consumption is far less consistent, and the conclusion that low levels of drinking produce these effects as well, albeit to a lesser degree, is far less convincing.

Low dose-effects would be possible if teratological effects were conceived in terms of a monotonic dose-response relationship with the etiological agent. But there are no monotonic dose-response relationships in teratology or pharmacology. Instead, every substance has a "threshold" or *no observable effect level* (*NOEL*) for every response (Hutchings, 1985). In teratology, dose-response relationships are generally "S" shaped—at relatively low doses, there is no observable effect. If the dose is increased, a threshold is exceeded and an effect is triggered. Relatively small increments above that threshold trigger larger effects, until every response capable of being affected is affected and the organism is either severely disturbed or killed.

In other words, just because alcohol is present in the system does not mean it will have an effect. The reason monotonic relationships between alcohol and an effect are sometimes found is that these relationships are products of an artifact inherent in the way drinking behavior is often characterized or in the way data are analyzed.

Some people drink every day; others drink only during the weekends. Some people consume no more than one or two drinks when they drink; others consume considerably greater amounts per drinking occasion. Because there are no reliable "biological markers" for alcohol consumption, clinicians and researchers have to rely on what their patients-subjects tell them about their drinking habits.

Leaving aside the problem of inaccuracies associated with self-reports (see Ernhart, 1991), researchers interested in alcohol's effects need a way to categorize drinking behavior. The simplest way of doing so is to ask people how much they drink during a typical week or month and then divide this amount by the appropriate number of days to arrive at an average number of drinks per day. Since a typical drink contains about 0.5 ounces of alcohol, this can also be expressed as average ounces or absolute alcohol (AA) per day, or AA/day. Inferences about the relationship between birth defects and alcohol consumption are then typically examined in terms of this *average* number of drinks or ounces per day.

Like all measures that attempt to simplify complex behavior, the average drinks index is a proverbial wolf in sheep's clothing—the wolf is there ready to pounce, but you can't see it. For example, the woman who consumes seven glasses of wine each Saturday night gets treated in the same way as the woman who drinks one glass a night every night, including Saturday. Both average one glass of wine per day, but their drinking patterns are very different.

Another reason many studies evaluating alcohol's in utero effects have led to erroneous inferences with respect to thresholds stems from their use of correlational analyses, such as multiple regression or partial least squares. These kinds of statistical analyses can lead to misleading conclusions because they do not include any provision for threshold levels below which alcohol has no effect. Instead, these tests assume linear relationships between dose and effect, thereby discounting the relatively greater impact on the study of the most heavily exposed children. Despite such assumptions, these tests are then used to make inferences concerning such thresholds.

Although there are several research reports stating that drinking an average of two drinks a day can cause "significant" effects on offspring, that average of two drinks often turns out to be the result of seven or more drinks on 1 day and the balance spread out over others. It is hardly ever two drinks a day, each day. The implications associated with characterizing drinking behavior in different ways are illustrated in Figure 1.1. These data are taken from a study comparing alcohol consumption on the 4 most recent days prior to the survey on which drinking occurred (Stockwell, Lang, & Lewis, 1995). The average alcohol consumption for all 4 days, whether drinking occurred on all 4 or not was calculated; as was the average daily consumption for those days on which drinking occurred; as well as consumption for the day on which the most alcohol was consumed.

As indicated by the figure, if five drinks or more is used as the criterion for

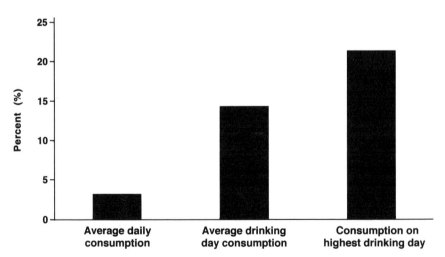

Figure 1.1.   Alcohol consumption during the four most recent drinking days, calculated as average consumption for drinking and nondrinking days, average consumption for drinking days only, and consumption on the highest drinking day of that 4-day period. $N = 373$. (Data adapted from Stockwell et al., 1995.)

abusive drinking, abusive drinking applies to only 3% of the 373 women in this study, using the average daily consumption statistic; whereas, if the focus is on the highest level of drinking during any one of those four days, 20.9% of the same group of women fall into this category (Stockwell, Lang, & Lewis, 1995).

Conceptually, alcohol abuse refers to drinking behavior that adversely affects an individual's health, behavior, or the society in which he or she lives, but does not necessarily involve impaired control over drinking. (An operational definition for alcohol abuse is offered in this chapter later.) If alcohol abuse progresses to the point that it does become obsessive/compulsive as well, it is called alcoholism or alcohol dependence (U.S. Department of Health and Human Services, 1993).

Although alcohol abuse is clearly an etiological factor in the full expression of the syndrome and for the individual anomalies mentioned earlier, unless someone took the time to look into the clinical literature, he or she would not realize this. One might expect physicians to do so. But as the Michigan survey (Abel & Kruger, 1998a) indicates, such is not always the case. Because the likelihood of a physician's encountering someone with the syndrome is less than one case out of 1,000 children seen (see Chapter 11), physicians can be forgiven for relying on secondary sources that often do not call their readers' attention to the kind of abusive drinking that always occurs in conjunction with the syndrome. Spohr is undoubtedly correct—many physicians have heard about FAS, and because what they have heard is fetal *alcohol* syndrome, not fetal *alcohol abuse* syndrome, they make the mistaken inference that one drink is all that is needed to produce the syndrome. If many physicians make this error, the general public cannot be expected to be any more prescient. This error would not be as likely to occur if the syndrome and its cognates were identified or referred to in terms of *alcohol abuse* instead of simply *alcohol*.

Changing the name to convey the idea that alcohol abuse is responsible still begs the question of how we operationally define alcohol abuse. One way of doing so is to base the definition on the relationship between the amounts of alcohol consumed and the resulting damage. This determination is more easily made in animal experimentation because unlike studies involving humans, animal studies involving animals permit researchers to control many of the conditions that affect this relationship.

Table 1.1 lists the doses most commonly used to study alcohol's prenatal effects in animals and the equivalent doses in humans. As the table indicates, in studying alcohol's effects in animals, we are invariably dealing with levels of alcohol exposure considered abusive if encountered in people.

A problem comparing the effects of alcohol dosages in different species, however, is that rates of absorption, metabolism, distribution, and elimination are not the same. For instance, to obtain a blood level of 3 µg/liter for some drugs requires administration of 200 mg/kg if the subject is a rabbit compared to only 1 mg/kg if the subject is a human (Abel, 1979). One pathway through the compari-

**Table 1.1. Alcohol Doses and Their
Drink Equivalents Typically Used
in Animal Studies**[a]

Animal dose	Human equivalent
2 g/kg/day	9 drinks/day
4 g/kg/day	18 drinks/day
6 g/kg/day	27 drinks/day
Animal liquid diet	Human equivalent
12 g/kg/day	54 drinks/day

[a]For a 60-kg male (about 130 lb).

son maze is to base equivalents on blood levels. Because the amount of a drug in the blood is generally the same as its effective concentration at its site of action, the effective dose is not the same as the administered dose. Table 1.2 gives examples of the kinds of blood alcohol levels (BALs) associated with different numbers of drinks consumed over a 5-hour period by a male weighing 60 kg (about 130 lb). Since blood alcohol levels resulting from consumption of a specific amount of alcohol are related to gender, these "drink equivalents" would be about 1 drink less for every 10 drinks for women (see later).

Returning to the criterion of "threshold," in the rat brain, damage only begins to occur when the blood alcohol level reaches 150 mg% (Bonthius & West, 1988; West, Kelly, & Pierce, 1987), and the overwhelming body of behavioral studies in animals have involved exposures resulting in blood alcohol levels of 200 mg% and above (Abel, 1984a).

If the blood alcohol threshold at which brain damage is produced in rats were to be translated in terms of human consumption, the level qualifying for "alcohol abuse" for someone weighing 130 pounds would be the equivalent of a daily binge of nine drinks over a 5-hour period (University of Michigan, n.d.). However, in most of these studies, the threshold blood alcohol levels were maintained over

**Table 1.2. Drink Equivalents
for Alcohol Consumption over
a 5-Hour Period**[a]

BALs	Drink Equivalents
150 mg%	9 drinks
200 mg%	11 drinks
300 mg%	15 drinks
400 mg%	20 drinks

[a]For a 60-kg male (about 130 lb).

several days and were, therefore, the counterpart of chronic bingeing over almost the entire course of gestation.

A Unifying Principle

The idea that it is alcohol abuse, and not simply alcohol, that causes *alcohol-abuse-related birth effects* (a term used hereafter to refer collectively to FAS, FAES, ARBDs, etc.) will be emphasized throughout this book as a unifying principle to explain not only the *ipso locitur* association between abusive drinking, fetal alcohol abuse syndrome, and fetal alcohol abuse effects, but also to show that the inconsistencies associated with lower levels of drinking are not inconsistencies at all but rather an emphasis on the trees instead of the forest. It is the scientific counterpart to Edgar Allan Poe's mystery of "The Purloined Letter," a story about a stolen document. The police suspect a government minister and search his home to no avail because the letter is turned inside out and stuck in a letter rack in full view. Frustrated, they turn to Detective C. Auguste Dupin, who says:

> "The business is very simple indeed, and I make no doubt that we can manage it sufficiently well ourselves, but then I thought Dupin would like to hear of it because it is so excessively odd."
> "Simple and odd," said Dupin.
> "Why, yes, and not exactly that either. The fact is we have all been a good deal puzzled because the affair is so simple, and yet baffles us altogether."
> "Perhaps it is the very simplicity of the thing which puts you at fault," said Dupin. (Poe, 1845/1986, p. 331)

Like the purloined letter, the relationship between drinking during pregnancy and birth defects should be "simple," but instead it "baffles us." It is right in front of us, yet we don't see it because we are distracted by the "average drinkers" all around us.

One indication that current research is in need of a unifying principle is reflected in the different ways researchers continue to operationally define the terms they use to characterize the low levels of consumption they believe cause FAS/ARBE. Some, for instance, defined *moderate* as an average daily consumption ranging upward from one and one-half drinks a day (Little, Asker, Sampson, & Renwick, 1986) to an average of three drinks a day (Kaminski, Franc, Lebovier, Du Mazubrun, & Rumeau-Roquette, 1981). A *drink* is defined as 12 ounces of beer, 5 ounces of wine, or 1.5 ounces of 80-proof distilled spirits. Although heavy drinking implies greater consumption that moderate drinking (Abel & Kruger, 1995), in many cases the operational definition of *heavy* is less than what others call moderate. For example, the threshold for heavy drinking has been defined in some studies as an average of 0.89 drinks a day (Day et al., 1989), 1 drink a day (Shiono, Klebanoff, & Rhoads, 1986), or 2 drinks a day (Virji, 1991).

The U.S. Substance Abuse and Mental Health Services Administration (SAMSA), on the other hand, defined *heavy drinking* as consumption of five drinks per occasion at least five times a month (SAMHSA, 1996, p. 91). The National Institute on Alcohol Abuse and Alcoholism (NIAAA) was less consistent in its definition but quite similar to the SAMSA definition, nonetheless. In its *Seventh Special Report to the U.S. Congress on Alcohol and Health,* for instance, it defined heavy drinking as the consumption of five drinks per occasion, at least once a week (NIAAA, 1990, p. 23). In its *Eighth Report* it defined it as two or more drinks a day (NIAAA, 1993, p. 5).

Emphasizing that ARBEs are due to alcohol abuse not only clarifies our understanding of the amounts of alcohol involved, it also allows us to examine previously reported studies with a more critical eye.

In their evaluation of children whose mothers drank during pregnancy, for instance, Jacobson and his co-workers (1993a) placed the threshold for alcohol-related damage at an average of 0.5 ounces of alcohol (1 drink) a day, but stated the effects they observed were undoubtedly the result of much higher consumptions per drinking day. "Because virtually none of the mothers drank every day, the average of 0.5 oz per day does not represent a typical dose; the women who drank above this threshold exposed their infants to a median of six drinks per occasion" (p. 181). If we recognize that it is the six drinks and not the one drink that are most likely responsible for the effects that were observed, it implies that future studies should focus directly on women who drink at the higher not the lower levels. This change in focus would save considerable time and money and result in a clearer relationship with those potential ARBEs being examined.

Ernhart's (1991) description of several women in one of her epidemiological studies was equally illuminating. Subject 901 was assessed an AA/day score of 0.55 (a little more than an average of one drink a day) when she was questioned during pregnancy, and 2.65 (about five drinks a day) when questioned about this same period 5 years later. However, during the first 3 months of her pregnancy, she reported drinking one gallon of wine and a half case of beer every Friday and Saturday evening. After that, she didn't drink for three months. Subject 643 had AA scores of 0.03 (less than an average of one-half drink a day) and 1.82 (about an average of three drinks a day) when questioned during her pregnancy and 5 years after it, respectively. But her drinking pattern consisted of a six-pack of beer every other day for the first three months of her pregnancy, and four to five cans of beer during the day, plus four to five cans of beer on every Friday, Saturday and Sunday evening after the first trimester.

As the Jacobson et al. (1993a) and Ernhart (1991) studies indicated—and these are only two of many such studies described in this book—the average drinks measure does not reflect the kind of abusive drinking mothers of children with FAS or FAE engage in. As Clarren pointed out,

Averaging daily consumption is certainly valid when comparing fetal outcomes in women with similar consistent drinking patterns—essentially women who drink a relatively constant amount over a consumptive period. But it should be intuitively obvious that a fetus exposed of [sic] 30 grams of alcohol (about 2.5 drinks) each day and a fetus exposed to 210 grams of alcohol (about 16 drinks) once per week would have very different patterns of exposure, both averaged to the same frequency…. By expressing consumption at [sic] an average score, the fetuses would be analyzed together and the actual results would be obscured. By using averaged daily consumption patterns as the index of consumption one ounce of absolute alcohol or more per day seems to be the threshold for teratogenesis … it should be clear that this is a bogus method of dose/response assessment. (Clarren, 1988, pp. 29–31)

I believe the point is clear: The "average drinks a day" statistic is illusory with regard to patterns of drinking that pose a danger to the unborn child. Statistically significant associations between relatively low levels of maternal drinking and some behavioral outcomes have been noted. But more often than not, these associations are statistically significant, as the Jacobson et al. (1993a) and Ernhart (1991) studies indicated, only by virtue of the inclusion of children of alcoholic or bingeing mothers, and, in some instances, by the inclusion of children with obvious FAS, whose mothers were children of "moderate" drinkers. It is the unusual cases that make these associations statistically significant. We have been sidetracked from this conclusion because of the ambiguity attached to the word *alcohol* and the message underlying it, in terms like fetal alcohol syndrome and fetal alcohol effect.

In its recent reformulation of the diagnostic criteria for FAS, the Institute of Medicine (1996) was quite explicit in stating that alcohol-related birth effects, however they are designated, are the results of "excessive drinking." I have rearranged the behaviors they characterize as "excessive" to form the more easily remembered acronym, *FLEAT*:

*F*requent episodes of intoxication
*L*egal problems related to drinking
*E*ngaging in physically dangerous behavior while drinking
*A*lcohol-related medical problems, such as liver disease
*T*olerance or withdrawal

These FLEAT traits are indicative of alcohol abuse not occasional drinking, and certainly not "an average consumption of 0.5, one or two drinks a day," with the implication of steady, rather than sporadic drinking. Although the IOM report leaves open the contingency that this etiology could be revised to include lower quantities of consumption if evidence supporting this conclusion were warranted, after more than 20 years of research into this possibility, it did not feel it was. "[A]lthough statistical associations between low to moderate levels of prenatal alcohol exposure … and effects on a variety of behavioral, educational, and psychological tests" had been reported, the IOM concluded that "these statistical associations are typically weak and the estimated average effects are usually small … (and) have little clinical significance for individual children" (IOM, 1996, p. 6).

An Operational Definition of Alcohol Abuse

Although the IOM declined to define what it meant by "excessive" in terms of levels of consumption, we can get some appreciation of what is involved by examining the case study literature. The levels of drinking typically described in these reports include consumption of over 14 drinks a day during pregnancy (Abel, 1990) and over 20 drinks (Azouz, Kavianian, & Der Kaloustian, 1993); a bottle of liquor a day (Beattie, Day, Cockburn, & Garg, 1983); one gallon of wine and a half case of beer every Friday and Saturday evening (Ernhart, 1991); three to four pints of liquor a day (Pierog, Chandavasee, & Wexler, 1977); two to three quarts of beer daily interspersed with an unknown amount of whiskey (Pierog et al., 1977); and 1.5 quarts of beer per day for 7 years (Wisniewski, Damboka, Sher, & Qazi, 1983). Many of these mothers have been described as drinking themselves "senseless" (Bierich, Majewski, Michaelis, & Tillner, 1976). The amount of alcohol consumption associated with FAS is obviously far greater than what is implied by drinking terms other than *alcohol abuse* or *alcoholism.*

In the alcohol abuser's world, heavy drinking is 10 times the two drinks many researchers arbitrarily use as their standard for it. Clinicians who treat alcohol abusers are incredulous that such definitions are seriously entertained. "Are researchers so naive," one such clinician rhetorically asks, "are they so ignorant to the real world out there, that they consider those patterns (i.e., two drinks a day) to be 'heavy drinking' " (Knupfer, 1987b, parentheses mine).

Given that alcohol abuse and not simply alcohol consumption is responsible for FAS and all other ARBEs, is there some level of drinking that can be used to operationally define what we mean by alcohol abuse? Although any such effort to set a standard may seem arbitrary, I believe it is now possible to do so based on the evidence that follows in this chapter and throughout the book.

Most researchers consider alcohol's effects on brain development to be its most devastating aspect, as well as the aspect most sensitive to measurement. A threshold estimate based on brain damage would therefore seem to be opposite for operationally defining alcohol abuse, at least in terms of its prenatal consequences.

Alcohol's impact on the brain has been studied in animals and humans and is detailed throughout this book, especially in Chapters 9 and 10. The threshold for the brain damage associated with alcohol exposure in animals, as previously noted, has been estimated at a blood alcohol level of around 150 mg%. As previously shown, this blood alcohol level would rise from bingeing nine drinks over a five-hour period, or six drinks over a two-hour period (based on the subject's weighing about 130 lb) (University of Michigan, n.d.). These estimates, however, are based primarily on males. Allowing for gender differences in determining the number of drinks necessary to achieve a comparable blood alcohol level in women (Frezza and colleagues, 1990) places this threshold at about eight drinks over the same 5-hour period or five drinks over the 2-hour period. In fact, both craniofacial features and cognitive deficits reflecting brain damage from in utero alcohol exposure in humans, have been associated with binges of five drinks or more (Jacobson et al., 1993a; Olsen & Tuntiseranee, 1995; Streissguth et al., 1994d). Animal and human research are convergent in this regard. Therefore, it would not seem unreasonable to place the threshold for ARBEs at five drinks, consumed over a 2-hour period once a week. This level of drinking is often described as bingeing. However, in a recent public opinion survey of drinking definitions, a large percentage of the respondents rated this level of consumption as heavy drinking if it occurred on weekends or in social contexts (Abel & Kruger, 1995). *Bingeing* and *heavy drinking*, therefore, will be used interchangeably in this book unless stated otherwise. However, since this level of consumption is associated with intoxication and a variety of behavioral problems when it occurs on a regular basis, it would seem reasonable to describe this level of drinking, if engaged in more than once a week, as alcohol abuse.

As noted earlier, these operational definitions are similar to those currently used by two U.S. government agencies in their operational definition of heavy drinking. It is also an amount slightly less than that originally recognized by the National Institute on Alcohol Abuse and Alcoholism as placing the fetus at "significant risk" for ARBEs (Abel, 1984a). The difference between FAS and other ARBES lies not in the amount of drinking, once this threshold has been exceeded, but in the frequency with which it is exceeded.

Validity

The validity of a concept is reflected in its ability to predict future events. When considering alcohol consumption, predictive validity refers to the accuracy with which clinicians or researchers can predict the future health or performance of someone who drinks.

From the standpoint of validity, we can be reasonably certain in our predictions that someone characterized as an alcohol abuser will develop liver damage and experience marital instability and poor job performance (U.S. Department of Health and Human Services, 1993). If she becomes pregnant, her children are likely to develop birth defects. We can be just as reasonably certain someone characterized as a moderate drinker will be more highly educated, have higher socioeconomic status, lower parity, stronger social networks, and typically will be living a healthier lifestyle than either alcohol abusers or abstainers (Mills &

Graubard, 1987; Skog, 1996). Where ARBEs are concerned, we can be reasonably confident alcohol abuse is involved, and even more confident moderate drinking is not. We cannot predict, however, whether a child whose mother drank "moderately" will go on to be president, priest, or profligate.

This chapter has outlined a number of reasons why I will use the term fetal alcohol abuse syndrome in lieu of fetal alcohol syndrome to denote the clinical condition described by Jones and Smith (1973). Likewise, alcohol-abuse-related birth effects has been adopted in lieu of fetal alcohol effects as a generic term for anomalies resulting from in utero alcohol exposure. The reasons for doing so are (a) these terms provide clinicians, researchers, and the general public with a much clearer insight into and direction for studying their etiology and for avoiding "glib diagnoses"; (b) renaming this pattern of anomalies fetal alcohol abuse syndrome and alcohol-abuse-related birth effects integrates these problems with the kinds of health and social problems traditionally associated with alcohol abuse; and (c) these terms have greater face and prognostic validity.

On the basis of animal and human research, using brain dysfunction as one of the most sensitive barometers of alcohol-related damage, the threshold level of consumption for producing alcohol-abuse-related effects is around five drinks per drinking occasion, two or more times a week. Although periodic consumption of this amount, e.g., once a week, may result in some abnormality, regular consumption at this level is more likely to be teratogenic. As pointed out by Knupfer (1984), although consumption of an ounce of alcohol a day is technically heavier than consumption of an ounce a week, the term heavy drinking implies something different, and "alcohol abuse" involves something different still—drinking at a level that has definite implications for the health of the drinker and her unborn child. The more frequent the episodes of heavy drinking, that is, alcohol abuse during pregnancy, the greater the potential abnormalities for the unborn child. While effects have been attributed to the kinds of low levels of exposure described as moderate, as the evidence reviewed here and "revisited" throughout this book clearly indicates this inference is unwarranted.

This does not mean lower levels of drinking do not affect the embryo/fetus. The changes in "fetal breathing movements" associated with one or two drinks clearly indicate the fetus does react to low levels of alcohol. But—and this is an important "but"—such reactions only prove the fetus is alive, not that it is suffering damage. Fetuses will also react to vibrations in the abdomen, but as yet no one has argued these reactions cause birth defects. As indicated throughout this book, there is no evidence, apart from that due to artifact, on which to conclude that low levels of consumption pose a danger to the well-being of the unborn child. Before turning to that evidence, we will take up the difficult issue of defining the criteria for what is and is not an alcohol-abuse-related birth effect.

CHAPTER 2

Diagnosis

Most human teratogens are first identified by physicians. This was the way that FAS was identified. In Seattle, Washington, an astute pediatric resident brought a number of unusual looking children to the attention of Drs. Ken Jones and David Smith. Because these children didn't conform to any known medical diagnosis, Jones and Smith realized they were dealing with an as yet unreported birth defect, which they subsequently called fetal alcohol syndrome (FAS) (Jones & Smith, 1973).

Once they knew what to look for, other physicians discovered similar cases in Australia, Belgium, Brazil, Canada, Chile, Croatia, Czechoslovakia, Denmark, France, Finland, Germany, Holland, Hungary, Ireland, Italy, Japan, Poland, Reunion, Scotland, South Africa, Spain, Sweden, Switzerland, and Taiwan. (Readers interested in the references associated with these and other reports can obtain them by request from the author.) The fact is that FAS has now been diagnosed in so many countries that despite the subtlety of it symptoms, physicians and biomedical researchers can become very astute in recognizing it once they know what to look for.

The key lies in its distinctive pattern of anomalies rather than any single anomaly. None of the individual abnormalities that collectively make up the syndrome are diagnostic; any one of these individual abnormalities may also occur in children born to abstinent mothers and mothers who use substances other than alcohol (Clarren et al., 1987; Hingson et al., 1982), or as part of syndromes with different etiologies (Zuckerman & Hingson, 1986).

Who Has FAS?

Differential diagnosis is essential from the perspective of patient care, research, and social programs. Early and accurate diagnosis may prevent unaffected

19

children from having to undergo lengthy, unpleasant, and costly evaluations. Equally important, an accurate diagnosis may lead to a better understanding of the failure of children with FAS to thrive, and the difficulties they experience in school. If parents know their child has FAS and know that children with this disorder do not respond well to traditional child-rearing practices, they may look for new ways to raise and educate them so that these children can better achieve their potentials.

A differential diagnoses is also essential from a research standpoint. If researchers are unable to agree on who has or does not have FAS, the following can occur:

Diagnosis will be haphazard.

FAS will go unrecognized.

Individuals with FAS will not receive adequate treatment.

People with similar but different disorders may be improperly treated.

Estimates of incidence and prevalence will be unreliable.

The cause(s) of the disorder will remain indeterminate.

Prevention will be illusory.

Although there are not several different paradigms for diagnosing FAS (Burd & Martsolf, 1989; Daehaene et al., 1981; IOM, 1996; Loser, 1995; Majewski, 1981; Rosett, 1980; Vitez, Koranyi, Gonczy, Rudas, & Czeizel, 1984), this chapter describes only three of these in detail. The first two paradigms have been in use for about 15 years; the last was proposed in 1996 by the Institute of Medicine. Despite differences among them, the key features in each are growth retardation, characteristic facial features, and abnormalities of the central nervous system.

The oldest of the formal diagnostic paradigms is presented in Table 2.1. This

Table 2.1. Criteria for Diagnosis of Fetal Alcohol Abuse Syndrome as Developed by the Alcohol Study Group

Prenatal and/or Postnatal Growth Retardation
    Weight, length, or head circumference below 10th percentile when corrected for gestational age
Central Nervous System Dysfunction
    Signs of neurological abnormality, developmental delay, or cognitive impairment
Distinctive Facial Features with at Least Two of the Following Signs:
    Short palpebral fissures
    Poorly developed philtrum
    Thin upper lip
    Flat midface
    Microphthalmia
    Head circumference below 3rd percentile

paradigm follows Jones and Smith's (1973) original description of FAS and was developed by the Fetal Alcohol Study Group of the Research Society on Alcoholism (Rosett, 1980) to bring standardization to the diagnosis. The terms in boldfaced letters refer to the three major categories of anomalies that define the syndrome. Individual anomalies listed under each of these main categories refer to examples of commonly occurring abnormalities representative of each category.

A clinical diagnosis of FAS in this minimalist paradigm is based on the presence of one characteristic, or in the case of facial dysmorphology, two, in each of the three major categories; the diagnosis does not depend on a history of maternal alcoholism during pregnancy, but is strengthened whenever it can be confirmed.

The major bias connected with this paradigm is that it is more inclusive than exclusive, thereby increasing the likelihood of a "false positive" diagnosis (overdiagnosis). In other words, the possibility of inaccurately labeling someone as having FAS is more likely to be increased than decreased when using this paradigm. This bias arises because to qualify for a diagnosis a patient need only have one characteristic in the growth and CNS categories, and two features in the facial dysmorphology category, no matter how mild those effects might be. Under this paradigm, an underdeveloped philtrum (the groove between the base of the nose and the upper lip) has the same importance as mental retardation and greater importance than organ pathology, which is not even considered to be diagnostic. Although cardiac and limb defects are relatively common in FAS (see Chapter 8, "Heart"; "Limb Joint Anomalies"), this paradigm does not include them or any other organ pathology.

The second paradigm, shown in Table 2.2, was devised by Majewski (1981, 1993) to quantify the severity of features associated with FAS. The same core group of symptoms as those making up the minimalist paradigm in Table 2.1 are found in Majewski's paradigm. In his case, however, physical anomalies are included as a formal component of the diagnosis, and individual anomalies are assigned a point score. The severity of the diagnosis is reflected in the total point count.

From a research standpoint, this checklist paradigm provides greater objectivity than the minimalist paradigm (Table 2.1) because it is much more explicit. As a result, a researcher has a more objective criterion for including or excluding an anomaly as pertinent. Because it is more rigorous than the minimalist paradigm, the checklist paradigm is also less subject to overdiagnosis. For example, a child could qualify for a diagnosis of FAS using the minimalist criteria paradigm if he or she weighed below the 10th percentile for gestational age at birth, had two characteristic facial features—for example, indistinct philtrum and thin upper lip—and had some kind of CNS dysfunction—for example, hyperactivity. Under the checklist paradigm, this same child would have a point score of 10 (4 for intrauterine growth retardation, 1 for indistinct philtrum, 1 for thin lip, and 4 for

Table 2.2. Majewski's Numerical Paradigm for Diagnosing FAS (Reformulated)

Points	Characteristic	Points	Characteristic
4	Prenatal growth retardation	2	Blepharophimosis
2/4/8	Statomotor/mental retardation	2	Clinodactyly of fifth finger
4	Microcephaly	2	Camptodactyly
4	Hyperactivity	2	Limited supination
4	Genitourinary malformation	2	Hip dislocation
4	Congenital heart defect	2	Hernia
2	Cleft palate	2/4	Genital anomalies
3	Short upturned nose	2	Muscular hypotonia
3	Abnormal palmar creases	1	Indistinct philtrum
2	Hypoplastic mandible	1	Thin lips
2	High arched palate	1	Hypoplastic endophalanges
2	Epicanthic eye folds	1	Sacred dimple
2	Ptosis		

hyperactivity), which is far below the 40-point criterion for a diagnosis of alcohol embryopathy (AE) III, this paradigm's counterpart to FAS.

Another of the strengths and, simultaneously, one of the weaknesses of Majewski's paradigm is that it is based on a relatively large homogenous population. Because Majewski examined each patient himself, he was able to be very systematic in developing a standardized and detailed list of anomalies characterizing the syndrome. But any checklist is only as good as the items it includes. In this regard, it is worth keeping in mind that Majewski's acumen—and that of every other clinician or researcher—depended on his interests, training, and experience. This may be one reason, for example, that postnatal growth retardation is not included in Majewski's paradigm, although it is a cardinal feature in the FAS Study Group's paradigm. Likewise, ancillary features, such as retinal tortuosity and optic nerve hypoplasia, are not mentioned as formal diagnostic features by Majewski or any other clinicians, but appear to be very common when children with FAS are examined by ophthalmologists (see Chapter 7, "Eyes").

Majewski also completely ignored sensory function, such as hearing loss, although other studies have found these problems to be commonly associated with FAS, so much so, that hearing loss, is considered as formally diagnostic by the IOM (see later).

That Majewski's patient population is comprised primarily of Caucasian children living in Dusseldorf, Germany, is also a weakness in terms of its applicability to children in other countries. Because the majority of cases of FAS in North America are either African American or Native American (see Chap. 11), recognizing the syndrome in these children may depend on deviations from norms that characterize these racial and ethnic groups rather than those derived from Majewski's population sample.

The IOM Diagnostic Paradigm

In 1996, the Institute of Medicine developed a diagnostic paradigm that departed markedly from its two predecessors in several ways, most notably by including maternal alcohol exposure as part of the diagnosis. The IOM's paradigm also included as part of the syndrome many features not specifically listed in the previous paradigms (e.g., agenesis of the corpus callosum, hearing loss) and attempted to provide guidelines for making a diagnosis.

The most innovative aspect of the IOM's paradigm is its division of FAS into three categories: Category 1—FAS with confirmed maternal alcohol exposure, Category 2—FAS without confirmed maternal alcohol exposure, and Category 3—partial FAS with confirmed maternal alcohol exposure. (Criteria for Category 1 FAS are listed in Table 2.3.)

The criteria cited in the IOM's Category 2 diagnosis come closest to those traditionally used in making a FAS diagnosis and are identical to Category 1's criteria, except for the absence of a confirmed maternal drinking history. Creation of this second category reflects the reality that as many as 50% of all children with FAS are in adoptive or foster homes when they are referred for diagnosis (Burd & Martsolf, 1989; Spohr, Williams, & Steinhausen, 1993; Streissguth & Randels, 1988), and that relevant information concerning the drinking behavior of their biological mothers is unavailable or unreliable because of the birth mother's denial of alcohol abuse.

The IOM also broke new ground by consciously introducing peripheral issues of patient care and research into the formulation of its Category 2 paradigm. The rationale behind the decision to do so, the IOM explained, was that it considered it unfair to deny patients the benefits of a clinical diagnosis of FAS because of lack of information about their mothers. Another rationale was that research investigations would be more solidly structured if based on the clearest possible diagnosis of FAS.

The IOM was also forthright in stating it had been strongly influenced by issues of services and reimbursement in formulating its Category 3 paradigm, which it called "partial FAS with confirmed maternal alcohol exposure," rather than "probable FAS." Calling it probable FAS, the IOM said, would denote uncertainty about etiology. Such uncertainty might then keep someone from qualifying for "*appropriate services and reimbursement for these services*" (IOM, 1996, p. 75; italics added), thereby closing doors for "*medical, social services, and other attention*" (IOM, 1996, p. 75; italics added). Although these reasons are laudatory, they are potentially pernicious because they set a precedent

Table 2.3. Institute of Medicine's (1996)
Diagnostic Criteria for FAS Category 1 (Reformulated)

A. Confirmed Maternal Alcohol Consumption
   Excessive drinking characterized by considerable, regular, or heavy episodic consumption
B. Characteristic Facial Features Include:
   Short palpebral fissures
   Characteristic premaxillary features, e.g., flat upper lip, flattened philtrum, flat midface
C. Growth Retardation
   Decreased birth weight for gestational age
   Failure to thrive postnatally not related to nutrition
   Disproportionate ratio of weight to height
D. CNS Abnormalities, including at least one of the following:
   Small head size
   Structural abnormalities, e.g., small brain, partial or complete absence of corpus callosum,
     decreased size of cerebellum
   Neurological hard or soft signs (age appropriate), such as impairment of fine motor skills
   Neurosensory hearing loss
   Incoordination
   Impaired eye–hand coordination

for making social and political concerns, not to mention medical reimbursement as factors in what traditionally have been objective guidelines for characterizing medical disorders. If adopted by other committees, further efforts to revise medical diagnoses for other disorders could be held hostage to social planning or reimbursement considerations.

The criteria the IOM decided on for its Category 3 diagnosis are presented in Table 2.4. Among the noteworthy features of this paradigm are its retention of maternal drinking and facial features as intrinsic to the diagnosis. In addition, an individual must have either small stature, a physically observable CNS anomaly, or some behavioral/cognitive disorder.

An added rationale for this category, the IOM said, was the need to have a diagnostic paradigm for identifying adults with FAS. Other paradigms were unable to do so reliably, it contended, because some of the salient characteristics associated with FAS in childhood, such as facial dysmorphia and growth retardation, often do not extend into adulthood. A Category 3 diagnosis could thus be made in the absence of good medical records of growth retardation or early infancy. However, this was its weakest rationale because the facial features so intrinsic to this diagnosis in children are usually not recognizable in adults. The paradigm is also far from explicit in its list of "Ps" and "Ds." For instance, what is "metacognition?" What are problems in "judgment?" How high is a "higher level?" The focus on "receptive" language is also dubious since most studies have found receptive language is intact (see Chapter 10).

**Table 2.4. Criteria for IOM's Category 3 Diagnosis:
Partial FAS with Confirmed Alcohol Exposure (Reformulated)**

A. Same excessive maternal alcohol as in Category 1.
B. Same facial features as in Category 2.

   Either C, or D, or E

C. Same growth retardation as in Category 1.
D. Same CNS abnormalities as in Category 1.
E. Evidence of complex pattern of behavioral or cognitive dysfunction unrelated to develop-
   mental maturity, or to family or home environment. The IOM's list of common "Ps" and
   "Ds" include the following:
   Difficulties in learning
   Poor in school performance
   Poor impulse control
   Problems in relating to others
   Deficits in language (understanding and speaking)
   Poor ability for abstract thinking
   Poor arithmetic skills
   Problems in memory, attention, or judgement

Reliability and Construct Validity

The hallmarks of any diagnostic paradigm are its reliability and validity, neither of which characterizes any of the paradigms examined in this chapter.

Reliability refers to the agreement among those making the diagnosis. Despite hundreds of case reports and hundreds of clinical research and epidemiological studies, the reliability of the various diagnostic paradigms for FAS has not as yet been tested. (Actually, it is not the paradigms that are tested, but the individuals who use them, the assumption being that raters have the same acumen.) Determinations of test-retest reliability can also take the form of how consistently individuals with FAS are identified over time. The latter criterion is more typical in FAS research but is frustrated because many of the features associated with FAS change in the normal course of development.

One of the largest group of patients with FAS to be followed over several years is the 44 German children diagnosed in early childhood, using the checklist paradigm (Table 2.2), who were then followed up on for 10–14 years by Spohr and colleagues (Spohr, Willins, & Steinhausen, 1994). At the time of follow-up, 70% (31/44) had only "mild" expressions of the syndrome, whereas 20% (8/44) could no longer be identified as having FAS. Only 10% of the original sample (5/44) were still recognizable as having FAS.

In a smaller study, using the minimalist paradigm (Table 2.1), Ernhart and her co-workers (1995) reported that seven out of the eight children whom they diagnosed as having FAS during infancy no longer warranted that diagnosis at four years of age.

Test-retest reliability is therefore not very high for FAS, but it is unclear whether this is because of inherent weaknesses in the paradigms, or because features may be more plastic than were previously thought.

Validity refers to whether or not what is being agreed on is relevant to the conditions being examined. (Issues regarding face validity were discussed in Chapter 1 and will not be repeated here.) Conceptually, the strongest evidence supporting the validity of the FAS diagnosis is its construct validity. Because facial characteristics arise from the same embryonic tissues that give rise to the brain, on the basis of construct validity, one would expect the more aberrant the facial features, the greater the insult to the brain and behavior—a relationship that has, in fact, been repeatedly noted in the context of FAS (Autti-Ramo, Gaily, & Granstrom, 1992; Iosub, Fuchs, Bingol, & Gromish, 1981a; Majewski, 1981; Streissguth, Herman, & Smith, 1978a).

What Is an Abnormality?

All of the diagnostic paradigms discussed in this chapter begin with the premise that FAS is characterized by a pattern of anomalies rather than any single anomaly. This premise is implicit in the concept of a *gestalt*, which means the whole is greater than the sum of its individual parts. In other words, each of the individual parts that go into the diagnosis may be slightly unusual, but meshed together, this collection of slightly unusual features has something unique about it. A fitting analogy could be taken from pointillism or abstract art. The points or forms in themselves are not unusual, but when put together in a particular way, they create a striking image. Because it is the gestalt that diagnosticians rely on when making a clinical judgment, the need to operationally define what is or is not an abnormality is less important in the clinical setting than it is in the research environment, where such definitions are typically a sine qua non.

In the laboratory, researchers are usually intent in breaking gestalts down to their individual parts. The goal is often to isolate each part of the gestalt and then figure out their recondite relationships. One of their first problems is deciding on whether a part is normal or abnormal.

Because biological definitions of *abnormal* more often than not rely on forcing continuous variables into categorical classifications, bias is inevitable. A well-known example of how biases determine our definitions of what is or is not abnormal is the criterion we use for labeling someone as mentally retarded.

In 1959, the criterion for mental retardation was a score on a standardized intelligence test that was one standard deviation or more below the average. In terms of the IQ test, the average score was 100, and one standard deviation below that average was a score of 85. On the basis of that criterion, the number of mentally retarded Americans was estimated at about 35 million (16% of the population). Because this was such an alarming estimate, the criterion was changed in 1973 from one to two standard deviations below the average, that is, from an IQ of less than 85 to one less than 70. This reduced the number of mentally retarded Americans to about 2.2 million (2.3% of the population) (Zigler & Cascione, 1984). Same people but a different criterion equaled fewer mentally retarded citizens. A shift in criterion for normality can obviously have a tremendous impact on what is defined as abnormal.

What researchers call abnormal is also often influenced by preconceptions and expectations. In the case of research dealing with the effects of prenatal alcohol exposure, deviation from the norm is typically defined in terms of a statistically significant difference between an experimental group and a control group. However, statistical significance does not necessarily mean biological significance, although as the previous example suggests, it can be interpreted as such. For instance, in discussing their finding that infants whose mothers drank moderately during pregnancy were less easily aroused than infants whose mothers did not drink, the authors interpreted this difference as a harmful effect associated with drinking. However, their criterion for "low arousal" was that these infants were "very easy to console, frequently self-quiet, and seldom get very upset or excited" (Streissguth, Barr, & Martin, 1983a). Rather than being negative attributes, most parents, I believe, consider these as signs of a "good" baby.

That statistical significance does not mean biological significance is reason enough to carefully scrutinize interpretations of any associations between drinking during pregnancy and prenatal outcomes. Such scrutiny is especially necessary when behavioral outcomes are being assessed because these interpretations, as noted in the context of self-quieting and excitement, are susceptible to the experimenter's personal biases. Unless these interpretations and the methodologies on which they are based are reviewed and discussed candidly and incisively, we will have no bases on which to agree whether the diagnostic paradigms we use for deciding who has a problem are valid or if the solutions for correction or prevention of that problem are reasonable or effective.

CHAPTER 3

Spontaneous Abortion

Although the paradigms for diagnosing FAS have become more detailed, there are many alcohol-abuse-related birth effects (ARBEs) that occur either independently of or in addition to the anomalies mentioned in these lists that warrant attention in their own right. (These anomalies will be examined in Chapters 3–13.)

Very high spontaneous abortion rates among alcoholic women have been reported in Hungary (18.8%) (Vitez & Czeizel, 1982), Germany (22%) (Seidenberg & Majewski, 1978), Denmark (23%) (Becker, Tonnesen, Kaas-Claesson, & Gluud, 1989), Scotland (46%) (Beattie, Day, Cockburn, & Garg, 1983), Russia (52%) (Shurygin, 1974), and France (81%) (Dehaene et al., 1977). In some of these studies, multiple pregnancy losses by the same women were likely included. For example, in the United States, women with a clinical diagnosis of alcohol abuse were twice as likely as controls to have experienced three or more spontaneous abortions (Sokol, Miller, & Reed, 1980). A survey of the clinical literature relating to FAS found that out of 90 mothers of children with FAS, 52% had had at least one spontaneous abortion, and the average rate of spontaneous abortion per mother was 2.2 (Abel, 1990).

Although alcoholic women and mothers of children with FAS have high rates of spontaneous abortion, their pregnancy rates are not necessarily reduced, as evidenced by the number of children they often give birth to (see Table 3.1).

The increased rate of spontaneous abortion among alcohol-abusing women may therefore be due to a higher number of pregnancies. When spontaneous abortions were considered in terms of alcoholic and nonalcoholic mothers, not individual pregnancies, the differences between alcoholic women and controls were no longer significant (Becker et al., 1989).

Most studies reporting high rates of spontaneous abortion among alcoholics are also problematic because the rates of spontaneous abortion among nonalcoholic women in the same studies (when presented) are often relatively high,

**Table 3.1. Birth Order
of Children with FAS**[a]

Birth order	% cases	Birth order	% cases
1	15	5	11
2	23	6	6
3	18	7	5
4	16	8 or more	5

[a]$N = 220$.

for example, 9.6% in Hungary (Vitez & Czeizel, 1982) and 8% in Denmark (Becker et al., 1989). Very little information is provided about the alcoholics in these studies. Their high spontaneous abortion rates may be symptomatic of other reproductive problems, as suggested by a Swedish study that found no differences in spontaneous abortion rates among a group of 92 alcoholic women whose alcohol consumption was about 12 drinks a day (Hollstedt, Dahlgren, & Rydberg, 1983a,b). One of the reasons for the difference in outcome was that unlike the previous studies, the alcoholics in the Swedish study did not differ from controls in socioeconomic status, marital status, previous diseases, or medical complications during pregnancies. The failure to find significant differences between alcoholics and nonalcoholics prompted the authors to conclude that in the absence of various social and health differences, alcohol ingestion, even at levels associated with alcoholism, may not precipitate spontaneous abortions. This was also the conclusion of an earlier study which found no differences in rates of spontaneous abortion between alcoholic women and those suffering from endogenous depression (Bark, 1979).

These latter two studies are noteworthy not because they are out of line with the previously cited studies that did find significant associations, but because they imply alcohol is not the only factor to consider in evaluating high rates of spontaneous abortion among alcoholics. Many female alcoholics also suffer from depression (Bark, 1979), and there may be some inherent biological condition(s) that these women share with depressive women that predisposes them for spontaneous abortion.

One medical condition associated with alcoholism and an increased risk for spontaneous abortion and other pregnancy complications not taken into account in any of the previous studies (or for that matter in the overwhelming majority of studies of ARBEs, including FAS), is cirrhosis (Scholtes, 1979). As far as the outcome is concerned, it doesn't matter if a pregnancy is lost due to alcoholism or alcoholism-induced cirrhosis. But if the cause is being sought, the difference is important.

Epidemiological Studies

Epidemiology is the study of the ways in which health-related conditions are distributed in human populations and the identification of factors influencing the occurrence of those distributions. Epidemiological studies concerned with frequencies and distributions are descriptive, whereas those using descriptive information to formulate and test hypotheses are considered analytic.

If the descriptive epidemiological literature relating to the effects of maternal drinking during pregnancy and spontaneous abortion is collectively scrutinized solely from the standpoint of alcohol consumption levels, no consistent relationship between the two is evident. About one-half of the studies report increased rates of spontaneous abortion related to drinking, while the other half reports no significant association (see Table 3.2).

However, as indicated in Table 3.2, if the focus is shifted from alcohol consumption levels to study site, there is almost total consistency in outcome, regardless of consumption level, or study design, for example, case-control, retrospective, or prospective strategy.

Table 3.2 also indicates that if the study was done in North America, then the results point to a significant effect on spontaneous abortion; if done in Europe or Australia, then the results indicate no adverse effect.

Because grouping studies in terms of drinking levels or design leads to inconsistency, while grouping studies by country leads to almost complete consistency, one inference to be made is that while drinking levels are the same in these studies, the "drinkers" are not. The corollary to this conclusion is that the women included in the drinking groups in American studies differ from their respective control groups in a way related to the outcome being studied, whereas these groups are balanced much more evenly in the Australian and European studies. Although this corollary cannot be proven or disproven, there is some evidence to support it. The discussion of studies from these different sites that follows highlights some of the important demographic differences—especially socioeconomic status—that may account for the disparity associated with study site.

American and Canadian Studies

In a very widely cited prospective study of alcohol's effects on spontaneous abortion, Harlap and Shiono (1980) reported a twofold increase in spontaneous abortions for women who consumed an average of one to two drinks a day during their second trimester of pregnancy. When the preliminary results of this study were first reported (Harlap, Shiono, & Ramecharan, 1979), maternal body weight was an important factor contributing to the rate of spontaneous abortions; "slen-

Table 3.2. Cross-Cultural Comparison of Studies Reporting Relationship Between Alcohol Consumption and Spontaneous Abortion

Country	% drinkers	% drinking 7 or more drinks/week	Significant increase	No significant increase	Type of study	Reference
Canada	30	4	×		r	Armstrong et al., 1992
United States	27	27	×		p	Anokute, 1986
	49	3	×		p	Harlap & Shiono, 1980
	57	6	×		c	Kline et al., 1980
		n.i.		×	p	Little, 1978
	50	5	×		r	Wilsnack et al., 1984
	35	3	×		c	Windham et al., 1989
Australia	54	n.i		×	p	Walpole et al., 1989
England	82	8		×	p	Griso et al., 1984
	51	n.i.		×	p	Davis et al., 1982
Finland	58	n.i.		×	c	Halmesmaki et al., 1989b
Italy	65	n.i		×	c	Parazzini et al., 1991
	34	13		×	c	Parazzini et al., 1994
	75	75		×	p	Cavallo et al., 1995
Scotland	92	6	×		p	Plant, 1985
Spain	18	n.i.		×	c	Dominguez-Rojas et al., 1994

Note: n.i. = no information; c = case control study; p = prospective; r = retrospective.
Source: E. L. Abel, Maternal alcohol consumption and spontaneous abortion: A review, *Alcohol & Alcoholism* (1997), 32, 211–219. Copyright by Williams & Wilkins. Reprinted by permission of the publisher.

der" women who drank were singled out as having a higher spontaneous abortion rate than others. When the final report appeared, maternal body weight was not even mentioned.

The absence of information about maternal body weight in the final report, given its fundamental relevance to pregnancy outcome and its apparent contribution in the original analysis, raises the obvious question: Why was maternal body weight ignored in the final redaction, especially when the decreased maternal body weights of the aborting women were probably the reason for their increased rate of spontaneous abortion? Omission of this information in the final publication coupled with its apparent contribution to the original analysis seriously compromises any conclusion one might draw from the reported findings.

This study is problematical for other reasons as well. Although over 32,000 women were sampled, the authors did not originally intend to examine drinking patterns, and there appears to have been considerable underreporting based on the fact that the number of women reported to be consuming an average of two drinks a day was only 0.5%, far less than the norm (Sokol, 1980).

Another widely cited American study also reported a relatively low threshold for alcohol-related spontaneous abortions (Kline, Shrout, Stein, Susser, & Warburton, 1980) but is likewise problematic. In this case-control study, women hospitalized for spontaneously aborting were compared with a control group in a prenatal outpatient clinic. Consumption of two to six drinks a week during pregnancy was estimated to produce a 2.35-fold increase in the likelihood of a spontaneous abortion. Although variables such as smoking, use of other drugs, and diet were taken into account, a larger percentage of the women in the alcohol group were on welfare. When the study was repeated with women in the alcohol group who were not on welfare, the previous relationship was no longer evident. (The role of poverty-related health status and undernutrition in such studies is examined in detail in Chapter 12.) The authors themselves raised the likelihood that, in their own words, "the group of women (who reported drinking twice a week in the first study may have) included those who on occasion drink a lot of alcohol" (Kolata, 1981). For instance, 62% of the cases drinking at least twice a week before pregnancy continued to drink at that level during pregnancy, although the trend for most women is (except very heavy drinkers) to decrease their alcohol consumption during pregnancy (Little, Schultz, and Mandell, 1976).

The probability that the relationships between the drinking levels reported in the previous two studies and an increase in spontaneous abortions is spurious and instead is dependent on poverty-related factors such as the health-status and undernutrition of the mothers being studied was suggested by a third study. That case-control study (Windham, Fenster, & Swan, 1992) likewise found an increase in spontaneous abortions associated with relatively low levels of consumption, an average of one or more drinks a day during the first trimester; but the association was strongest among "uninsured women" (a circumlocution for poverty stricken).

Although a prospective study from Oklahoma City reported an increase in spontaneous abortions associated with drinking during pregnancy among mainly white women of similar socioeconomic status, the data presented in Table 3.2 from that study do not support the author's conclusion. Nor do they support another of the author's conclusions that the smokers in his study had a 100% chance of nonlive births compared to nonsmokers (Anokute, 1986).

The Canadian study listed in Table 3.2 was likewise problematic because the overall spontaneous abortion rate in previous pregnancies was almost 22%, while the rate among abstainers was 20.5%. These very high baseline rates of spontaneous abortion suggest inherent problems in ascertainment or an unexplained but important bias in the overall study.

While the primary purpose of another study was to assess drinking among women, the study also included questions regarding spontaneous abortions and stillbirths. Based on their retrospective analysis, the investigators estimated the threshold for spontaneous abortion or stillbirth was estimated at six or more drinks per day consumed at least three times per week (Wilsnack, Klassen, & Wilsnack, 1984). Although the authors did not distinguish between spontaneous abortions and stillbirths, their results suggested a relatively high threshold for these effects, more in line with the data from studies relating to alcohol abusers than to women who drink an average of one drink a day.

Interestingly, the one exception to the general pattern in North America linking drinking and an increase in spontaneous abortion involved women enrolled in a health maintenance organization (Little, 1978). This exception is similar to that of the Swedish study (Hollstedt et al., 1983a) mentioned earlier in which no significant association between maternal alcoholism and spontaneous abortion rates was found when alcoholic women did not differ from nonalcoholics in health. Although participation in a health maintenance organization does not preclude differences in health or socioeconomic status among the women participating in the study, if differences did exist, they would support the inference that the relationship between drinking during pregnancy and an increase in spontaneous abortions is influenced by factors in addition to alcohol consumption.

European and Australian Studies

In contrast to the populations examined in the American studies, the populations studied in Europe and Australia seem to be much more socioeconomically homogeneous. Interestingly, when there appear to be class differences between subjects, there is a stronger association between drinking and spontaneous abortions.

Four case-control studies, one from Spain, one from Finland, and two from Italy, did not find any relation between alcohol consumption and spontaneous abortions (Dominquez-Rojos et al., 1994; Halmesmaki, Valimalci, Karonen, & Ylikorkala, 1989b; Parazzini et al., 1991, 1994).

The Parazzini et al. (1994) study is noteworthy because all miscarriages were confirmed by uterine curettage and pathology examinations. Women in the control group were recruited from women who delivered at term. All cases and controls were interviewed by trained interviewers using a standard questionnaire. The questionnaire asked patients about the number of days per week each type of alcoholic beverage was consumed in the week prior to and during the first trimester of pregnancy, average number of drinks per day, and duration of drinking in years. None of these alcohol-related indices was significantly related to spontaneous abortion rates.

Nearly all of the European and Australian prospective studies have likewise found no significant associations between drinking and spontaneous abortion.

Walpole, Zulrick, and Pontre's (1989; Australia) prospective study did not find any increase in the rate of spontaneous abortions related to total alcohol intake; but in two other studies conducted in France, when women who miscarried were examined in terms of different alcoholic beverages, those who were heavy beer drinkers (an average of two or more a day) were more likely to have had a spontaneous abortion than those that did not (Dehaene et al., 1977; Kaminski, Rumean-Rouquette, & Schwartz, 1976). The authors pointed out that these heavy beer drinkers were more likely than wine drinkers to smoke more than a pack of cigarettes a day; they were also likely to be of different ethnic origins, unmarried, and in a lower socioeconomic class. The fact that these women differed significantly from control women in several ways in addition to their alcohol consumption is congruent with the previous argument that it is the drinker and her living conditions, as much as the drink, that accounts for the significant epidemiological increased spontaneous abortion rates associated with drinking during pregnancy.

An interesting study from Finland examined the effects of alcohol administered to women in treatment for threatened first- or second-trimester abortions. A total of 239 women were routinely treated with betaminentics; 136 of these women also received oral and intravenous alcohol. Alcohol was administered as brandy (30–40 ml) four to five times a day, and "additional doses were liberally offered if a patient sensed uterine contractions." Some women also received intravenous infusions of alcohol. Treatment lasted from 3 to more than 22 days. Alcohol-treated patients consumed an average of 3.8 drinks a day. After discharge, 53% of the women who received alcohol treatment in the hospital continued to drink at home to arrest uterine contractions. Alcohol treatment had no significant effects on spontaneous abortions (Halmesmaki & Ylikorkala, 1988).

The one European study which did find a significant association between spontaneous abortions and drinking during pregnancy was correlational in nature (Plant, 1985). When the relationship was reexamined after controlling for diet and smoking, the correlations, which were very weak to begin with, remained very weak, for example, 0.09.

Studies in Animals

Studying animals enables researchers to examine questions about causality in a more direct way than is possible in clinical or epidemiological studies. These studies support the conclusion that very high blood alcohol levels, such as one might expect in conjunction with alcohol abuse, are capable of producing spontaneous abortions. The blood alcohol threshold for these increases is around 200 mg%, although in some cases, blood alcohol levels (BALs) have been considerably higher (Clarren et al., 1987; Ellis & Pick, 1980; Scott & Fradkin, 1984; Stuckey & Berry, 1984). To achieve a blood alcohol level of about 200 mg%, comparable to the level that produces spontaneous abortions in animals, a 130-pound pregnant woman would have to drink about 11 drinks over a 5-hour period (see Table 1.2). A blood alcohol level this high would be associated with extreme stupor in someone not accustomed (i.e., tolerant) to this level of intoxication (animals are rendered comatose); hence, it would not likely be achieved by the overwhelming majority of drinkers. Although some individuals have survived with blood alcohol levels ranging from 500 mg%–780 mg% (Lindblad & Olsson, 1976), a blood alcohol level of 260 mg% is the lower lethal limit for most people (Maling, 1970).

Conclusion

Although maternal alcohol abuse is associated with an increased risk for spontaneous abortion, it is uncertain whether this association is directly due to alcohol; a secondary effect of maternal illness, such as cirrhosis; or some other underlying reproductive problem variously described as "habitual," "recurrent," or repetitive abortion (Glass & Golbus, 1978), which is only coincidentally, not causally, related to drinking itself.

On the other hand, the consistency of the studies in non-human primates and dogs with regard to threshold BALs for spontaneous abortion are impressive. If they have any bearing on humans, they give a certain validity to Wilsnack's estimated threshold in humans of six drinks a day for several days a week (a level defined operationally as alcohol abuse in Chapter 2).

As indicated by Table 3.2, epidemiological studies reporting increases in spontaneous abortion rates associated with very low levels of drinking during pregnancy were singular in that virtually every study reporting such a relationship was conducted in the United States or Canada; those that did not find a significant link between the two were conducted in Europe or Australia. This singular pattern cannot be simply explained as a difference in the percentage of heavy drinkers in North America compared to that of other countries (see Chapter 11).

CHAPTER 4

Perinatal Problems

Stillbirth

Around the turn of the century, W. C. Sullivan (1899) reported that over half of the 600 children born to 120 alcoholic women inmates in a Liverpool prison were stillborn or died in early infancy, a rate 2.5 times higher than for infants born to sober relatives of these women. Sullivan attributed this increase to alcoholism because the longer these alcoholic women remained in prison during their pregnancies, the lower the stillbirth rate. In arriving at this conclusion, Sullivan did not consider the fact the imprisoned women were not only prevented from drinking but also received more medical attention and better food than those not living in prison.

Recent studies examining the relationship between maternal alcoholism and stillbirths are inconsistent. One case-control study (Vitez & Czeizel, 1982) found a slight but statistically significant increase in stillbirths associated with maternal alcoholism (2.6% for alcoholic women vs. 1.2% for controls), whereas another did not (Hollstedt et al., 1983b).

In France, Kaminski et al. (1976) found an increase in stillbirth rate associated with consumption of three or more drinks per day, but only among heavier beer drinkers. There was no comparable relationship for heavier wine drinkers. Because beer consumption is far less common than wine consumption and is correlated with lower socioeconomic status in France, the authors speculated the increase in stillbirths among heavier beer drinkers may have been related to their poverty rather than beer consumption. A second study by Kaminski's group evaluating three different populations of women replicated the earlier result in only one population.

Retrospective studies involving analyses of data from the 1980 United States National Natality Survey and 1980 National Fetal Mortality Survey found a

37

significant and opposite result to that reported by Kaminski, that is, stillbirth rates were lower among drinkers than among abstainers (Little & Weinberg, 1993; Praeger et al., 1983).

A study reported by Marbury and co-workers (1983) found smoking was a critical factor affecting alcohol's link to stillbirths. Although the authors found a significant increase in stillbirths among women consuming 14 or more drinks per week, the association ceased to be statistically significant after the authors controlled for confounding variables, such as smoking and parity.

Prospective studies have failed to uncover any association between alcohol consumption and stillbirth rates among women clinically characterized by alcohol abuse (Sokol et al., 1980). Consumption of an average of three (Gibson, Baghurst, & Colley, 1983) or five or more drinks a day (Davis et al., 1982; Griso et al., 1984; Plant, 1985) has likewise not been linked to any significant increases in stillbirths.

The conclusion from these studies is that drinking during pregnancy does not increase the risk for stillbirths.

Preterm Birth

Gestational age is the most important factor affecting neonatal mortality: Although preterm birth (<37 weeks gestation) occurs in only 9.8% of all live births, it accounts for 57.7% of all infant deaths.

Gestational age is also the most important factor contributing to decreased birth weights. A possible reason why children with FAS weigh considerably less at birth than other children (see Chapter 6) is that they are born prior to term. Because preterm birth is such an important factor for a child's subsequent development, the potential role of maternal drinking in preterm delivery has been intensively studied, especially because about half (52%) of all children with FAS described in the clinical case literature were born preterm (Abel, 1990).

Association with FAS

Preterm births were found to occur more often among children with FAS in two studies. In France, 46% of a group of children with FAS were preterm compared with 29% for non-FAS children (Dehaene et al., 1981). However, the preterm rate in the general population was about 7% (Peacock, Bland, & Anderson, 1995). This means the fourfold increase in this patient population was far from representative of the general population. A study from Sweden also noted a high rate of preterm birth among children with FAS, but little was noted about the mothers of these children (Olegard et al., 1979).

Because cirrhosis is associated with alcoholism, studies relating preterm births to drinking during pregnancy, especially among alcoholics, should control for this factor. As in the case of spontaneous abortions, cirrhosis is also one of the most important factors increasing the likelihood of preterm birth (Scholtes, 1979). Other than mentioning the fact that some mothers may have the disease, no studies have considered cirrhosis when preterm births have been examined in the context of FAS/ARBEs.

Association with Maternal Alcohol Abuse in Absence of FAS

Although a high rate (34%) of preterm births was noted in a French retrospective study examining children born to alcoholic women (Dehaene et al., 1977), these children were initially referred for evaluation because of a malformation. Children with malformations are often born preterm. If the malformation resulted from alcohol, it would still be an alcohol-related birth effect, but not one directly related to alcohol consumption.

A Swedish study that examined preterm delivery rates among alcoholic women compared preterm births prior to and after drinking. No significant change in preterm deliveries was associated with drinking (Hollstedt et al., 1983b).

Little, Streissguth, Barr, and Herman (1980) compared 50 alcoholic women who drank during pregnancy with another group of 50 alcoholic women who remained abstinent during pregnancy and a third group of 50 women who had no history of alcoholism and who were essentially abstinent during pregnancy. Average gestational age for children in all three groups was well above 37 weeks, and differences were not statistically significant.

A retrospective study from the United States found a statistically significant increase in preterm births associated with drinking six or more drinks per day, three times per week (Wilsnack et al., 1984). This result is in contrast to another study evaluating the effects of occasional binges (five or more drinks per occasion) that did not find any significant effect on preterm birth (Tolo & Little, 1993).

Retrospective studies evaluating preterm birth must be considered in light of the frequently noted observation that unfavorable outcomes are generally more common in retrospective compared with prospective studies. In the context of alcohol's relation to preterm birth, the contrast between retrospective and prospective studies is reflected in a series of studies conducted in France by Kaminski and her co-workers (1981). When collected retrospectively, the frequency of preterm birth was doubled among moderate and heavy drinkers; when collected prospectively, drinking during pregnancy had no significant impact on preterm birth.

A prospective study of over 12,000 women, of whom 204 were alcohol abusers, found no evidence alcohol abusers were more likely to have experienced a preterm delivery (Sokol et al., 1980).

Association in the Absence of Alcohol Abuse

Table 4.1 lists prospective studies that examined the relationship between preterm birth and maternal alcohol consumption. As indicated by this table, far

Table 4.1. Epidemiological Studies Evaluating Relationship
Between Maternal Alcohol Consumption and Preterm Births

Increased occurrence	No effect	
Berkowitz et al., 1982	Bell & Lumley, 1989	Mills et al., 1984
Hingson et al., 1982	Bonati & Fellin, 1991	Ogston & Parry, 1992
Kaminski et al., 1981*	Borges et al., 1993	Peacock et al., 1995
Little et al., 1986	Coles et al., 1985a	Primatesta et al., 1993
Lumley et al., 1985	Davis et al., 1982	Rostand et al., 1990
McDonald et al., 1992	Gibson et al., 1983	Russell, 1977
Olegard et al., 1979	Jacobson et al., 1984	Shiono et al., 1986*
Ouellette et al., 1977	Kaminski et al., 1978*	Sokol et al., 1980
Rosett et al., 1983	Kapamadzija & Horvat, 1991	Tolo & Little, 1993
Shiono et al., 1986*	Lazzaroni et al., 1993	van den Berg, 1977
Sulaiman et al., 1988	Marbury et al., 1983	Verkerk et al., 1993
Tennes & Blackard, 1980		

*The same studies reported *both* decreases or no changes depending on inclusion of confounding
variables in the analyses.
Source: E. L. Abel & J. H. Hannigan, "J-shaped" relationship between drinking during pregnancy and
birth weight: Reanalysis of prospective epidemological data, *Alcohol & Alcoholism* (1995) *30*, 172–179.
Copyright by Williams & Wilkins. Reprinted by permission of the publisher.

more studies have reported no effect of maternal drinking on preterm birth than
have reported finding such an effect (22 to 12).

Many of the studies reporting increased preterm births did not take into
account potential confounding factors, such as socioeconomic status, previous
history of preterm births, malformations, and so on, so even here the evidence for
an increase in preterm births is weak.

A major factor contributing to preterm birth is low socioeconomic status
(Peacock et al., 1995). Women who work at manual jobs and are unmarried, and
women who are undernourished are especially at risk for preterm births (Peacock
et al., 1995).

Race, which is confounded with socioeconomic status (SES), is also related
to preterm birth. For example, African-American children are twice as likely to be
born preterm as Caucasian children (17.6% vs. 8.2%) (Hoque et al., 1987). Preterm
births also occur more often among Native Americans than Caucasians (Grossman, Krieger, Sugarman, & Forquera, 1994). When SES or race are taken into
account, previously significant associations between alcohol consumption and
reproductive outcomes often cease to be significant (Marbury et al., 1983). Smoking is also related to increased prematurity (Abel, 1984b). Because smoking is
highly correlated with drinking (Ernhart, Morrow-Tlucak, Sokol, & Martier, 1988;
Jacobson, Jacobson, & Sokol, 1994a; Olsen, Pereira, & Olsen, 1991; Sokol et al.,
1980; Wright et al., 1983), it is also possible that many of the outcomes linking

drinking to preterm birth are more likely attributable to smoking or to an interaction between drinking and smoking.

Even when potential confounding factors are ignored, the effects of alcohol, though statistically significant, are biologically trivial. In the Hingson et al. (1982) study, for instance, drinking prior to pregnancy accounted for no more than 0.5% of the effect on preterm birth; drinking during pregnancy had no statistically significant effect on this outcome. Tennes and Blackard (1980) estimated that drinking during pregnancy accounted for only 2% of the effect in their study. In their prospective study of 952 women in Dundee, Scotland, Sulaiman, Florey, Taylor, and Ogston (1988) found a significant increase in preterm birth, but alcohol accounted for only 2.5% of this effect.

Although no longer the case, alcohol was once clinically used to postpone labor (Abel, 1981). This would imply that rather than precipitating labor, alcohol consumption should actually delay it. However, alcohol's effects on labor have since been dismissed as a placebo effect (Abel, 1981), so these studies cannot be used to make any inferences regarding alcohol's effects on preterm labor.

In summary, the relationship between maternal alcohol consumption and preterm birth is tenuous and even when statistically significant, the association is weak.

Intrapartum Problems

Children with FAS experience a number of intrapartum complications that could, in themselves, result in problems related to development. Breech birth, for example, occurs in about 3% of all births (Barden, 1975), but occurs in about 15% (Majewski et al., 1976) to 35% (Abel, 1990) of all cases of FAS. The percentage may be even higher because fetuses in the breech position are often delivered by Cesarean section, which also occurs with a relatively high frequency in FAS (e.g., 36%, Abel, 1990). When twins are differentially affected with ARBEs, including FAS, it is the twin in the breech position who is primarily affected (Riikonen, 1994). Because breech birth is associated with many of the behavioral effects of FAS, such as hyperactivity and mental retardation (Abel, 1984a), the higher prevalence of these behavioral effects in children with FAS may be due to their having been born as breech babies rather than the direct effects of alcohol on the nervous system.

Whether the increased rate of Caesarean sections is related to breech birth or not, its higher incidence among women who give birth to children with FAS is noteworthy because of the involvement in such births of anesthetics and analgesics which exhibit cross-tolerance to alcohol (Han, 1969). As a result, alcohol abusers will require higher doses to produce maternal narcosis or analgesia than nonabusers (Han, 1969). Assuming alcohol abusers are unlikely to deliver their children by the Lamaze method, children born to alcohol-abusing women, will receive higher doses of obstetrical medication. Among the behavioral effects associated with such medications are newborn depression; altered EEG activity; poorer performance on newborn test measures, such as orientation to novel stimuli; and increased irritability and altered motor activity, lasting several days after birth (Abel, 1984a). In short, all of the newborn behavioral effects reported in conjunction with maternal drinking during pregnancy may be due to intrapartum exposure to obstetric medication rather than directly related to maternal alcohol abuse. When taking into account whether or not obstetric medication was administered equally in these studies, consideration should also be given to dosage.

Neonatal Withdrawal

A relatively mild neonatal withdrawal symptomatology has been reported for children with FAS, and for children without FAS who were born to alcoholic women. Among its characteristics are jitteriness and tremulousness (Coles, Smith, Fernoff, & Falek, 1984; Coles, Smith, Lancaster, & Falek, 1985b; Fried & Makin, 1987; Haddad & Messer, 1994; Harris, Osborn, Weinberg, Look, & Junald, 1993; Iosub, Fuchs, Bingol, & Gromisch, 1981; Landesman-Dwyer, Keller, & Streissguth, 1978; Ouelette, Rosett, Rosman, & Weiner, 1977; Pierog et al., 1977; Riikonen, 1994; Scher, Richardson, Goble, Day, & Stoffer, 1988), increased muscle tone (Pierog et al., 1977), increased respiratory rates (Pierog et al., 1977), hyperacusis (Pierog et al., 1977), exaggerated reflexes (Chernick, Childiaeva, & Ioffe, 1983; Coles, Smith, & Falek, 1987b; Ioffe, Childiaeva, & Chernick, 1984), and sleep disturbances (see later). While observable in a few cases, these symptoms are of an entirely different magnitude and severity compared with those associated with neonatal withdrawal from narcotics (Zelson, 1975).

In some instances, these effects have been noted as late as 10 days (Haddad & Messer, 1994) or even as long as one month after birth (Coles et al., 1985b; Ioffe et al., 1984; Streissguth et al., 1994a). The persistence of these effects implies that they are not likely to be symptomatic of withdrawal.

Although a study in mice speculated that prenatal exposure to alcohol can result in neonatal withdrawal and related postnatal mortality, there is little evidence to support this speculation. The basis for the interpretation was the observation of a delay in postnatal mortality in neonatal mice whose mothers were maintained on a liquid alcohol diet for a few days after giving birth as compared with neonates whose mothers were taken off the diet one day prior to parturition (Middaugh & Boggan, 1995). As the authors note, this hypothesis presumed that the offspring were consuming alcohol through nursing, thus delaying withdrawal. This possibility is highly implausible but cannot be dismissed outright.

Placenta Pathology and Size

The placenta begins to develop at the time of implantation, around 6 to 7 days after conception. This organ not only cements the embryo/fetus to the mother, but it also mediates the exchange of nutrients, gases, and waste substances between the two. Anything that affects the placenta's structure or cellular activity can therefore be expected to impact adversely on the embryo/fetus.

Premature separation of the placenta from the uterus, a condition called *abruption*, was mentioned as the cause of death in two children born to alcoholic women (Olegard et al., 1979). Two early studies found evidence that premature placental separation occurred more frequently among heavy drinkers (Kaminski et al., 1976; Sokol et al., 1980). However, little else has been reported concerning the role of abruption in conjunction with maternal drinking. Because this is a life-threatening situation, the absence of such reports implies that abruption is an unlikely factor contributing to ARBEs.

Pathology

Gross pathology is not usually visible or evident in the placentas of alcohol-abusing women (Lapatto & Raisanen, 1988; Sokol et al., 1980). When pathology is seen, it is typically related to nutritional problems or diseases with a known etiological relationship to placental pathology rather than alcohol abuse. In these instances, alcoholism is a correlate not a cause of placental pathology. Histological examination of 23 placentas from infants whose mothers drank 28 to 54 drinks a day, revealed considerable damage in the form of chorioamnionitis, infarction, villous dysmaturity, and villitis (Baldwin, MacLeod, & Benirschke, 1982). Interestingly, only half of these women had children with FAS. Where background information was available, the socioeconomic status of these women was always low and increased vasculitis and chorioamnionitis were attributed to their living conditions.

A scanning-and-transmission electron microscopic study of placentas from five alcohol abusers (5 or more drinks per drinking occasion) found signs of hyperplasia of villous capillaries and endarteritis—a narrowing or obliteration of small blood vessels that is often the result of proliferation of cells into the lumen or fatty degeneration of arterial tissues—as compared with controls (Amankwah & Kaufmann, 1984). These kinds of effects are generally associated with maternal diseases rather than alcohol abuse (Amankwah & Kaufmann, 1984).

The effects of very high levels of alcohol exposure on placental pathology in animals are equally inconclusive. A single intraperitoneal injection of a high dose of alcohol early in gestation resulted in placental necrosis in mice, characterized by large cysts, infarctions, and fibrinoid accumulation. The decidua basilis of the placenta (the part of the placenta that is maternal in origin) also contained inflammatory cells and large vacuoles (Padmanabhan, 1985). The animals in this study were not pair-fed, so some of this damage may have been due to nutritional factors, but the damage was so extensive that it seems more likely to have been the result of alcohol toxicity. Similarly degeneration and toxicity, including increased presence of large vacuoles in the basal zone and signs of inflammation (infiltration by polymorphonuclear leukocytes) were observed in placentas from rats that consumed alcohol in their drinking water (Eguchi et al., 1989; Kennedy, 1984).

Given its toxicity, a massive dose of acetaldehyde (100 mg/kg, administered intraperitoneally) not surprisingly produced placental lesions and decreased weights (Sreenathan, Singh, & Padmanabhan, 1984). This level of exposure is so improbable outside of the laboratory that its relevance is dubious.

Size

Placental weight is highly correlated with birth weight. Marked changes in the ratio of the placenta's weight relative to birth weight often reflect subsequent problems at and after birth. Increases in placental weight relative to birth weight, for instance, are often associated with low Apgar scores, respiratory distress syndrome, neurological disorders, and neonatal death; decreased placental weight relative to birth weight is associated with low birth weight and below-average postnatal growth (Maprurira, Msamati, & Banadda, 1992).

As in the case of placental pathology, little has been reported concerning human placental size in conjunction with maternal alcohol abuse. What has been reported in inconclusive. For example, while decreased placental weights were associated with maternal alcohol abuse in a prospective study in which nine mothers gave birth to children with FAS (Andersson, Halmesmaki, Koivusalo, Lapatto, & Ylikorkala, 1989), nearly all of the women smoked; the decrease, therefore, may have been due to smoking, alcohol, their combination, or to some other related factor. Decreased placental weight was associated with drinking during pregnancy in two other retrospective studies (Kaminiski et al., 1976; Lapatto & Raisanen, 1988), but not in a large prospective study (Sokol et al., 1980).

When examined superficially, studies of placental weight in animals seem equally inconsistent. Many studies have reported no significant changes associated with maternal alcohol treatments, whereas others have reported enlargement and occasionally decreases in weight. These apparent inconsistencies are not random outcomes, but instead reflect the time during pregnancy when alcohol exposure occurs. This relationship was first noted by Aufrere and LeBourhis (1987) and is detailed in Table 4.2.

As Table 4.2 indicates, when alcohol exposure begins prior to or during the first trimester of pregnancy, placentas are enlarged; exposure during midpreg-

Table 4.2. Placenta Size Effects in Animals Treated with Alcohol During Different Periods of Gestation

Prior to or during first two weeks of pregnancy		Midpregnancy		Mid- to last week of pregnancy	
Increases	Exceptions	No Efffect	Exceptions	Decreases	Exceptions
Aufrere & LeBourhis, 1987	Greeley et al., 1990	Henderson et al., 1981		Greizersteln & Aldrich, 1983	Wunderlich et al., 1979
Baran, 1982	Leichter & Lee, 1984	Kennedy et al., 1986		Kennedy, 1984	
Eguchi et al., 1989	Snyder et a., 1986	Samson et al., 1979		Padmanabhan, 1985	
Fisher et al., 1985					
Ghishan et al., 1982					
Gordon et al., 1985					
Henderson et al., 1981					
Leichter & Lee, 1984					
Marquis et al., 1984					
Sanchis et al., 1986					
Singh et al., 1989					
Tanaka et al., 1988					
Weiner et al., 1981					
Witek-Janusek, 1986					
Zidenberg-Cherr et al., 1988					

nancy does not produce significant changes in placenta size; exposure during the middle and last week of gestation results in decreased size.

Some investigators have attributed alcohol-related placental hyperplasia to compensatory growth initiated to maintain fetal growth in the face of alcohol-induced hypoxia (Gordon, Streeter, & Winick, 1985). Although this is plausible, it does not explain the decreases in placental size or absence of changes that occur when alcohol exposure takes place during mid- or late-pregnancy, unless demands for oxygen are much greater during the latter part of pregnancy.

Function

The placenta performs a number of metabolic and endocrine functions that have a potential bearing on the etiology of FAS/ARBEs.

One consequence of alcohol-induced placental damage, for instance, may be a decrease in some of its metabolic functions, such as decreased lactate production. After glucose and amino acids, lactate production by the placenta is an important energy substrate for the fetus (Burd et al., 1975). The fetal growth spurt, for example, is paralleled by an increase in placenta lactate production (Burd et al., 1975). At least one study has shown that in isolated placentas exposed to alcohol, lactate levels were actually slightly increased (Rice et al., 1986).

Because decreased placental lactate production is an unlikely explanation for alcohol's effects on the fetus, free fatty acid production may be an important mechanism mediating fetal damage. This mechanism is discussed more fully in Chapter 13. For now, it is worthwhile noting that fatty acid ethyl esters (FAEE) may be produced by the placenta as a consequence of its low alcohol dehydrogenase (ADH) activity. Instead of metabolism by this oxidative pathway, alcohol may instead be metabolized by a nonoxidative pathway by way of fatty acid ethyl ester synthase, which is present in the human placenta at term (Bearer, Gould, Emerson, Kinnunen, & Cook, 1992), resulting in production of free fatty acids and FAEE (Laposta & Lange, 1986). The placenta only produces these FAEEs in the presence of alcohol (Bearer et al., 1992). These FAEEs bind to mitochondria and can uncouple oxidative phosphorylation, resulting in many of the effects associated with cellular damage due to prenatal alcohol exposure (see Chapter 13).

The placenta is also a major source of progesterone and lactogen during pregnancy, but little attention has been focused on these placental hormones in conjunction with alcohol abuse during pregnancy. One study reported an alcohol-related decrease in progesterone production in term human placentas in vitro, which was attributed to inhibition of the progesterone's substrate (Ahluwalia, Smith, Adeyiga, Akbasak, & Rajguru, 1992). Lactogen production has not been found to be significantly altered by alcohol (Halmesmaki et al., 1986).

Most of the attention focused on the placenta has involved its role in passive and active transport of nutrients from the mother to the fetus, especially during the last trimester of pregnancy when most of the fetus's growth occurs. Passive transport of diffusible molecules involves their movement across a concentration gradient and is dependent on uterine and umbilical blood flow. Alcohol decreases blood flow on both sides of sheep placenta for up to two hours, resulting in a decrease in glucose supply to the fetus (Falconer, 1990). A similar effect occurred in rats (Jones, Leichter, & Lee, 1981). (Effects on placental transport are discussed in connection with specific nutrients, for example, glucose and folate, and the various mechanistic explanations accounting for ARBEs in Chapter 13.)

Although placental pathology is associated with alcohol abuse, this relationship is only indirect. On the other hand, changes in placental size appear to be a direct consequence of alcohol abuse. The extent to which these changes directly impact the embryo/fetus awaits clarification.

The fetus adapts to decreases in nutrients by slowing its growth rate, either through a direct retardation in the rate of cell division or through reducing the concentration of growth factors or growth-related hormones. Depending on the extent of oxygen deprivation, the growth rate may likewise be slowed or cells may die. In either case, disproportionate growth rates in various organs may occur. Disproportionate head circumferences and body weights at birth reflect the adaptations that the fetus makes in coping with altered nutrients and oxygen at critical periods in its development.

CHAPTER 5

Miscellaneous ARBEs

Immune Function

Depressed immune function is not considered diagnostic of FAS, despite the fact that children with FAS have very high rates of upper respiratory tract infections and recurrent serious otitis media (SOM). Recurrent SOM is the most commonly encountered infection in children with FAS (see Table 5.1). Urinary tract infections, meningitis, tumors, and myasthenia gravis, an autoimmune disorder, have also been found in conjunction with FAS (Church & Gerkin, 1988; Dahl-Regis & Jayan-Trought, 1986; Johnson, 1981; Knight, Marmer, & Steele, 1981; Steinhausen, Nestler, & Spohr, 1982). Convergent studies in animals clearly support these associations.

SOM, characterized by fluid accumulation in the inner ear, is often caused by a bacterial infection originating in the upper respiratory tract. The frequency of its occurrence in patients with FAS is indicated in several studies in Table 5.1. In the study reported by Church and Gerkin (1988), 8 out of 13 children with FAS and recurrent SOM recovered after receiving antibiotics; the other 5 required myringotomies and ventilation tubes (cf. also Streissguth, Clarren, & Jones, 1985).

Altered susceptibility to infection is also reflected in the decreased lymphocyte response to mitogen stimulation and in an increased eosinophil count in children with FAS who were matched for age, sex, and gestational age with control children (Johnson et al., 1981).

Studies in animals prenatally exposed to alcohol have noted comparable susceptibilities to infection. For example, alcohol-exposed offspring are more likely than controls to develop perforated corneas in response to pseudomonas, a gram negative opportunistic bacterium, and the days to perforation are also shorter (see Figure 5.1).

To some extent, the increased responsiveness to infection may be due to a

Table 5.1. Prevalence of Serous Otitis Media (SOM)
in Patients with FAS

Study site	Sample size	No. with SOM (%)	Reference
Denver	14	13 (93%)	Church & Gerkin, 1988
Detroit	22	17 (77%)	Church et al., 1997
Seattle	9	5 (56%)	Streissguth et al., 1991
Little Rock	3	7 (54%)	Johnson et al., 1981

decreased fever response (Yirmiya, Pilati, Chiappelli, & Taylor, 1993). A suppressed fever response is potentially important with respect to bacterial infections because fever raises body heat above the optimal temperature supporting bacterial growth, thereby reducing the virulence of such infections.

Decreased contact hypersensitivity, decreased local graft versus host reactions, and increased parasitic infection rates have also been noted in conjunction with prenatal alcohol exposure in animals (Gottesfeld, 1996).

The increased susceptibility to bacterial infections associated with prenatal alcohol exposure in humans and animals has been attributed to retarded development of the thymus, impaired lymphocytic responses, and decreased T-cell proliferation and B-cell antibody formation (see Chapter 13).

Neoplasms

Brain tumors are the second most common neoplasms in children (leukemia being the first). About 200 to 300 children develop such tumors each year in the United States (Starshak, Wells, Sty, & Gregg, 1992).

Several clinical studies have reported neoplasms (ganglioneuroblastoma, neuroblastoma, rhabdomyosarcoma, nephroblastoma, hepatoblastoma, endodermal-sinus tumor, sacrococcygeal teratoma) in children with FAS. In most cases, these neoplasms have appeared in early childhood, but there are also case reports in which they appeared in adolescents (see Abel, 1990).

Apart from these sporadic case studies, there is little evidence that alcohol is a transplacental carcinogen. A case-control study of risk factors for hepatoblastoma in children did not find any evidence that maternal alcohol consumption was a contributing factor (Buckley et al., 1989). The link to prenatal alcohol exposure is even more tenuous when considering what is otherwise known about some tumors, such as hepatoblastomas. These tumors are generally found in children with above-average birth weights (Buckley et al., 1989), whereas children with FAS are nearly always characterized by low birth weight (see Chapter 6).

Studies of tumorigenesis in animals prenatally exposed to alcohol are incon-

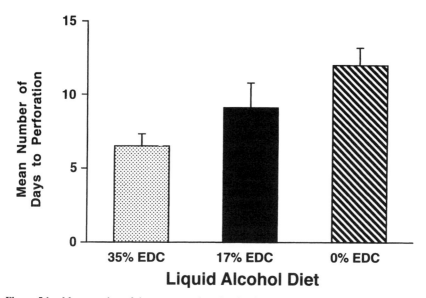

Figure 5.1. Mean number of days to corneal perforation in 50-day-old rats prenatally exposed to alcohol, after treatment with pseudomonas bacteria. EDC = Ethanol derived calories. (Adapted from Hazlett, Barrett, Berg, & Abel, 1989).

clusive. One study found an increase in pituitary tumors (Gottesfeld, Trippe, Wargovich, & Berkowitz, 1992), while another found a decrease in liver tumors (Kahn, 1968). An increase in pancreatic tumors was observed when alcohol and nicotine-derived nitrosamine, a potent carcinogen, were combined prenatally (Schuller, Jorquera, Reichert, & Castonguay, 1993). An increased number of tumors was also noted when mice were challenged with Rous sarcoma virus within 24 hours of birth (Haughton, Mohr, & Ellis, 1981). At present, there is no reason to believe the association between FAS and spontaneous childhood tumors is anything but coincidental.

Myopathy

Muscle weakness and gross muscle pathology have not been widely studied in the context of FAS, although general weakness, incoordination, strabismus and related ocular anomalies (see Chapter 7), cardiac anomalies, and increased rates of hernias (see Abel, 1990, for references concerning hernias) are all associated with FAS.

Adickes and Shuman (1983) described three children with FAS as having advanced muscular weakness. Biopsies of skeletal muscle tissue revealed an advanced stage of muscle cell degeneration. Myocytes in general were small and exhibited various cellular irregularities. Similar anomalies were observed in three patients with FAS in studies by Loser and his coworkers (Loser, Themann, Welim, & Dittrich, 1988). Because the kinds of anomalies found in these children are associated with major physical weakness, the fact they are rarely mentioned outside of these reports indicates that they are not commonly encountered in FAS.

Studies in animals, however, have found decreased weights of selected skeletal muscle groups (Ihemelandu, 1984) and myopathies similar to those seen in the children described earlier, such as myofibril dysplasia, myofibril disorganization, and decreased myofibril volume (Adickes, Mollner, & Lockwood, 1990).

Neural Tube Defects (NTDs)

Neural tube (closure) defects (NTDs) such as anencephaly, spina bifida, and meningomyelocele are major causes of infant mortality and morbidity. Because of their epidemiological and embryological similarities, NTDs have been regarded as a single etiologic entity (Sever, 1995), despite considerable evidence for multi-causality and heterogeneity (Sever, 1995).

NTDs are mentioned in about 2.4% of the case literature studies for FAS (see Abel, 1990; Steinhausen & Spohr, 1986) but are uncommon in related clinical or epidemiological studies. Reports of neural tube defects in siblings born to an alcoholic mother (Castro-Gago, Novo, & Pena, 1987; Dehaene et al., 1977), and the absence of this defect while one of these mothers was being treated for alcoholism supported the possible involvement of alcohol in this disorder.

However, neural tube defects have not been noted in other studies of siblings with alcoholic mothers and is not observed in nonhuman primates exposed to relatively large amounts of alcohol in utero (Clarren & Bowden, 1982; Clarren et al., 1987; Scott & Fradkin, 1984). Therefore, its association with FAS awaits clarification.

A factor associated with NTDs that has only recently begun to be appreciated is they are often "clustered" in time and place (Sever, 1995). Clustering implies that environmental and possibly occupational factors are important etiological considerations in NTDs. The increased incidence of NTDs in FAS may therefore be only coincidental.

Although exencephaly is rarely observed in connection with FAS, it has been observed in a nonhuman primate (Siebert et al., 1991) and in rats, mice, and hamsters prenatally exposed to high doses of alcohol (Kotch & Sulik, 1992a; Samson et al., 1979; Webster, Walsh, McEwen, & Lipson, 1983; Wynter, Walsh, Webster, McEwen, & Lipson, 1983) or acetaldehyde (O'Shea & Kaufman, 1981). It has also been produced in vitro using very high concentrations of alcohol

(Wynter et al., 1983). One study found 90% of all fetuses with exencephaly were females (Padmanabhan, Wasfi, & Craigmyle, 1994).

Considerable compensation or reversibility of these defects may occur in rodents, depending on when embryos are examined. For example, mouse fetuses exposed to acetaldehyde on gestation days 7–9 and examined on gestation day 10 had a much higher incidence of neural tube defects (25%) compared with those exposed on the same days and examined on day 12 of gestation (2%) (O'Shea & Kaufman, 1981). Because neural tube defects are not common in animals or children prenatally exposed to alcohol, these results may be peculiar to acetaldehyde. However, these results suggest the possibility that repair mechanisms may be involved in these and other anomalies, and that teratogenic effects may involve insult to these mechanisms, along with the original insult to the tissues whose development was arrested.

Because folic acid supplementation prior to conception and during early gestation reduces the occurrence of NTDs (Sever, 1995), some researchers have asked whether heavy preconceptual and gestational drinking may contribute to an increase in NTDs due to effects on folic acid. However, a large prospective study from Roubaix, France, did not find significant differences in serum folate levels associated with alcohol consumption in pregnant test subjects, after controlling for such factors as smoking and parity, both of which are related to heavy drinking (Larroque et al., 1992). Because most of the women in this study were beer drinkers, the authors speculated that the heavy drinkers were not folate deficient because they supplemented their folate intake with beer, which contains relatively high levels of this nutrient, thereby correcting what might otherwise have been a folate deficiency.

Infant Mortality

The infant mortality rate (mortality before the first year of life) in the United States is about 10.0 infant deaths per 1,000 live births, or about 1% of all live births. Race is a major factor in infant mortality, being higher among African-American infants (18.3 per 1,000 live births) than among Caucasian infants (8.9 per 1,000 live births). The leading cause of infant death among African-American children is sudden infant death syndrome (SIDS)—the sudden and unexpected death of an infant or young child without apparent cause. Among Caucasian infants, the leading cause of infant mortality is congenital anomalies (Praeger et al., 1983).

Sudden Infant Death Syndrome (SIDS)

Although three studies have noted an increase in the frequency of sudden infant death syndrome (SIDS) associated with FAS or FAE (Church, Gerkin, &

McPherson, 1986) or with maternal drinking during pregnancy (Hoffman, Dames, Hillman, & Krongrad, 1988; Southall, 1987), all three present problems of inter-pretation because the mothers of these SIDS children were primarily of low socioeconomic status and many were also smokers.

Infant mortality is inversely correlated with a mother's educational attain-ment. Rates among college graduates are much lower than rates among women with less than eight years of schooling (7.0 vs. 12.8 per 1,000). Maternal education level is proxy for socioeconomic status; the lower the socioeconomic status (educational attainment), the higher the infant mortality rate. Because mothers of children with FAS are overwhelmingly of low socioeconomic status (see Chapter 11), this result may reflect their social condition rather than their drinking behavior. Smoking is a correlate of low socioeconomic status and heavy drinking and is independently a major contributor to SIDS (Southall et al., 1987).

In one of the studies reporting a statistically significant relation between maternal drinking and SIDS (Hoffman et al., 1988), SIDS children were also characterized by low birth weight. The infant mortality rate in general for low-birth-weight infants (term weight of less than 2,500 g) is 94.5 deaths per 1,000 live births, 22 times higher than the 4.3 per 1,000 rate for infants weighing 2,500 grams or more at birth. Low-birth-weight infants comprise only 6.8% of all live births, but account for 61.1% of all infant deaths (Praeger et al., 1984). When the SIDS children whose mothers drank during pregnancy were compared with control low-birth-weight children, maternal drinking did not increase the risk for SIDS (Hoff-man et al., 1988).

Given the various risk factors independently associated with SIDS in these studies, the reported associations between maternal alcohol consumption and SIDS are tenuous at best (Kandall & Gaines, 1991).

Other Epidemiological Studies

Two methodologically weak retrospective studies involving relatively few children have reported increased postnatal mortality rates among children with FAS or in children whose mothers were alcoholics (Jones, Smith, & Streissguth, 1974; Olegard et al., 1979). These findings were not corroborated by a large-scale prospective epidemiological study (Sokol et al., 1980).

Studies in Animals

Increased postnatal mortality in animals prenatally exposed to alcohol has been noted in several studies (Abel, 1978; Abel & Dintcheff, 1978; Henderson & Schenker, 1977; Middaugh & Boggan, 1991). Because offspring in these studies remained with their biological mothers after birth, the increase in infant mortality could have been due to residual effects on lactational performance or maternal behavior. However, increased mortality still occurred when these confounding factors were eliminated by fostering offspring to nontreated adoptive mothers (Abel, 1978; Abel & Dintcheff, 1978; Middaugh & Boggan, 1991).

The reasons for the increased mortality in these animals may be due to their previously mentioned longer latencies to begin suckling and their lower sucking pressures, associated with prenatal exposure. Another possible explanation was their previously mentioned difficulty maintaining body temperature, which made them lethargic so that they failed to elicit maternal care if they strayed out of the nest (see Chapter 6, "Postnatal Growth Retardation"). Because there is no "intensive care unit" to assist these animals, they may die as a result of neglect or because they did not receive enough milk.

Studies in animals also indicated that the combination of prenatal exposure to alcohol and other drugs, such as marijuana or cocaine, can also increase postnatal mortality, and the increase may be greater than that associated with either drug alone (Abel, 1985; Church, Holmes, Overbeck, Tilak, & Zajac, 1991).

CHAPTER 6

Growth Retardation

Prenatal Growth Retardation

The previous chapters examined alcohol-related birth effects often associated with maternal alcohol abuse during pregnancy, but not listed in any of the diagnostic paradigms mentioned in Chapter 2. Now we will turn to a discussion of the main contributions to the pattern of anomalies associated with FAS in one or more of the diagnostic paradigms, beginning with growth retardation.

Growth retardation is one of the hallmarks of fetal alcohol abuse syndrome. It may occur prenatally and therefore be recognizable at birth, or postnatally, when it is described as "failure to thrive."

One criterion for prenatal growth retardation with respect to FAS is a birth weight less than the 10th percentile when corrected for term. A normal birth weight for a child born in the United States, regardless of race, is about 3,370 grams (7 lb, 7 oz) (Wegman, 1987). The average birth weight of a term infant with fetal alcohol abuse syndrome is 2,290 grams (5 lb, 1 oz) (Abel, 1990).

A second criterion is low birth weight, defined as a term birth weight below 2,500 g. Because the average birth weight of a child with FAS is 2,290 grams, this child is growth retarded at birth, according to this criterion. In fact, about 53% of all term FAS births meet this latter clinical criterion (Abel, 1990) compared with 7% of the general population (Wegman, 1987).

Low birth weight itself is associated with a host of subsequent problems, including increased perinatal mortality, postnatal growth retardation, delayed reflex and motor development, sleep disturbances, lower IQ, speech problems, poor sucking reflex, poor school performance, and many other effects (Abel, 1984). Because many of the effects associated with low birth weight are identical to those associated with FAS, it becomes a moot point whether they are independent consequences of prenatal alcohol exposure or the sequelae of growth retardation. The end result is the same; the issue is only important from the standpoint of the mechanisms involved.

One crude way of estimating the level of consumption necessary to produce a child with low birth weight is as follows: The median birth weight in America is about 3,370 g, and the criterion for low birth weight is 2,500 g, therefore, the difference is 870 g. If birth weight decreases by 200 grams for every two drinks (see later), then a 130-lb woman would have to consume a minimum of eight to nine drinks a day in a 5-hour period to place her child in the low-birth-weight range (see Chapter 1, Table 1.2).

We can carry out the same kind of extrapolations using data from any epidemiological study. For instance, Kaminski (Kaminski, Rumeau, & Schwartz, 1978; Kaminski et al., 1981) estimated birth weight decreased by 60 grams from normal for every three drinks a woman consumed a day. Because the average birth weight of an infant with FAS is typically about 1,080 grams below normal (see earlier), this would imply the level of consumption resulting in this much of a decrease is about 54 drinks a day! Similarly, the decrease of 165 grams associated with consumption of from three to five drinks a day reported by Mills and coworkers (Mills et al., 1984) would put maternal consumption for FAS at about 21 to 35 drinks a day! These extrapolations are congruent with the conclusion reached in Chapter 2: The focus of our attention should be on alcohol abuse during pregnancy rather than on relatively low levels of drinking.

Whatever impact drinking has on birth weight, this impact is greatest during the last three months of pregnancy. Rosett and his co-workers (Rosett, Weiner, Zuckerman, McKinlay, & Edelin, 1980) reported alcoholic women who abstained or markedly reduced their drinking before the third trimester gave birth to infants whose birth weights were not decreased as much as the infants of those women who continued to drink during pregnancy (Little, 1977).

The effects of high doses of alcohol on the birth weights of animals likewise indicates that exposure during the last third of pregnancy has the greatest impact on birth weight (Abel et al, 1979). A study using a mouse model found that extending the duration of alcohol exposure up to the time of delivery, in contrast to terminating alcohol exposure a day prior to delivery, resulted in an additional 10% decrease in birth weight (Middaugh & Boggan, 1995). In discussing this surprising result, the authors pointed out that this additional day of exposure late in pregnancy represents about 5% of the total gestational period (20 days) in the mouse and is comparable to two additional weeks of alcohol exposure in a human pregnancy (266 days).

As with most of the characteristics of FAS, racial factors affect birth weight and therefore represent a source of potential error in clinical diagnosis. For example, American children of African descent are twice as likely as Caucasians to fall into the low-birth-weight category of 2,500 grams simply by virtue of race. Low birth weights are also much more common among Native Americans than Caucasians (Grossman et al., 1994).

From a research standpoint, potential distortions in the association between maternal drinking and birth weight may occur outside of alcohol abuse merely because different drinking groups contain disproportionate numbers of African-American and Caucasian children. Since African-American children weigh about 150–200 grams less at term than Caucasian children (Dombrowski, Berry, Johnson, & Salai, 1994), if one drinking group contains proportionately more African-American children than a control group, that group is more likely to be identified as growth retarded. It is unlikely that an African-American child would be clinically misdiagnosed as FAS on the basis of this underlying racial difference in birth weight, but in a research study in which the impact of relatively low levels of drinking during pregnancy are being assessed, racial differences can account for the same 200-gram decrease that is typically associated with maternal drinking during pregnancy.

The Constitutionality Factor

In the absence of FAS, maternal alcohol abuse has a surprisingly minor impact on birth weight. For example, Little and Streissguth (1978) found that birth weights of children born to alcoholics who drank during pregnancy were on the average 493g below those of children born to controls. However, the birth weights of children born to alcoholic women who were abstinent during pregnancy were an average of 258g less than children born to nonalcoholic controls. Differences between the two alcoholic groups were not related to years of problem drinking or months of abstinence before conception. Similarly, a large prospective study in Cleveland of over 12,000 primarily poverty-stricken, African-American women found alcohol abusers gave birth to infants that weighed only 190 g less than nonabusers (Sokol et al., 1980).

One inference from these studies is that there is a "constitutionality factor" responsible for much of the decrease in birth weight associated with drinking during pregnancy. In other words, women who become alcohol abusers may have unique physiological characteristics that not only predispose them to alcohol abuse but also affect the intrauterine growth of their children.

In addition to gestational events, the mother's genome and the preconceptual environment can affect fetal growth. The correlation in birth weight between half-siblings with the same mother, for instance, is 0.58 compared with a correlation of 0.10 for half-siblings with the same father (Morton, 1955). Preconceptual conditions are likewise a factor because the risk of delivering a growth-retarded baby is increased if a mother's prepregnancy body weight is low. Women with a history of delivering one growth-retarded infant are more likely to give birth to growth-retarded babies in subsequent pregnancies (Sparks & Cetin, 1992). Furthermore, mothers who were born with low birth weights are more likely to give birth to their own low-birth-weight children (Sparks & Cetin, 1992).

The Law of Confounding Determinism

The weaker the association between two variables, the greater the impact of confounding factors. This is the underlying premise of what can be called the *law of confounding determinism*. As indicated throughout this book, this law applies to most of the epidemiological and clinical studies involving prenatal exposure to alcohol. One of its most common occurrences is the spuriously significant association between low levels of alcohol consumption and birth weight. For example, in the list of epidemiological studies examining the relationship between drinking during pregnancy and birth weight presented in Table 6.1, there are far more studies that have either found no significant effects of alcohol on birth weight, or, surprisingly, a slight increase in birth weight relative to abstention or near abstention.

These studies differ along many dimensions, such as methodology—for example, retrospective versus prospective design—study populations, levels of alcohol consumption, and so on, but none of these differences can consistently account for birth weight disparity except one, smoking.

If the data from the prospective studies listed in Table 6.1 are standardized in terms of drinking levels (equivalent average drinks per day), then the relationship between drinking and birth weight established by this data can be depicted by Figure 6.1. When no distinction is made between smokers and nonsmokers, alcohol consumption during pregnancy is associated with a statistically significant effect (SE) on birth weight, beginning at an average daily consumption of two drinks. When analyzed with respect to whether or not the mother smoked, smoking accounted for more than three times the effect on birth weight than alcohol did (26% vs.7%) (nonetheless, the interaction between smoking and alcohol is not statistically significant). However, when analyzed after first stratifying for each smoking condition separately, consumption of an average of two drinks a day during pregnancy has no significant effect on birth weight—unless it occurs in conjunction with smoking.

The impact of smoking during pregnancy relative to low levels of drinking illustrates the law of confounding determinism. Smoking is far more consistently associated with decreased birth weights than are low levels of drinking, but that effect is concealed unless the role of drinking is examined separately for smokers and nonsmokers. This conclusion is nothing new, but European epidemiologists, unlike their American counterparts, have adopted a strategy better suited to analyzing the relationship between drinking and smoking in light of this relationship.

In any research study exploring the effects of a particular condition, the most important factor affecting the validity of that study is the extent to which the experimental and control groups are equal except for the condition being evaluated. It is impossible to equate all the factors affecting humans that could possibly

Table 6.1. Epidemiological Studies Evaluating Relationship Between Maternal Alcohol Consumption and Birth Weight

Decreased birth weight	No effect or increased birth weight	
Brooke et al., 1989*	Bell & Lumley, 1989	Lazzaroni et al., 1993*
Chernick et al., 1983	Bonati & Fellin, 1991	Little & Wendt, 1991*
Coles et al., 1985a	Borges et al., 1993	Lumley et al., 1985*†
Da Costa Pereira et al., 1993	Coles et al., 1985a	Marbury et al., 1983
Day et al., 1989‡	Davis et al., 1982	Ogston & Parry, 1992*
Fried & O'Connell, 1987	Day et al., 1989‡	Primatesta et al., 1993*
Hingson et al., 1982	De Nigris et al., 1981	Rostand et al., 1990
Ioffe & Chernick, 1987	Ernhart et al., 1985a	Russell & Skinner, 1988
Kaminski et al., 1981	Gibson et al., 1983	Sulaiman et al., 1988
Kline et al., 1987*†	Godel et al., 1992	Tennes & Blackard, 1980
Kuzma & Sokol, 1982	Greene et al., 1991b	Tolo & Little, 1993
Larroque et al., 1993*	Griso et al., 1984	van den Berg, 1977*
Little, 1977	Hingson et al., 1982†	Verkerk et al., 1993*
Little et al., 1986*	Jacobson et al., 1984	Walpole et al., 1990, 1991
Lumley et al., 1985†	Kaminski et al., 1981	Yla-Outinen & Tuimala,
Mills et al., 1984*	Kariniemi & Rosti, 1988	1984
Olsen et al., 1983	Kline et al., 1987*†	Zuckerman et al., 1989
Ouellette et al., 1977		
Plant, 1987		
Rosett et al., 1983		
Russell, 1977		
Smith et al., 1986*		
Sokol et al., 1980		
Streissguth et al., 1981		
Virji, 1991		
Wright et al., 1983		

*Studies included in parametric analyses of mean birth weights see Fig. 6.1.
†The same studies reported *both* decreases or no changes in birth weight, depending on inclusion of confounding variables in the analyses.
‡Day et al., (1989) is listed in both columns.
Source: E. L. Abel & J. H. Hannigan, "J = shaped" relationship between drinking during pregnancy and birth weight: Reanalysis of prospective epidemological data, *Alcohol & Alcoholism* (1995) *30*, 172–179. Copyright by Williams & Wilkins. Reprinted by permission of the publisher.

influence the outcome being evaluated. Therefore, one alternative is *randomiza-tion*, whereby all of the potential factors that could confound the relationship are randomly distributed between the experimental and control groups. When exploring the relation between drinking and birth weight, however, the potential involvement of smoking is hardly ever adequately taken into account. The reason is that different groups of smokers are not equally represented among different groups of drinkers. Smoking is very highly correlated with drinking; that is, heavy drinkers also tend to be heavy smokers. Likewise, abstainers tend to be nonsmokers

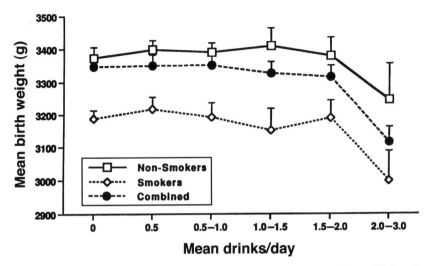

Figure 6.1. Relationship between drinking during pregnancy and mean birth weight (± SE). Data for each drinking level were obtained from an analysis of the previously published prospective studies listed in Table 6.1. These levels were integrated as closely as possible into the categories used in the figure. Studies that stratified drinkers by smoking status (nonsmokers = squares; smokers = diamonds) are presented as such. The "combined" condition (filled circles) includes the two conditions. *Source*: E. L. Abel and J. H. Hannigan, "J-Shaped" Relationships between drinking during pregnancy and birth weight: Reanalysis of prospective epidemiological data, *Alcohol & Alcoholism* (1995a), *30*, pp. 172–179. Copyright by Williams & Wilkins. Reprinted by permission of the publisher.

(Ernhart et al., 1988; Jacobson et al., 1991a; Olsen et al., 1991; Sokol et al., 1980; Wright et al., 1983). Thus, whenever people are divided into groups on the basis of their drinking behavior, there will be one subgroup of heavy drinkers who are also heavy smokers and another subgroup of abstinent or "light" drinkers who are nonsmokers, but there will not be very many women who fall into the categories of heavy drinker-nonsmoker, light drinker-heavy smoker, or groups in between. Because most statistical tests assume continuums and random distribution of smokers and drinkers, the fact that these kinds of statistical analyses almost never find statistically significant evidence for an interaction between drinking and smoking because the analysis violates the basic principle of sample size—there are never enough women in the intermediate drinker–smoker combinations to analyze.

In any study using traditional statistical analyses, especially where associations between such independent variables as drinking and outcome measures as birth weight are very weak, sample size is critical. Unless the number of people or animals in a study is large enough, the presence or absence of statistically significant associations will be in doubt. A large sample size is especially important to make sure that if no effect is found, it is very likely that an actual effect was not missed. In statistical parlance, the smaller the sample size, the lower the *statistical power* of the tests. And the lower the statistical power, the greater the impact of the law of confounding determinism. Only by stratifying women into smokers and nonsmokers and then looking for relationships between drinking and birth weight during pregnancy can the influence of drinking be assessed independently of the confounding influence of smoking. This is the strategy typically employed by European epidemiologists (Olsen et al., 1991; Verkert et al., 1993; Wright et al., 1983), whereas American epidemiologists tend to rely on analyses that violate the randomization principle.

Besides smoking, it may be apposite to stratify women on the basis of the kind of alcoholic beverages they drink. For example, in France, FAS/ARBEs are invariably associated with beer drinking rather than wine drinking (see Chapter 4).

Several epidemiological studies have likewise noted significant increases in preterm births or decreases in birth weights only among beer drinkers (Dehaene et al., 1977; Kaminski et al., 1981; Kline, Stein, & Hutzler, 1987; Kuzma & Sokol, 1983; Larroque et al., 1995; McDonald et al., 1992). (The role of socioeconomic status in FAS/ARBEs is examined at length later in this book, see Chapter 12.) At this point, it is enough to note that significant relationships between drinking during pregnancy and various outcomes may not be clarified unless groups are first stratified on the basis of factors otherwise confounded with drinking.

Studies in Animals

Studies in animals are directed almost exclusively at evaluating the effects of very high blood alcohol concentrations, which often exceed 200 mg% (Abel, 1984a). Not surprisingly, these kinds of in utero blood alcohol levels result in consistent decreases in fetal or birth weights (Abel, 1984a; Hannigan, Abel, & Kruger, 1993a). To achieve a comparable blood alcohol level, a 130-lb woman would have to consume 5 drinks over a 2 hour period, or 11 drinks over a 5-hour period (see earlier).

Studies employing such high blood alcohol levels are far removed from the kinds of blood alcohol levels one might expect to encounter in prospective epidemiological studies, but they do provide valuable insights into the kinds of biological effects one might encounter in the case of alcohol-abusing mothers who give birth to children with fetal alcohol abuse syndrome.

Animals subjected to these very high blood alcohol levels eat much less than untreated animals and gain much less weight during pregnancy (Abel, 1978; Abel & Dintcheff, 1978). In that regard, they are not very different from mothers who give birth to children with FAS (Abel, 1984a). In addressing the obvious question of whether alcohol's effects on fetal or birth weight are the direct result of alcohol use or an indirect result of decreased food intake, researchers working with animals often employ an experimental strategy known as *pair-feeding*. In this procedure, control animals are given food and fluid equivalent to that consumed on the previous day by alcohol-treated animals. As a result, animals in all pair-fed conditions are allotted the same amount of food and fluid as those given alcohol. An independent group can also be given ad libitum access to food and water so that the effects of the pair-feeding procedure itself can be assessed.

Pair-feeding inevitably results in lower birth weights than those occurring in animals with unrestricted access to food and water. However, even when animals are pair-fed, animals that receive alcohol at high doses typically give birth to newborns that weigh less than their pair-fed controls. This result implies that the combination of alcohol and decreased food intake has a greater impact on birth weight than decreased food intake alone. Again, alcohol's effects are never evaluated independently of other factors.

It is also worthwhile to point out that although pair-feeding provides an important nutritional control group, placing animals on the kind of restricted meal feeding associated with pair-feeding is a stressful experimental treatment in and of itself. Animals being fed in this way consume most of their restricted diets as soon as they receive them rather than throughout the night, as is the case for rats with unrestricted access to food. This restricted feeding pattern alters circadian rhythms in hormones and brain amines, which is indicative of stress (Weinberg, 1984).

Although investigations of the impact of large doses of alcohol on fetal and birth weights are de rigeur in animal experimentation, in some instances, lower doses have been included in study designs intended to provide threshold estimates for alcohol's effects. These relatively rare studies have invariably found no significant decreases in fetal or birth weights associated with administrations of 1 or 2 g/kg of alcohol or consumption of liquid diets containing 17% ethanol-derived calories (Abel, 1996a). Interestingly, in some of these studies, fetal or birth weights of alcohol-exposed animals appear slightly heavier than controls, although no such statistical comparisons were undertaken.

The results of a study directly evaluating the effects of relatively low doses of alcohol (0.15 or 0.3 g/kg) on pregnant rats is shown in Figure 6.2. Note the slight (but nonstatistically significant) increase in birth weight associated with low doses and the typical decrease associated with the relatively high doses (3.0 g/kg).

One implication of this study is that if extrapolated to the epidemiological literature, the interesting possibility arises that when very light or occasional drinkers are combined with abstainers, or when light or occasional drinkers are treated as controls, differences between heavy drinkers and controls may be artifactually increased (Little & Wendt, 1991).

When Is a Decrease in Birth Weight a "Defect?"

Although decreases in birth weight are often considerable when encountered in the context of FAS, apart from FAS the decreases are typically small and

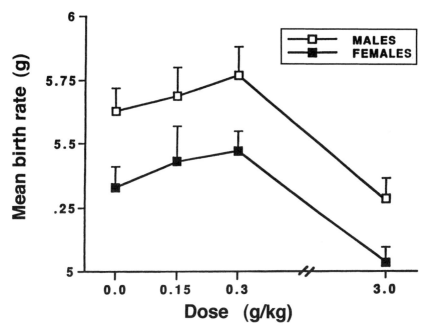

Figure 6.2. Effects of relatively low doses of alcohol administered on gestation days 8–20 on the birth weights of male and female rats. *Source*: E. L. Abel, Effects of prenatal alcohol exposure on birth weight in rats: Is there an inverted U-shaped function? *Alcohol* (1996b), *13*, pp. 99–102. Copyright by Elsevier Science Ltd. Reprinted by permission of the publisher.

biologically meaningless. A decrease of 100–200 grams from a norm of 3,370 grams has no known biological importance and certainly does not qualify for the emotionally laden word, *defect*, as in alcohol-related birth defect. Calling such a meaningless decrease a defect reflects slavish attention to statistical significance rather than biological importance. The unchallengeable fact is that the decreases associated with drinking during pregnancy at levels other than alcohol abuse are trivial and totally without any clinical relevance—and epitomize the law of confounding determinism.

Postnatal Growth Retardation

Based on the U.S. Center for Health Statistics' growth standards for the total population of the United States, most children with FAS are shorter than the average child of the same age (Streissguth, Clarren, & Jones, 1985). Figure 6.3

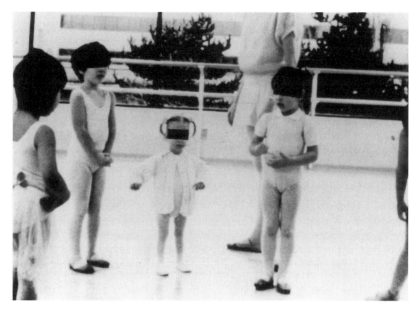

Figure 6.3. Height comparison of girl with FAS with girls of the same chronological age. (Photo courtesy Dr. C. Loock.)

illustrates how dramatic this decreased stature can be. The children pictured are all about the same chronological age. The smallest girl was diagnosed with FAS.

Since many children with FAS whose growth has been monitored in follow-up studies have been either Native American or African-American children, there is a possibility that their shorter statures may be related to racial or socioeconomic backgrounds.

For instance, based on U.S. population standards, the first group of children ever to be diagnosed with FAS had body weights no greater than 50% for their heights at 9–10 years of age. However, more than half of these children were Native Americans (Streissguth et al., 1985). All of these children came from low socioeconomic backgrounds and spent their early years in what the authors described as "tumultuous" environments: Six lived intermittently with biological mothers who continued to drink; only one lived in a "stable foster home." Child neglect was documented for five of these children. In some cases, primarily in girls, catch-up growth began to occur around puberty (Streissguth et al., 1991).

Another study of adolescents and adults with FAS or ARBEs (most of whom were Native Americans) found short stature to be their "most differentiating characteristic." About 50% of the 61 cases had heights two standard deviations below the mean, while 24% had normal heights. Body weights were not as severely affected: Only 12% had body weights two standard deviations below the mean, while 37% had normal weights or weights above normal for height (Streissguth & Giunta, 1988).

Follow-up studies of children with FAS in Germany have likewise found short stature to be common. Because the children in these, where much of the research in FAS has been conducted, were primarily Caucasian, the possibility that racial factors uniquely influenced the observations was lessened. But the role of preconceptual parental weight and height still remains problematic. Like the Seattle study, the German studies also noted catch-up growth mainly in girls, beginning around puberty (Spohr & Steinhausen, 1987; Spohr et al., 1993, 1994).

Postnatal Growth in the Absence of FAS

In contrast to these follow-up observations of children with FAS, epidemiological studies of mothers whose drinking during pregnancy did not result in FAS have found catch-up growth is the rule rather than the exception, except when low socioeconomic status is involved.

In Seattle, a slight decrease in height, weight, and head circumference at birth, which was attributed to prenatal alcohol exposure, and which was less than effects due to smoking, was observable at 8 months of age (Barr, Streissguth, Martin, & Herman, 1984; Sampson, Brookstein, Barr, & Streissguth, 1994) but not at 18 months, at school age (Sampson et al., 1994), or at 14 years of age (Sampson et al., 1994) in a group of primarily white middle-class children. Similarly, there was no evidence of postnatal growth retardation at 12 months of age (Fried & O'Connell, 1987; O'Connor, Brill, & Sigman, 1986), 24 months of age (Fried & O'Connell, 1987), or 4–5 years of age (Greene et al., 1991b) in similar studies. Several noteworthy exceptions include a study from Atlanta that found that while weight was within the normal range, height and head circumference were reduced in a group of 6-year-old children from low-income, African-American backgrounds, whose mothers drank during pregnancy (Coles, Brown, Smith, Platzman, & Erickson, 1991). The other exception is that Russell and co-workers (Russell, Czarneci, Cowan, McPherson, & Mudar, 1991) reported that height was significantly reduced in a group of similarly exposed children. The reason this latter study is also noteworthy is that to arrive at this conclusion the authors relied on a statistical criterion of 0.10 for their inference. This criterion is far above that normally used in the scientific community for decisions concerning statistical significance.

Another noteworthy exception is the series of studies from Pittsburgh that reported persistent decreases in growth at 8 months of age (Day, Richardson, & Robles, 1990), 18 months (Day et al., 1991), 36 months (Day et al., 1992), and 6 years (Day, Richardson, Geva, & Robles, 1994) in a group of low-income, African-American children who did not have FAS, but whose mothers drank during pregnancy. In Detroit, Jacobson and colleagues, (Jacobson et al., 1994a) found postnatal growth (weight, size, and head circumference) was delayed at 6.5 months of age in African-American children whose mothers consumed an average of four drinks a day or more.

The first point to consider in evaluating these reports is that, as in the case of most of the epidemiological studies of the effects of drinking during pregnancy, despite being statistically significant, the effects associated with drinking are biologically trivial, which some investigators readily admit: "[These differences are] small and would not be of clinical significance for any individual child" (Day et al., 1994). In the Jacobson (Jacobson et al., 1994a) study, not only was the effect without clinical significance, but maternal alcohol consumption accounted for no more than 3% of their clinically irrelevant finding and, at 13 months of age, the erstwhile association between drinking and postnatal weight ceased to be even statistically significant.

In discussing their studies on postnatal growth, Day et al. (1994) made the important point that persistent growth deficits associated with prenatal alcohol exposure have mainly been found when the children were from low-income families (average income for 41% of the women in their studies was $400 or less per month), whereas comparable effects are rarely seen in "more advantaged" populations. The authors, however, did not speculate on what the differences might be; but they stated that about 50% of the children in their studies were consuming less than the recommended daily allowance (RDA) for dairy products, 46% were below the RDA for protein, and 60% and 34% were receiving less than the RDA for fruits/vegetables and grains (Day et al., 1992). The authors also state that the women they studied were also more likely than not to have smoked and used illicit drugs during pregnancy and they continued to be heavier smokers after it (Day et al., 1992, 1994). Despite their own caveats, the authors came to the dubious conclusion that nutritional factors did not affect the relationship between alcohol and growth measures, and they did not attribute the differences in growth to any of the other differences in the drinking and nondrinking groups.

Studies in Animals

Studies in animals are equally inconsistent as to the effects of prenatal alcohol exposure on long-term postnatal growth, although these inconsistencies may in some cases be related to amounts of exposure. For example, rat offspring whose mothers were given 6 gm/kg of alcohol per day during pregnancy—very close to the maximal dose rats can tolerate—weighed less than controls well into adulthood (Abel, Church, & Dintcheff, 1987), while rats exposed to lower doses exhibited "catch up" growth (Abel, 1978).

A series of interesting studies in mice found that when alcohol was consumed during pregnancy in amounts resulting in blood alcohol levels of about 250 mg%, offspring only began to exhibit postnatal growth retardation around the time of weaning (about postnatal day 21) rather than at birth (Middaugh & Boggan, 1991, 1995). This effect was only seen when alcohol consumption occurred during the latter part of pregnancy (Middaugh & Boggan, 1991).

Feeding efficiencies in animals experiencing postnatal decreases in body weight due to prenatal alcohol exposure have not found any evidence that these decreases are due to assimilation or metabolic factors (Abel, 1984a). Increasing milk availability and quantity in animals by raising animals in small litters has also had no significant remedial impact on postnatal weight gain (Lee & Leichter, 1980). However, animals prenatally exposed to high blood alcohol levels (200 mg%) have weaker sucks than control animals, and, therefore, they may not receive as much milk as controls (Rockwood & Riley, 1986). A weak sucking reflex has also been observed in some infants with FAS (Riikonen, 1994; Van Dyke, Mackay, & Ziaylek, 1982) and in infants born to alcoholic mothers (Martin, Martin, Streissguth, & Lund, 1979; Ouellette et al., 1977; Stock, Streissguth, & Martin, 1985). In addition, more than 20 case studies mention feeding difficulties in conjunction with FAS (Abel, 1990).

Another possible explanation for the postnatal growth retardation associated with prenatal alcohol exposure in rats is an increased inability to maintain body temperature in response to cold (Zimmerberg, Carson, Kaplan, Zuniga, & True, 1993). As a result of their increased temperature loss, these animals may become lethargic if they wander from the nest. This lethargy, in turn, may cause them to elicit less maternal attention and could result indirectly in growth retardation (Zimmerberg et al., 1993).

The most likely explanation for the failure to thrive and the permanent growth deficit, however, is alcohol's inhibiting effects on protein and DNA accretion (indices of cell size and cell number, respectively) during fetal development (Abel, 1984a). Although decreased cell size is reversible, decreased cell number is not. The long-range implication is that growth retardation will be permanent because once cell division has ended, it cannot be compensated for by later cellular increases.

CHAPTER 7

Craniofacial Anomalies

In 1988, a convicted murderer, Robert Francis, contended he had FAS and that his condition should be considered a mitigating factor in sentencing him for torturing and then shooting someone who informed against him. The psychiatrist who testified Francis had FAS, however, never tested Francis's ability to reason. He also said Francis's IQ was in the normal range, and he had not looked for any physical evidence of brain damage, adding he was basing his diagnosis solely on Francis's facial characteristics (*Francis v. State*, 1988). Because he believed Francis had facial features compatible with the syndrome, the psychiatrist felt that there was no need for tests, no need to prove a history of prenatal alcohol exposure, no need to determine Francis's growth history, and no need to determine his cognitive abilities. He simply assumed anyone with FAS facial features must be brain damaged, and, therefore, that person's ability to control violent behavior must also be impaired.

The fact that this diagnosis of FAS was based solely on facial features reflects the singular importance attributed to this aspect of FAS by some clinicians. Although one might question the psychiatrist's pronouncements in this case, the important point is this: On the basis of Francis's facial features, the psychiatrist rendering the diagnosis was willing to make the added inference that Francis was also suffering from personality traits attributable to the same cause or causes responsible for his unusual facial features.

The Francis case is noteworthy for at least three reasons. The first is the clinician's total reliance on facial features for the diagnosis. Despite the fact the clinical definition and diagnosis for FAS emphasizes a pattern of defects, the facial features associated with FAS are nevertheless regarded by some clinicians as the syndrome's sine qua non: "No one can receive an FAS diagnosis without an experienced clinician's assertion that the face, when taken as a whole, appears to be the FAS face" (IOM, 1996, p. 72).

The second noteworthy feature is that facial features that characterize FAS are not static. Even experienced dysmorphologists would have had difficulty determining if Francis had FAS on the basis of his adult facial features. "The natural history of FAS is such that some of the hallmark indicators (of facial dysmorphia) used during infancy or childhood are not maintained into adolescence or adulthood" (IOM, 1996, p. 75). This is the reason the Institute of Medicine created a distinct diagnostic category called "alcohol-related neurodevelopmental disorders" (IOM, 1996, p. 77) for behavioral problems in which there is a history of alcohol exposure but no characteristic facial features (see later).

The third noteworthy aspect of the Francis case is that even if the diagnosis were accurate, it cannot be relied on for inferences about someone's character. Facial anthropometry or physiognomy, as it was once called, has been a subject of considerable interest since the 17th century. It was especially prominent in the 19th century when, like phrenology, it was a part of the new "Science of Mankind," which relied on facial and head analysis as a barometer of character. Studies based on these theories provided a foundation for biobehavioral theories that inferred the potential for criminal behavior from facial features and provided a scientific basis for later eugenic policies aimed at population control (Gould, 1989). In light of the sordid history connecting facial features and behavior, we must be vigilant not to read too much into an "unusual" face, especially when it is connected with a socially "disapproved" background, such as one involving maternal alcohol abuse. Although very severe dysmorphic features are generally associated with intellectual deficits in a large number of syndromes, including FAS (Autti-Ramo et al., 1992; Iosub et al., 1981; Majewski, 1981; Streissguth, Herman, & Smith, 1978a), intellectual deficits and antisocial personality are not one and the same. Some people with FAS may indeed be involved in the criminal justice system either as offenders or victims because their neurodevelopmental disability places them at higher risk for problems involving impulsivity, poor judgment, language and learning, or memory disorders. However, there will also be individuals without FAS (and their advocates), invoking the diagnosis of FAS as a mitigating factor for antisocial behavior. To avoid skepticism about this disorder, a diagnosis of FAS should be made by an impartial expert who is familiar with the spectrum of anomalies that characterize FAS and "partial FAS." The Francis case clearly illustrates the kinds of misdiagnoses that can arise either from a sole reliance on craniofacial features or a lack of experience in syndromal recognition.

The reason for the correlation between distinctive facial abnormalities (the key word here is *distinctive*) and decreased intelligence is that the face and brain arise from the same embryological structures. As noted in Chapter 3, this correlation is the basis for the syndrome's construct validity. The idea that a criminal or antisocial personality can likewise be gleaned from someone's facial physiognomy was disproved long ago (Gould, 1982), but it is still with us as reflected in the Washington State Council on Crime and Delinquency's (1991) recent recommendations regarding FAS. Prison wardens, the council suggested, ought to be trained in dysmorphology to enable them to identify which of the inmates in their charge have FAS and possibly to take appropriate remedial action—whatever that might be. The opposite side of the coin is that children with these features could also be labeled as potential criminals; once stigmatized as such, the diagnosis could create a self-fulfilling prophecy.

The FAS Face Is a Gestalt

Whenever clinicians make a diagnosis, it is axiomatic that they will attach special significance to those conditions with which they have most experience. Stromland (1985), a pediatric ophthalmologist, for example, has so often observed ophthalmological anomalies within the eyes of her FAS patients that she considers them diagnostic; Garber (1982) feels the same about curvature of the cornea (see below). Clarren, a pediatric dysmorphologist, didn't mention either condition (Astley & Clarren, 1995), and because he was the dysmorphology expert on the Institute of Medicine's panel (see Chapter 2), these features were not specifically mentioned in the IOM's diagnostic paradigm (IOM, 1996).

Clarren, however, made the important point that it is the "gestalt" or "general clinical impression" rather than any individual characteristic that renders the FAS face distinctive (Astley & Clarren, 1995). Clarren likens this gestalt, which is primarily localized to the central area of the face (see Table 7.1), to a "T," with the eyes as the "T's" horizontal bar (IOM, 1996).

The facial features associated with FAS can be best appreciated by comparing the two children in Figure 7.1A, B. These children were 11-month-old (at the time the photos were taken) dizygotic twins, born to an alcoholic mother (they will be discussed in greater detail later in this book). For now, it is enough to

Table 7.1. Characteristic Facial Features in Children with FAS

Short palpebral fissures (short eye slits)
Flat, broad nasal bridge
Short upturned nose
Indistinct philtrum (groove between nose and upper lip)
Hypoplastic or narrow upper vermillion (thin upper lip)
Maxillary hypoplasia (flattened midface)

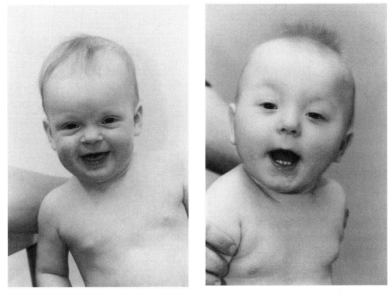

Figure 7.1A, B. Eleven-month-old dizygotic twins born to a mother who drank "10 bottles of beer almost daily." The twin on the left (**A**) is normal; the twin on the right (**B**) has various craniofacial features related to FAS, such as hypertelorism, short palpebral fissures, elongated philtrum, and a thin upper lip. (Photos courtesy of Dr. Raili S. Riikonen. Used with permission.)

note the differences between the two. Twin 7.1B has no distinctive facial features. Twin 7.1A has many of the facial features listed in Table 7.1—short palpebral fissures, long philtrum, thin upper lip, maxillary and mandibular hypoplasia, along with hyperteleorism (widespread eyes), and low set ears.

The fact that one twin has FAS facial dysmorphia and the other does not indicates that there is reasonably strong evidence for genotypic susceptibility to alcohol's in utero effects. On the other hand, it is still worth keeping in mind the possibility that some of the syndrome's phenotypic features are also influenced by genotype apart from alcohol exposure. For instance, diagnosticians who do not have experience with aboriginal populations may attribute aboriginal facial features to FAS because some of them resemble the facial characteristics of the syndrome: "The facial dysmorphology in native children with FAS can be somewhat confusing as many aboriginal children have epicanthus and a depressed nasal bridge. This appears to occur so commonly in aboriginal children that the physicians I work with feel it is simply a genetic variant and is not representative of fetal alcohol syndrome" (Dr. Jo Nanson, personal communication, 1995). The same caveat applies to other minority groups as well (see later).

How Distinctive Is the FAS Face?

Although recognition of the FAS physiognomy is not as yet based on objective biological markers, we must assume those specifically trained to recognize the distinctive facial gestalt are the most qualified to determine if a condition is indicative of FAS or some other disorder. Even for the nonexpert, there appears to be a close similarity in the appearance of these children, as evidenced in the faces of children in Figure 7.2.

Some of the facial features associated with FAS resemble those observed in other conditions that are the results of phenylketonuria or maternal exposure to solvents like toluene (Pearson et al., 1994) or drugs like marijuana (Hingson et al., 1982), as examples. However, a trained dysmorphologist is more likely to be aware of the subtle differences between FAS and other conditions, and he or she is therefore able to render a more accurate diagnosis than a clinician lacking comparable training and experience. Likewise, a trained dysmorphologist is more likely to be able to differentiate malformations from the deformations such as compression, that can occur as a result of mechanical factors in the uterus. At birth, some compression-related features can resemble FAS. But a major difference between deformations and malformations is that the former do not persist long after birth.

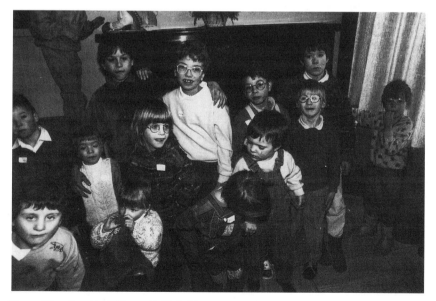

Figure 7.2. German children with FAS. (Photo courtesy Dr. H. Loser. Used with permission from Vandenhoeck & Ruprecht.)

This difference may not be appreciated by those untrained to make such distinctions. Misattribution at birth in this regard may be likely, especially if the mother has a history of alcohol abuse.

Because recognition of the facial characteristics of FAS requires training and experience and is based on a gestalt, it is unlikely that the diagnosis of FAS eventually will be reduced to a mathematical formula based on distances between various facial features (Clarren et al., 1987; Escobar, Bixler, & Padilla, 1993; Sokol, Chik, Martier, & Salari, 1991; Vitez, Koranyi, Gonczy, Rudas, & Czeizel, 1984).

The idea that a "one size fits all" formula will identify children with FAS is unrealistic, even more so when extended to include fetal measurements by ultrasound (Escobar et al., 1993). Ward pointed out that

> it is unlikely simple linear, angular, and circumferential measurements will ever be able to model accurately the complex, three-dimensional structure of the head and face ... (so) interpretation of any facial measurements derived from supposedly fixed points (points of registration) is problematic.... Small errors in measurement technique or landmark identification can inadvertently move a measurement from the "normal" to "abnormal" range. (Ward, 1989, pp. 47–48).

Thomas and his co-workers concurred: "accurate measurements of three-dimensional objects cannot be made directly from two-dimensional images. Points on the cranioface can only be precisely localized by systems that collect three-dimensional data, much as depth perception is possible with binocular but not monocular vision" (Thomas, Hintz, & Frias, 1989, p. 110). Other considerations include overall body size; for example, proportionately smaller people may be "plotted out" as microcephalic (Ward, 1989).

That the results of these morphometric analyses have not been impressive supports the conclusion the facial features associated with FAS constitute a gestalt that cannot be reduced to mathematical formulas. As the next section indicates, while dysmorphologists agree on the gestalt, they do not always agree on which individual features create that gestalt.

Characteristic Facial Anomalies in the FAS Gestalt

Periocular Area

The most distinctive physical features contributing to the FAS face occur around the eyes and nose. (The most common of the periocular anomalies are listed in Table 7.2.)

Although shortened palpebral fissure size—the distance between the inner and outer canthus (see Aase, 1990, Figures 7.1 and 7.2)—is the most commonly mentioned of all the facial anomalies associated with FAS (Abel, 1990) and was

Table 7.2. Periocular
Anomalies Associated
with FAS

Most Commonly Mentioned
  Short palpebral fissures
  Epicanthic folds
  Blepharophimosis
Less Commonly Mentioned
  Antimongoloid slant
  Asymmetry of eyelids
  Hyperteleorism
  Hypoteleorism
  Ptosis
  Strabismus

prominently mentioned by the FAS Study Group and the IOM in their diagnostic paradigms (see Chapter 3), short palpebral fissure size may be common only in some patient populations. For instance, short palpebral fissure size was such a rare occurrence in Majewski's FAS population of Caucasian children (0%–11%) (Majewski, 1981) that he did not even include it in his list of diagnostic features (Majewski, 1993). Other German clinicians have likewise found little evidence that palpebral fissures are shortened in conjunction with FAS (Bierich et al., 1976; Spohr & Steinhausen, 1987).

The FAS Study Group and IOM paradigms emphasizing this particular feature were based primarily on African-American and Native American children with FAS, whereas European paradigms like Majewski's were based primarily on Caucasian cases. Because there are significant differences between blacks and whites in palpebral fissure sizes (Fuchs, Isoub, Bingol, & Gronusch, 1980), impressions involving this part of the face may be affected by racial backgrounds. One corollary to this conclusion is that epidemiological and clinical studies using palpebral fissure size as an outcome variable need to match groups on the basis of race, gender, and age before looking for associations between maternal drinking and palpebral fissure size. Evaluation should also take into account possible microcephaly because short palpebral fissure size for some children may reflect a smaller head size rather than some specific effect on palpebral fissures. Short palpebral fissures are often proportionately related to microcephaly because short palpebral fissures reflect small eyes, which are an outward manifestation of the brain.

Dysmorphologists also differ in the importance they attribute to epicanthic folds—the crescent-shaped skin folds in the inner corner of the eye that obscure the inner portion of the upper and lower lids in the inner canthus. This facial feature is prominently mentioned in conjunction with FAS in European studies. Majewski (1993), for instance, estimated that this feature occurred in about 55% of his FAS cases. Steinhausen and his co-workers (Steinhausen et al., 1982) reported an even higher rate of 68%. The IOM (1996), however, only considered epicanthic folds an auxiliary feature of the syndrome, perhaps because epicanthic folds are common in certain Native American groups (Aase, 1990). In other words, North American diagnosticians may simply dismiss the occurrence as a genetic variant rather than a characteristic feature associated with FAS (see Nanson's comment, earlier). Aase (1990), however, noted that there were subtle differences between hereditary and FAS conditions. In FAS, for instance, the epicanthic fold joins the lower lid at the inner canthus, while in the hereditary condition it joins both lids (see Aase, 1990, Figure 4.4.7).

Another noteworthy difference between the facial features emphasized in the American and European diagnostic paradigms is the frequency with which blepharophimosis—a decrease in the size of the upper eyelid that restricts the space between the two eyelids—is mentioned. Majewski (1993) estimated the rate of occurrence for this anomaly at around 31% in his patients, but the same anomaly was not mentioned at all in the FAS Study Group or IOM paradigms. Furthermore, it was rarely mentioned in any case reports or epidemiological studies from North America.

The reasons for the differences in attribution between the U.S. and European paradigms for palpebral fissure size, epicanthic folds, and blepharophimosis need to be resolved. If the essence of a "syndrome" is the regular occurrence of certain features, how can maternal alcohol abuse, for example, lead to short palpebral sizes in the United States and not Germany?

A number of other periocular anomalies are less commonly mentioned in connection with FAS and are not considered diagnostic of the syndrome. Nevertheless, these features have a relatively high prevalence in FAS in European and North American studies. For example, ptosis (drooping eyelid) has been observed in 51% of Majewski's FAS patient population (1993), and in 14%–24% of other FAS patient populations (Abel, 1990; Miller, Israel, & Cuttone, 1981; Steinhausen et al., 1982; Stromland, 1985). Ptosis may be bilateral (Jones, Smith, Ulleland, & Streissguth, 1973; Miller et al., 1981; Stromland, 1985) or unilateral (Miller et al., 1981; Stromland, 1985) (as shown in Figure 7.3). Other features mentioned in conjunction with FAS, but not contributing or detracting from the FAS facial gestalt, are listed in Table 7.1.

Eyes

Although the eyes are an extension of the brain, they are usually discussed in the context of facial features. This section deals primarily with readily observable features. Functional disorders are discussed in the context of the syndrome's neurodevelopmental features (see Chapters 9 and 10).

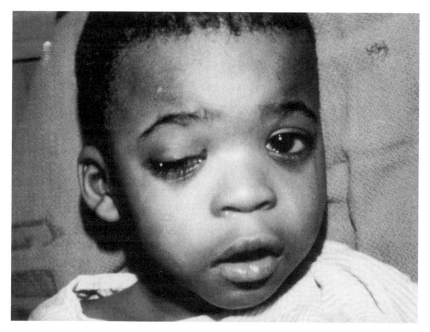

Figure 7.3. Young male with unilateral ptosis. Other facial features visible in this photo are epicanthic folds, hypoplastic philtrum, hypoplastic nasal bridge, and hyperteleorism. (Photo courtesy of Dr. Phillip Spiegel. Used with permission.)

In humans, the eyes begin to develop around the fourth week of gestation and continue to develop until about the 15th week. Because maturation occurs over a relatively long period, the opportunity for injury due to alcohol is considerably greater than it is for organs whose development takes place over a much shorter time period. Although anomalies affecting the eyes are commonplace in FAS, their presence or absence does affect the FAS facial gestalt.

One of the most common physical anomalies affecting the eyes is tortuous retinal vasculature (anomalies in the width and distribution pattern of the arteries and veins coursing over the retinal surface of the eye). This anomaly, however, is not part of any diagnostic paradigm and will probably escape notice unless patients with FAS are examined by an ophthalmologist or a diagnostician who is alert to its frequency of occurrence. Stromland (1985), a pediatric ophthalmologist, found as many as 49% of her patients with FAS had retinal tortuosity. Even higher prevalence rates have been reported by others, for example, 7 out of 8 cases (Cardones, Brancato, Venturi, Bianchi, & Magni, 1992) and 4 out of 6 cases (Hinzpeter, Renz, & Loser, 1992; Root, Reiter, Andriola, & Duckett, 1975). Other researchers have found it a relatively infrequent occurrence (Church & Gerkin,

1988; Miller et al., 1981). It is also absent in nonhuman primates prenatally exposed to alcohol (Clarren, Astley, & Bowden, 1988).

Abnormal curvature of the eye has been found in 40%–65% of FAS cases in three studies (Church & Gerkin, 1988; Miller et al., 1981; Stromland, 1985). Garber found abnormal corneal curvature in 91% of the Navajo Indian school children with FAS whom he examined, a prevalence so high he felt it to be diagnostic for the syndrome (Garber, 1982). Whether the same high prevalence occurs in children of other racial backgrounds has not yet been determined.

Strabismus, an inability of the eyes to focus parallel to one another, is also common in FAS, with a prevalence rate of 20%–27% (Abel, 1990; Majewski, 1993; Steinhausen et al., 1982). Frequencies as high as 43% and 56% have also been reported (Miller et al., 1981; Stromland, 1985). Both esotropia (eyes turn inward, a condition sometimes called "crossed eyes") (Jones et al., 1973; Miller et al., 1981) and exotropia (eyes turn out) (Walpole & Hoelig, 1980) are associated with FAS. Strabismus results from a disturbance in cranial nerve function and fine motor control of the rectus muscles, rather than a malfunction in the eye itself. A third and less common condition called amblyopia, sometimes called "lazy eye" or "perceptual blindness," refers to an inability to coordinate eye movements. The latter may occur when one of the eyes becomes dominant, and the brain does not respond to information from the other eye so as to avoid double vision.

Nystagmus (jerky eye movements) has been noted in some cases of FAS (Miller et al., 1981; Stromland, 1985) but with much less frequency. Nystagmus can occur in the horizontal or vertical planes, but it is not necessarily associated with altered visual acuity (Aase, 1990). Other visual anomalies infrequently mentioned in children with FAS include cataracts, corneal opacity (Garber, 1982; Miller et al., 1981; Stromland, 1985), Duane's retraction syndrome (restricted adduction) (Holzman, Chrousos, Kozma, & Traboulsi, 1990), Peter's anomaly (Miller et al., 1981), astigmatism, hyperopia, photophobia, corneal atresia, and glaucoma (Church & Gerkin, 1988).

Nose

In FAS, the nose is often described as being short and upturned, the bridge, low and broad. About one third of the 22 African-American children with FAS studied by Church et al. (1997) had deformed nares. The upturned appearance of the nose may give a false impression that the distance between it and the upper lip is elongated. In some cases, the nose tends to become very large after puberty (Streissguth et al., 1985).

In contrast to the frequency with which nasal features are mentioned, there was only one report mentioning any nasal disorder, in this case persistent rhinorrhea, associated with FAS (Johnson, 1979). However, persistent rhinorrhea arises as a result of upper respiratory problems, as does serous otitis media, which is very common in FAS (see Chapter 8 "Immune Function").

Oral Features

Anomalies involving the area around and inside the mouth are very common in FAS. (The most commonly mentioned of these are listed in Table 7.3.)

An indistinct philtrum (the groove extending from the bottom of the nose to the top of the upper lip) is considered by the FAS Study Group (Rosett, 1980) and the IOM (1996) as one of the most common features of the syndrome (see Figures 7.1A and 7.3). A related characteristic is an upper lip that is very thin and lacking the "cupid's bow" shape. Another feature characteristic of FAS is a hypoplastic mandible (in about 91% of all cases of FAS) (Majewski, 1993).

Throat, Pharynx, and Dentition

The throat is rarely mentioned in connection with FAS, although two reports mentioned FAS cases with a thin epiglottis and small trachea (Finucane, 1980; Lindor, McCarthy, & McRae, 1980). In one of these reports, two neonates with FAS had such small tracheas that they had to be anesthetized so as to intubate them (Finucane, 1980).

Feeding difficulties (dysphagia) have been mentioned in at least 20 cases of FAS (Abel, 1990). Harris and her co-workers (Harris et al., 1993) related that one of the 12-month-old children with FAS they studied gagged on anything other than pureed food and would only eat pureed or junior baby foods at 18 months old. During his first postnatal year, the child also had a history of vomiting and constipation (Riikonen, 1994). These feeding problems may reflect fine motor dysfunction. In this instance, the dysfunction takes the form of impaired coordination of the tongue and pharynx (Aase, 1990). The weak sucking reflex observed in some infants with FAS (Riikonen, 1994; Van Dyke et al., 1982) may reflect brain stem and autonomic nervous system dysfunctions and fine motor dysfunction.

Table 7.3. FAS-Related Anomalies Involving the Area around the Mouth

Indistinct or flat philtrum
Thin upper lip
Absence of "cupid's bow" in upper lip
Maxillar hypoplasis
Mandibular hypoplasia
High arched palate
Cleft palate
Cleft lip
Abnormal dentition

Other features occurring regularly in FAS, which are not diagnostic, are high-arched palates (about 45%) (Majewski, 1993; Steinhausen & Spohr, 1986) and cleft palate and/or lip (about 9%–18%) (Abel, 1990; Church et al., 1997; Majewski, 1993; Steinhausen & Spohr, 1986). Werler and his co-workers (Werler, Lammer, Rosenberg, & Mitchell, 1991) found that cleft lip with or without cleft palate was associated with maternal alcohol consumption of an average of five or more drinks a day. As in the case of other malformations, the alcohol-related increases in cleft lip and cleft palate may arise as a result of an exacerbation of an underlying familial sensitivity to these anomalies (Saxen, 1975). For instance, cleft lip and cleft palate occur with greater frequency in Finland, at a rate of 1.5 to 1.7 cases per 1,000, but this rate was not found to be related to alcohol consumption, implying environmental causes (Saxen, 1975). Another possible reason for this disparity, however, is a difference in the dental services provided in these countries.

Malocclusion, the misalignment of the upper and lower jaws, are not uncommon in North American cases. In some instances, malocclusions may, be serious enough to require surgery (Webb, Hochberg, & Sher, 1988). These anomalies, however, are rarely mentioned in European case or clinical studies, although they were noted in 30% of the 44 adolescents with FAS studied by Spohr and colleagues (Spohr et al., 1993).

A wide variety of dentition problems, however, are commonly encountered in FAS cases and clinical studies in both North America and Europe: crossbite and overbite (Church et al., 1997; Webb et al., 1988); hypoplastic teeth and enamel and frequent caries (Steinhausen & Spohr, 1986; Webb et al., 1988); and missing teeth, rotated teeth, overjets, crooked teeth (Church et al., 1997). In some instances, these dental problems have been treated with extractions or dental appliances, such as braces.

Despite their potential seriousness, dentition problems are rarely mentioned in case studies and may in fact be present in only certain populations of patients with FAS. For example, most patients with FAS who have malocclusions are from a low socioeconomic background. No attempt was made to compare the dental problems of these patients with controls from the same racial or socioeconomic backgrounds. One of the few studies to make such a comparison matched 19 patients with FAS, all but one of whom were Native Americans, with 20 controls from the same racial background. Dental anomalies were noted in both groups, and the differences were not statistically significant (Riekman & Paedo, 1984).

Ears

Physical anomalies involving the outer ear are often alluded to in connection with FAS (Abel, 1990). Majewski (1993) estimated the prevalence of dysplastic ears in patients with FAS at about 42%. Spohr and Steinhausen (1987) placed the estimate at 59%. In two studies in the United States, the prevalence was found to be 22% (Church et al., 1997; Hanson, Jones, & Smith, 1976).

The most commonly mentioned anomalies are low set ears, posteriorly rotated ears, prominent ears, and poorly formed pinnae. Low set ears (see Figure 7.1A) may arise due to incomplete embryonic migration of the ear anlage. Posterior rotation of the ear is commonly associated with low set ears because migration and maturation of the embryonic tissues involved are the same as those involving migration of the ear as a whole (Aase, 1990). Some authors have attributed such anomalies as low set ears to an illusion resulting from the presence of other anomalies—micrognathia or receding or bulging forehead, for example—which create the impression of ear anomalies (Pfeiffer, Majewski, Fischbach, Bierich, & Volk, 1979).

Comparable outer ear anomalies are also very common in other syndromes, so their appearance is considered supportive rather than diagnostic of FAS or any other syndrome (Aase, 1990). (Hearing loss and middle ear function are described in Chapter 9).

Currently, we do not have objective clinical methods for measuring microphthalmia, ear size, or dentition problems. Developing such standards may provide greater objectivity with respect to these individual anomalies, but the FAS diagnosis is based on a gestalt. Standardization of these anomalies will likely have relatively little bearing on the clinical diagnosis of FAS in individual patients.

Studies in Animals

Many of the facial features associated with FAS have been observed in animals exposed to high blood alcohol levels (200 mg% and above). Sulik and her co-workers (Sulik, Johnston, & Webb, 1981) found that they could produce such anomalies by administering two relatively large doses of alcohol on a single day of gestation (see Figure 7.4), comparable to a "binge" during early pregnancy in humans (although one day of pregnancy in the mouse is not the equivalent of one day in a human pregnancy).

Clarren and Bowden (1982) produced facial anomalies similar to those associated with FAS in a nonhuman primate model 30 to 40 days after conception by using a bingelike regimen of alcohol administration once a week. Peak blood alcohol levels were as high as 450 mg%. Facial abnormalities in the nonhuman primate offspring included a flattened philtrum, small ears that were posteriorly rotated, a wide nose, and a retrusive maxilla.

Outer ear anomalies, for example, low-set or absent ears (Webster et al., 1983), and cleft lips and palates (Ellis & Pick, 1980; Giknis, Damjanov, & Rubin, 1980) have been observed in mice and dogs exposed to high doses of alcohol prenatally, but such reports are limited and have not been observed in nonhuman primates similarly exposed to high doses of alcohol.

Studies in animals suggest that dental anomalies and susceptibility to dental caries may be increased as a result of prenatal alcohol exposure. In one study,

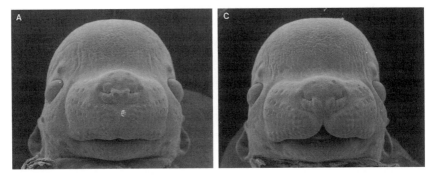

Figure 7.4. Fourteen-day-old mouse fetuses from alcohol-exposed (A) and control (C) mothers. Note the absence of a philtrum in A. Facial characteristics were induced by acute alcohol exposure during what corresponded to the third week of human gestation. (Photo courtesy of Dr. Kathy Sulik. used with permission.)

almost all (94%) of a group of mice prenatally exposed to a high dose of alcohol had a missing third molar, compared with no cases for controls (Stuckey & Berry, 1984). This anomaly, however, is not one of those noted in conjunction with FAS. Another study found that exposure to alcohol during gestation resulted in an increased frequency of dental cavities in animals when they were challenged by cariogenic bacteria (Lee-Chuan, Cerklewski, & Soeldner, 1985).

Although studies of alcohol's effects on facial features in animals should be used to validate occurrences in humans, they should not be relied on to formulate diagnostic paradigms for humans. Microphthalmia, for instance, is relatively common in animals prenatally exposed to high blood alcohol levels (Sulik & Johnston, 1983; Sulik et al., 1981; Webster et al., 1983) but is uncommon in FAS. Based on early reports of microphthalmia in animals prenatally exposed to alcohol, the FAS Study Group specifically mentioned it when developing its diagnostic paradigm (Rosett, 1980), but the rare occurrence of microoophthalmia in FAS (Abel, 1990) underscores the importance of caution in formulating diagnostic paradigms based on observations in animals.

Thresholds

Although maternal alcohol abuse can produce facial features associated with FAS, consumption of less than five drinks per occasion has not been reliably linked to the production of abnormal facial features.

This conclusion is based on three studies: Clarren and his co-workers (Clarren et al., 1987) sent facial photographs of 42 children to seven experts in the identification of FAS. The judges were in agreement with one another for four of the children, all of whom had mothers who consumed more than an average of eight drinks a day during pregnancy. They were also in agreement when it came to children of nondrinking mothers. However, they were not in agreement when it came to their ratings of children whose mothers drank less than eight drinks a day; that is, they rated 38% of the children whose mothers did not drink during pregnancy as having possible features associated with the syndrome. Clarren and his co-workers concluded that the faces of children exposed to substantial amounts of alcohol are highly indicative of that exposure, but facial features are not distinctive in the context of moderate drinking. Olsen and Tuntiseranee (1995) conducted a prospective study in which they ascertained maternal drinking behavior during early pregnancy, took photographs of children at birth and at 18 months of age, and had the photographs subsequently rated by "blind" observers. Statistically significant associations between facial features and drinking were found only for those children whose mothers drank five or more drinks on occasion during the first trimester. Comparable results were reported by Abel and his co-workers (Abel, Martier, Kruger, Ager, & Sokol, 1993) with respect to facial anomalies and positive scores on the Michigan Alcoholism Screening Test (MAST).

Based on their prospective study of facial features in children whose mothers drank during pregnancy, Ernhart and her co-workers (Ernhart et al., 1987) estimated the threshold for producing such anomalies at an average of six drinks a day. In agreement with these findings, Halmesmaki and her co-workers (Halmeski, Raivio, & Ylikorkala, 1987) found no relation between consumption of around four drinks a week during the first trimester of pregnancy and unusual facial features (Mills & Graubard, 1987; Tennes & Blackard, 1980). In the Ernhart et al. study (1987), when the authors projected their findings to the total pregnancy population, they estimated the increased risk of facial anomalies would be detectable in only 2% of all pregnancies (i.e., the heaviest drinking population). .

In contrast to these findings, and in spite of the inability of experts to agree on whether facial features in the absence of FAS are so discernible they can be attributed to maternal drinking during pregnancy, Day and her co-workers (Day et al., 1989) estimated the threshold for producing facial features characteristic of FAS at one drink a day on an average over the first 2 months of pregnancy. The implication of this estimate is hardly credible in light of the previous studies or in light of the millions of Italians, Spaniards, and Greeks whose mealtime alcohol consumption is commonplace. If the Day et al. (1989) findings actually reflected daily drinking rather than frequent binges during the measurement period, we would be confronted with an interesting paradox: the faces of the "abstinent" mothers' children would be unusual because more than 50% of all pregnant women in the industrialized world drink during pregnancy (see Chapter 11). In other words, if one drink a day during pregnancy resulted in these features, readers of this book lacking these features would be "abnormal"! However, as Day and her colleagues report in a subsequent study, 30% of the women whose average intake was estimated at an average of one drink a day, reported drinking five or more drinks on occasion during their first trimester (Day et al., 1991). In other words, the average drinks threshold is an artifact.

Long-Term Effects

Although the facial features associated with FAS are readily discernible in children, once these children reach puberty, their facial features undergo numerous changes and are usually no longer recognizable as FAS in adolescence and adulthood. "In some adults," Spohr noted, "the faces of the affected individuals had normalized so much that early childhood photographs were needed to confirm the diagnosis" (Spohr, 1996, p. 214).

The most persistent features making up the FAS faces in adolescence and adulthood, along with other features still observable, are listed in Table 7.4 (Lemoine & Lemoine, 1992; Spohr, 1996; Spohr et al., 1993; Streissguth et al., 1991). Interestingly, one of the most common features mentioned in this list—prominent noses, is not observed in younger people with FAS.

Conclusion

If facial features are to be used as part of the diagnostic criteria for FAS, this diagnosis should be based on the gestalt or constellation of multiple features and not on any single feature or menu of features. Although there are individual facial features frequently associated with FAS during childhood, they vary in different populations. When it comes to recognizing the facial dysmorphia of FAS, the whole is greater than the sum of its parts. During adulthood, typical facial features

**Table 7.4. Characteristics of FAS
in Adolescents and Adults**

Craniofacial Features
    Short palpebral fissures
    Thin upper lip
    Large nose with prominent nasal bridge
    Large chin
Growth Retardation
Microcephaly
Cognitive Deficits

become more difficult to discern and, in some instances, may not be discernible at all.

Although similar anomalies occur in animals prenatally exposed to alcohol, the blood alcohol levels needed to produce these effects are very high, for example, above 200 mg%. Whereas studies in animals are invaluable for determining mechanisms of action by which alcohol produces these effects, some anomalies commonly associated with prenatal exposure to alcohol in animals, for example, microphthalmia, are not common outcomes of such exposure in humans.

Although there is no consensus regarding a threshold amount of drinking during human pregnancies for producing facial effects, the lowest estimate is an average of six drinks a day throughout at least the first trimester of pregnancy. However, as noted throughout this book, these averages tend to obscure the bingeing pattern of alcohol consumption that more likely result in such anomalies. This means that if the average is 6 drinks a day, consumption levels may be as high as 40 drinks on a drinking day, which falls in line with the consumption levels associated with FAS in chapter 2. This level of drinking is convergent with animal studies and supports the essential argument of this book: It is alcohol abuse (regular consumption of 5 or more drinks per drinking day more than once a week) and not occasional or moderate drinking that leads to the anomalies associated with FAS/ARBEs.

CHAPTER 8

Alcohol-Abuse-Related Malformations

As noted by the Institute of Medicine, "Virtually every malformation has been described in some patient with FAS" (IOM, 1996, p.77). Although the presence or absence of these malformations does not influence the diagnosis, many of these abnormalities are so commonly encountered in conjunction with FAS that their occurrence in this context must be more than coincidental.

The IOM labels these malformations alcohol-related birth defects (ARBDs) to distinguish them from anomalies affecting the CNS; the IOM combines these latter anomalies with cognitive abnormalities and labels them *alcohol-related neurodevelopmental disorders (ARNDs)*.

Although the IOM's use of ARBDs is relatively specific, referring to malformations in this way is confusing because ARBD continues to be used by others to refer to any anomaly associated with in utero alcohol exposure, including neurodevelopmental disorders. To avoid such confusion, these malformations will be labeled *alcohol-abuse-related malformations (ARMs)* in this book. To avoid further confusion, the IOM's term will be placed in parentheses for frame of reference.

Although the IOM clearly states ARMs (ARBDs) and neurodevelopmental abnormalities, which it terms alcohol-related neurodevelopmental disorders (ARNDs), are the product of the same abusive drinking that leads to FAS or partial FAS, it differentiates between the two so as to identify alcohol-impaired individuals who exhibit abnormalities in the absence of the facial gestalt from those with FAS or partial FAS. Because neurodevelopmental abnormalities are much more common than major malformations in the context of in utero alcohol exposure, the IOM felt creation of a specific category of behavioral anomalies was important from the standpoint of qualifying individuals for social services. This distinction has been adopted in this book, except that, in keeping with this book's major unifying principle and the IOM's own diagnostic criteria (see Chapter 3), the acronym refers more appropriately to alcohol-abuse-related neurodevelopmental disorder.

In creating these diagnostic categories, the IOM acknowledged that many of the effects it included as ARMs (ARBDs) and ARNDs were, to some extent, based on animal research. But as previously illustrated, many of the effects commonly associated with prenatal alcohol exposure in animals are not commonly associated with prenatal alcohol exposure in humans. As argued throughout this book, the greatest strength of animal research lies in the validity it gives to clinical and epidemiological findings and its unique contributions to investigators of biological mechanisms responsible for the outcomes being studied, rather than the other way around.

Limb and Joint Anomalies

Limb and joint anomalies are the most common structural anomalies in FAS, occurring in about 18% of all cases (Abel, 1990). If flexion problems and related movement problems were included in this estimate, the prevalence of this disorder in FAS would be even higher. Among the anomalies frequently mentioned in this context are clinodactyly (see Figure 8.1A), camptodactyly, nail dysplasia (see Figure 8.1B), and radioulnar synostosis (see Figure 8.1C). Punctate epiphyses, also called stippled epiphyses or chondrodysplasia punctata, are unusual calcium deposits usually seen in the lower extremities; they have also been noted in FAS, as have hip dislocation, shortened limbs/digits, clubfoot, cervical spine fusion, scoliosis, polydactyly, syndactyly, exostoses (bony protrusions), shortened fingers, and missing limbs (amelia or digits) (see Abel, 1990, for references).

Anomalous palmar crease and dermal ridge patterns have also been mentioned in the context of FAS (Majewski, 1981; Spohr et al., 1993). Simian creases (see Figure 8.1D) occur in about 6% of FAS cases, as compared with about 1.3% in the general population (Tillner & Majewski, 1978).

Alcohol-related increases in skeletal defects have been reported in several epidemiological studies (Aro, 1983; Foster & Baird, 1992; Ogston & Parry, 1992), but the relationships are problematic. A Canadian study (Foster & Baird, 1992) found only when maternal alcohol consumption was so severe that it was noted in the medical chart was alcohol abuse associated with a very high incidence of skeletal anomalies (6 out of 8 cases, compared with the general population, 217/651).

Animals prenatally exposed to alcohol exhibit many of the same skeletal anomalies seen in connection with FAS, but the types of anomalies vary depending on species and strain. Although skeletal anomalies, such as polydactyly, syndactyly, and ectrodactyly, occur occasionally in rats (Mankes, Battles, LeFeore, van der Hoeven, & Glick, 1992) and miniature pigs (Dexter et al., 1980) exposed to alcohol in utero, they are not as common in these species as they are in some strains of mice, such as $C_{57}B1$ mice (Boggan, Monroe, Turner, Upshurk, &

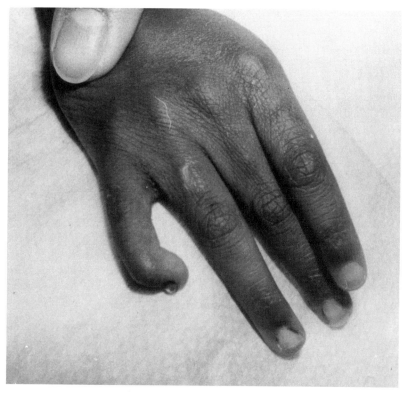

A

Figure 8.1A–D. (**A**) Clinodactyly of fifth finger in patient with FAS. (**B**) Nail dysplasia in patient with FAS. (**C**) Radiograph of radioulnar synostosis of elbow in patient with FAS. (**D**) Abnormal palmar creases in patient with FAS. *Note* the simian crease (horizontal crease in center of hand). (All photos courtesy of Dr. Phillip Spiegel. Used with permission.)

Middaugh, 1989; Gilliam, Kotch, Dudek, & Riley, 1989; Randall & Anton, 1984; Webster et al., 1983; West, Hodges, & Black, 1981). The most sensitive time of exposure for producing these anomalies are days 9–10 of gestation in the mouse (Webster et al., 1983). The blood alcohol levels involved are very high, for example, 400 mg%. Although increased skeletal anomalies have been reported in conjunction with lower blood alcohol levels (Chernoff, 1977; Zidenberg-Cherr et al., 1988), blood alcohol levels were assessed at arbitrary sampling times, when it was convenient for the researchers to obtain samples, rather than at the animal's peak blood alcohol level. Anomalies of the rib cage have also been observed in mice prenatally exposed to alcohol (Chernoff, 1977), but this effect is far less common than those previously mentioned.

Retarded skeletal development, on the other hand, is relatively common in all

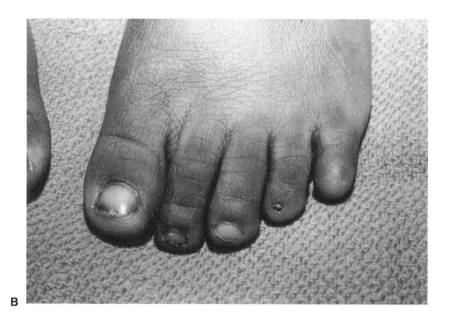

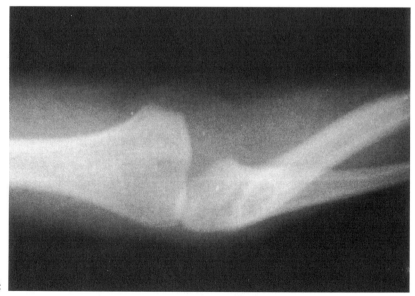

Figure 8.1. (*Continued*)

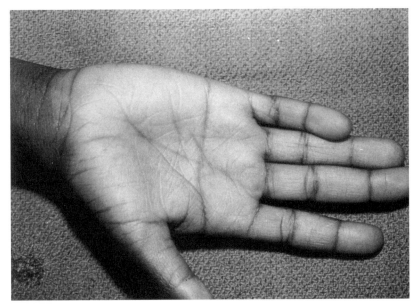

Figure 8.1. (*Continued*)

strains of animals prenatally exposed to alcohol (Lee & Leichter, 1980, 1983; Mankes, Hoffman, LeFebre, Bates, & Abraham, 1983; Miralles-Flores & Delgado-Baeza, 1992; Stuckey & Berry, 1984). Retarded skeletal development has been related to decreased bone ossification and volume (Miralles-Flores & Delgado-Baeza, 1992) stemming from alcohol-induced bone calcium loss (Lee & Leichter, 1983), and, indirectly, to stress-induced changes in the hypothalamic-pituitary-gonadal axis (Portoles et al., 1988; Root et al., 1975).

The very high blood alcohol levels of 400% or more needed to produce these anomalies in animals (Gilliam et al., 1989; Randall & Anton, 1984) are very close to the LD50 (lethal dose that kills half the animals to which it is administered) of 690 mg% in mice (Maling, 1970). Mothers that survive remain comatose for at least five hours (Beauchemin, Gartner, & Provenza, 1984), and resorption rates are very high among those that survive (Kotch, Dehart, Alles, Chernoff, & Sulik, 1992), raising the possibility these and other anomalies are the result of alcohol-induced maternal toxicity. The fact the same kinds of skeletal anomalies can be produced by a wide variety of agents, including sodium valproate, acetazolamide, carbon dioxide, and cadmium (Kotch et al., 1992), which have very little in common with one another or with alcohol, likewise raises the possibility the changes are not directly pharmacological. Even if dose related, a possible interpretation is the dose-response relationship could be due to graded increases in maternal toxicity.

Heart

The prevalence of cardiac anomalies in FAS is relatively high, possibly because of the types of cases that are specifically referred for medical attention. In other words, cardiac cases may not represent an unbiased sampling of FAS cases. (This is also true of rates of other malformations associated with FAS.)

Septal heart defects are the most common cardiac anomaly associated with FAS. Rates vary from 26% (Sandor, Smith, & Macleod, 1981) to 76% (Dupuis et al., 1978). The more common type of lesion involves the ventricles rather than the atria (Abel, 1990). In many cases, these apertures are tiny and close on their own, without surgical intervention. Estimates of cardiac anomalies, without regard for the type of anomaly, may be especially high in German patient populations, between 29% and 63% (Loser et al., 1988; Majewski, 1993), because the cardiac diagnosis of *herzinsuffizienz* is liberally applied, often without any substantive corroborating evidence (Payer, 1988).

Other cardiac problems occurring in between 0.9% and 2.7% of all FAS cases are tetralogy of Fallot and pulmonary stenosis (Abel, 1990). Less common are polyvalvular disease, pentalogy of Fallot, abnormal right aortic arch, hypoplastic pulmonary artery, pulmonary aplasia, atrioventricular canal, idiopathic hypertrophic subaortic stenosis, coarctation of the aorta, double outlet right ventricle, dextrocardia, ventricular hypertrophy, and mitral valve prolapse (see Abel, 1990, for references).

Very high rates of ventricular septal defects and other anomalies have been induced prenatally in mice exposed to blood alcohol levels above 200 mg% (Chernoff, 1977; Giknis et al., 1980; Webster, Germain, Lipson, & Walsh, 1984). In mice, the highest rates of damage occur following intraperitoneal injection on gestation days 8 and 9 (60% and 75%, respectively); injection on gestation day 10 results in a frequency of about 15%. Exposure to alcohol on gestation day 7 does not result in heart defects in the mouse (Webster et al., 1984). The frequency of occurrence in animals is genetically related; some strains are affected more/less than others (Giknis et al., 1980). In chick embryos, susceptibility to alcohol-related cardiac anomalies ranges from 4.0% to 34%, depending on strain (Bruyere & Stith, 1993).

Bruyere and Stith (1994) speculated that alcohol may induce structural anomalies in the heart and elsewhere by decreasing cardiac hemodynamics because they found a temporary interruption of blood supply to the pregnant rat uterus caused intracardiac abnormalities in the embryo. Decreased cardiac output resulted in a decrease in total circulating blood volume and transient episodes of ischemia in the embryo. If these results were followed by rapid tissue reperfusion, they could result in overproduction of reactive oxygen radicals. Because the embryo had very little antioxidant activity, it was very vulnerable to the cytotoxic effects of these reactive radicals. (For further discussion, see Chapter 13.)

Lung

Lung structure and function have been ignored in the context of FAS. The implication is that there is little evidence of abnormalities. Respiratory distress syndrome (Ioffe & Chernick, 1987) and decreased lung surfactant (Halvorsen, Gross, & Sokol, 1985) have been noted in some infants born to alcoholic mothers, but the general absence of such reports indicates that these are atypical, although decreased lung surfactant has also been reported in animals prenatally exposed to alcohol (Zagorul'ko, Fisik, & Tikus, 1991). Interestingly, the incidence of respiratory distress syndrome in a group of prematurely delivered neonates was significantly decreased if their mothers had received maternal intravenous alcohol to delay delivery (Barrada, Virnig, Edwards, & Hakanson, 1977).

Human fetal lung fibroblasts incubated with alcohol underwent a marked inhibition in collagen synthesis (or an increase in collage degradation), which resulted in decreased protein synthesis (Thanassi, Rokowski, Sheehy, Hart, & Absher, 1980), an effect that would be expected to result in decreased size. Such a decrease has not been seen in humans, but studies in rats have found hypoplastic lungs (O'Gorman & Bannigan, 1991).

Kidney and Urological Anomalies

Although a number of kidney.and urological anomalies, for example, hydronephrosis, hypoplastic kidney, and renal agenesis, have been associated with FAS (see Abel, 1990, for references), the impression that there is a high rate of kidney anomalies among patients with FAS is misleading, and it appears to be due to the previously mentioned (re: the heart) overemphasis on problems that require treatment.

In one of the few clinically based experiments to examine kidney anomalies, Taylor and her co-workers (Taylor, Jones, Jones, & Kaplan, 1994) compared a group of 51 children with FAS with 39 others whose mothers had been heavy drinkers during pregnancy (4 or more drinks a day) and a control group. All subjects were given renal ultrasounds. There were no significant differences in structural renal abnormalities among the three groups. Although kidney sizes in the FAS group and the other group of prenatally exposed children were smaller than normal for chronological age and height, the size difference had no biological importance. Based on their findings, the authors concluded that there was no need to screen children prenatally exposed to alcohol for renal anomalies.

Although functional renal damage (impaired renal acidification and associated metabolic acidosis) in the absence of gross pathology has been noted in some children with FAS (Assadi & Ziai, 1986), there have been few reports of comparable dysfunction in most children with FAS, so this anomaly appears to be a relatively isolated problem coincidental to FAS.

The impression that there is a high prevalence of kidney defects associated with FAS also may have arisen from experiments with some strains of mice (C_{57}Bl/6J) that develop a high incidence of kidney anomalies following in utero alcohol exposure (Boggan, Randall, & Dodds, 1979). Other strains (LS and SS) seem relatively unaffected in this regard (Gilliam et al., 1989). There are isolated reports of kidney anomalies in rats (Mankes et al., 1992) and beagles (Ellis & Pick, 1980), but such reports are also uncommon.

Alcohol-induced renal anomalies in mice always take the form of hydronephrosis or hydroureter. Because these anomalies are seen in animals with and without obstructions in the urogenital system (Boggan et al., 1989), they arise from some as yet unidentified condition. Although the frequency of alcohol-related renal anomalies varies between strains, the consistency of their occurrence in C_{57}BL mice is impressive (Boggan et al., 1979, 1989; Gage & Sulik, 1991; Giknis et al., 1980; Mankes et al., 1983; Randall & Anton, 1984).

Liver

Surprisingly, there are few case reports of liver damage in patients with FAS and little consistency among those which do report such anomalies, suggesting that these reports are probably a coincidence rather than a strong correlate of FAS. Among the hepatic anomalies most frequently mentioned are hepatomegaly, hepatic fibrosis, and hepatic deposition. Most of these reports come from isolated patient populations (see Abel, 1990, for references).

Because the activity of alcohol dehydrogenase, the enzyme involved in metabolism of alcohol, is increased following chronic alcohol consumption (Lieber, 1991), some investigators have questioned whether a comparable increase in the activity of this enzyme also occurs in animal offspring prenatally exposed to alcohol. Results of their work have been inconsistent. Increases (Ledig, Tholey, Kopp, & Mandel, 1989), decreases (Duncan & Woodhouse, 1978), and no changes (Sanchis & Guerri, 1986) in enzyme activity have all been reported. Effects on aldehyde dehydrogenase, the enzyme that metabolizes acetaldehyde, are also inconsistent (Burke & Fenton, 1978; Ledig et al., 1989). These inconsistencies imply that in utero alcohol exposure does not affect these enzyme activities either pre- or postnatally.

Pancreas

There are no reports of gross pancreatic pathology in connection with FAS. However, there are several studies that suggest prenatal alcohol exposure may result in resistance to insulin's actions on fetal cellular glucose transport; insulin resistance may also persist after birth (see Chapter 13).

Hypothalamic-Pituitary-Adrenal Axis (HPA)

With very few exceptions (Coulter, Leech, Schaefer, Scheithauer, & Brumbach, 1993), there is little evidence of structural damage to the pituitary or adrenal glands associated clinically or epidemiologically with maternal drinking during pregnancy. A rare instance of pseudo-Cushing syndrome in an infant who was exposed to alcohol by means of breast milk (Binkiewicz, Robinson, & Senior, 1978) indicated that the human hypothalamic-pituitary-adrenal (HPA) system can be activated at a very early age. There is, however, no evidence of altered HPA function associated with FAS (Root et al., 1975). Although a brief report suggested that infants prenatally exposed to alcohol had an overly reactive HPA response to stress (blood sampling) (Jacobson, Jacobson, Bihun, Chisdo, & Sokol, 1993b), the results were far from conclusive.

Studies in animals, on the other hand, have found prenatal alcohol exposure has the potential to affect HPA activity, and this effect carries over into adulthood. Much of this literature has recently been reviewed by Kim, Osborn, & Weinberg (1996). Unless and until comparable effects occur in humans, data and hypotheses generated in the context of animal models need to be carefully considered as to their pertinence. Such considerations are particularly relevant in the context of corticosteroids because the main corticosteroid in humans is cortisol, whereas the main corticosteroid in animals is corticosterone. Important differences in their regulation or effects (see Jerrels & Pruett, 1994) may preclude generalizations between species. (Studies in animals evaluating the potential involvement of corticosteroids in the response to stressors and immune function are discussed in Chapter 13.)

Thyroid

Because congenital hypothyroidism and FAS have many features in common, such as altered growth, delayed development of the skeletal system and such brain areas as the cerebellum, impaired auditory function, and so on (Gottesfeld & Silverberg, 1990), thyroid function was assessed in several cases of FAS (Castells, Mark, Abaci, & Schwartz, 1981), but no evidence of clinical hypothyroidism was observed. An epidemiological study examining the possible link between altered thyroid function and ARBDs likewise found no evidence supporting such a relationship (Hannigan, Martier, & Naber, 1995b).

As in the case of the HPA axis, although there is no clinical or epidemiological evidence indicating a link between thyroid function and prenatal alcohol exposure in humans, there is considerable evidence for such a link in animals (see Chapter 13).

Reproductive Organs

The external genitalia are sometimes abnormal in both males and females with FAS (see Abel, 1990, for references), but these anomalies are not common. In their large prospective study of over 32,000 births, in which they looked for 60 different anomalies, Mills and Graubard (1987) found no significant relation between drinking and any anomaly, except those involving the genitourinary system. When individual genitourinary malformations were considered, the increase was attributable to malformations of the sex organs. The authors argued that the increase in sex-organ anomalies was biologically significant because such anomalies had been reported by other investigators (see Abel, 1990), although, at the same time, they ignored their own failure to corroborate previously reported increases in many other organs, such as the heart and limbs. However, the authors did acknowledge the possibility that the increase in sex-organ anomalies in their study may have been due to chance, as a result of the large number of comparisons they made.

Sokol and his co-workers (1980) also reported a statistically significant increase in the frequency of genitourinary anomalies, for example, hypospadias, among alcohol abusers relative to controls. However, alcohol-abusing women were also eleven times more likely to have experienced some kind of infection during the study period, and these infections may have contributed to the statistically significant increase.

Thresholds

Although malformations are commonly associated with FAS and hence with maternal alcohol abuse during pregnancy, most studies have not reported an increased rate of malformations apart from FAS, except when the study population includes alcohol abusers, that is, women regularly consuming five or more drinks on occasion (Hollstedt et al., 1983b; Rosett et al., 1983; Werler et al., 1991). Studies with relatively few alcohol abusers or alcoholics have generally not found any statistically significant link between malformations and maternal drinking at lower levels of consumption (Gibson et al., 1983; Griso et al., 1984; Hingson et al., 1982; Kaminski et al., 1978, 1981; Lumley et al., 1985; Marbury et al., 1983; Mau, 1980; Tennes & Blackard, 1980). Even when such studies included a few alcohol-abusing women, malformation rates were not reliably increased. (In the Tennes and Blackard [1980] study, for instance, four women reported consumption of 11 to 40 drinks within an 8-hour period during their first trimester of pregnancy.)

Although a few studies have reported significant associations between malformations and relatively low levels of consumption, these findings are problematic. For example, Davis et al. (1982) reported a slight increase (1.2%)in anomalies in children born to mothers who drank relative to abstainers, but the increase did not differ from the background rate of 1.6% for the geographical area in the United Kingdom where the study was conducted. Another unusual aspect of the study was that the increase in anomalies was only seen among women in the lowest alcohol consumption group (average about 1 drink per week). From the standpoint of face validity or construct validity, the inference that malformations were increased as a result of prenatal alcohol exposure was dubious.

Similarly, the very slight increase (0.11-fold) in congenital anomalies associated with low levels of maternal alcohol consumption reported by Day et al. (1989) related only to "minor malformations"—which were not described—and did not take into account the frequency of those anomalies in the predominantly poverty-stricken African-American population being studied.

Studies reporting significant associations between drinking during pregnancy and "minor malformations" typically look for any and every possible anomaly. Each anomaly is then examined for statistical significance, with no correction made for multiple analyses, a bias that increases the likelihood of positive relationships occurring by chance. Some studies also fail to consider the contributions of confounding variables to these associations (thereby falling victim to the law of confounding determinism, see Chapter 3), and, more often than not, the overwhelming majority of these studies do not indicate the extent to which alcohol contributed to these associations. Those that do find that the contribution is almost negligible.

Among the reasons anomalies are not frequently encountered outside of FAS is that alcohol is not a very potent teratogen. Very large quantities of alcohol must be consumed for malformations to occur. Based on the clinical and epidemiological evidence—and the experimental evidence in animals—the threshold for these anomalies is a minimum of five drinks per drinking occasion consumed regularly during the first trimester of pregnancy.

CHAPTER 9

Neurodevelopmental Abnormalities

Structural and Sensory

Microcephaly

Neurodevelopmental abnormalities are among the most important components of fetal alcohol abuse syndrome. Information relating to these abnormalities is now voluminous; therefore, it has been divided into two chapters for purposes of presentation, beginning with microcephaly, the most readily observable of this family of neurodevelopmental disorders. It is important to bear in mind, however, that all of these abnormalities are biologically linked—they all arise from disturbances to the ectoderm, the outer surface layer of the trilaminar embryonic structure, which also gives rise to the skin, teeth, and nails. Because disturbances in these structures all arise from the same tissue layer, it is not surprising that abnormalities in these different parts of the body are clustered into what might otherwise be called an *ectodermal syndrome*. The fact that structures like the heart arise from the mesoderm, the middle layer of the trilaminar layer, is a possible reason that abnormalities in those organs are less common in FAS and should not be included as a formal component of FAS. Distinctions relating to specific embryological tissue origins provide construct validity for a syndrome—structures originating together are damaged together.

There are two critical periods in human growth when the brain is especially vulnerable to insult. The first occurs during the first trimester, between the 12th and the 20th weeks of gestation, and is characterized by a rapid rate of nerve-cell proliferation. The second occurs during the third trimester and lasts up to 18 months postnatally. This latter phase is called the brain *growth spurt* and is characterized by overall growth, extensive dendritic arborization, growth of axons, myelination, increased synaptogenesis, gliogenesis, and maturation of neurotransmitter systems.

Microcephaly (decreased head circumference below the 3rd percentile) occurs in about 80% of young children with FAS (Loser, 1995; Streissguth, Brookstein, Sampson, & Barr, 1993) and is a reliable consequence of maternal alcohol abuse, that is, regular consumption of five or more drinks per drinking occasion. Microcephaly is also one of the most persistent characteristics of FAS. Although catch-up growth occurs in adolescence in some instances, microcephaly often remains a visible indication of FAS (Streissguth et al., 1991). Microcephaly is also a reliable effect of maternal alcohol abuse, even when it is not associated with FAS (Godel et al., 1992; Kyllerman et al., 1985; Russell et al., 1991), but the link with lower levels of consumption is very inconsistent. Statistically significant associations with low levels of drinking have been reported in some studies (Chernick et al., 1983; Day et al., 1989; Rosett et al., 1983; Sulaiman et al., 1988) but not in others (Ernhart et al., 1985a; Fried & O'Connell, 1987; Greene et al., 1991b; Mills & Graubard, 1987; Tennes & Blackard, 1980). Even when statistically significant, however, consumption rarely accounts for as much as 3% of the decrease in head size.

In discussing these inconsistencies, Ernhart (1991) raised the *argumentum ex silentio* as evidence against any significant relationship. Many studies designed to examine growth and development, Ernhart contended, could have easily included a measure of head circumference. Given the interest in head circumference as an index of brain damage, it seemed unlikely that these measurements were not performed. Ernhart considered the absence of such reports strong evidence against any relationship. "This possibility," Ernhart reflected, "decreases somewhat the confidence one may have in inferences drawn across studies of an effect for head circumference as such" (1991, p. 141).

Ernhart raised the equally valid and even more disturbing possibility that much of what has been published regarding the effects of relatively low levels of drinking is a biased presentation of facts. While a statistically significant result is published, studies employing equally rigorous procedures that fail to find statistically significant associations may not be submitted or accepted for publication, thereby creating the distorted impression that what might otherwise be an unusual outcome is instead accepted as a reliable consequence of drinking during pregnancy.

Studies in Animals

As in the case of maternal alcohol abuse in humans, high blood alcohol levels, for example, 150 mg% and above, reliable produce microcephaly in rats when exposure occurs during the postnatal brain growth spurt, a developmental period in rats equivalent to the late second and third trimesters of pregnancy in humans. For our hypothetical pregnant 130-pound woman to achieve a comparable blood alcohol level, she would have to ingest about six drinks over a 2-hour period, or nine drinks over a 5-hour period (see Table 1.2) on a regular basis during the latter part of her pregnancy.

Exposure to this level of alcohol produces an irreversible microcephaly in rats (Bonthius & West, 1988; West et al., 1987), resulting from decreased neuronal cell densities in somatosensory cortex (Miller & Potempa, 1990), hippocampus (West, Hanire, & Cassell, 1986), and cerebellum (Goodlett, Marcussen, & West, 1990). Microcephaly in these studies is not solely a reflection of decreased body weight because it occurs even when brain weight is expressed as a ratio of body weight.

Prenatal alcohol exposure at this high level in rats and mice (Henderson, Hoyumpa, McClain, & Schenker, 1979; Lopez-Tejero, Ferrer, Llobera, & Herra, 1986; Miller, 1986), guinea pigs (Abdollah & Brien, 1995), beagles (Ellis & Pick, 1980), and miniature swine (Dexter, Tumbleson, Decker, & Middleton, 1980), corresponding to exposure during the first or early second trimester of pregnancy in humans, can also result in microcephaly, but unlike exposure during the growth spurt, the decrease is usually related to an overall decrease in body weight (Henderson et al., 1979; Lopez-Tejero et al., 1986).

Structural Anomalies

One of the brain structures most frequently affected in FAS is the corpus callosum, a thick bundle of nerve fibers that connects the two halves of the brain and serves as the main pathway through which information relating to the body is shared. Structural damage to the corpus callosum can take the form of agenesis, or thinning (Mattson et al., 1992; Mattson & Riley, 1996), which can in turn result in a widening of the third ventricle (Starshak et al., 1992). An enlarged ventricle is serious because increased ventricular size produces physical pressure on surrounding brain cells, causing their destruction. However, neither agenesis of the corpus callosum or enlarged ventricles occur in every case of FAS (Gabrielli et al., 1990).

Agenesis of the corpus callosum is relatively uncommon in the general population, occurring once in every 1,000 births (Mattson et al., 1994). Interestingly, this is also the same frequency with which FAS occurs in the general population (Abel, 1995), and FAS may be the most commonly known cause of this anomaly (Mattson & Riley, 1996). Thinning of the corpus callosum has also been observed in children who do not have FAS, but whose mothers were described as alcoholics or heavy drinkers (Mattson et al., 1994; Mattson & Riley, 1996). However, slight thinning of areas of the corpus callosum is a normal variation that should not necessarily be considered indicative of dysgenesis (Starshak et al., 1992).

Although agenesis of the corpus callosum has been observed in animals prenatally exposed to alcohol (Chernoff, 1977), it is relatively uncommon in this context (Wainwright et al., 1985; Zimmerberg & Scalzi, 1989). However, behavioral studies of position preference or directionality, which are related to corpus callosum function, have been reported in animals (Zimmerberg & Scalzi, 1989), suggesting that subtle physical changes have occurred.

The cerebellum is another area of the brain that frequently undergoes damage in connection with FAS. Comparable neuroanatomical anomalies have been found in nonhuman primates exposed to regular bingelike episodes of alcohol exposure (Astley, Weinberger, Shaw, Richards, & Clarren, 1995).

Postmortem examination of 16 children with FAS found 4 with a dysgenesis of the cerebellum (Clarren, 1986). Magnetic resonance imaging (MRI) of children with FAS has likewise found instances of gross neuroanatomical peculiarities in the cerebellum (Mattson et al., 1992, 1994; Sowell et al., 1996). A positron emission tomography (PET) study of four children with FAS, ages 4 to 6, found this area of the brain had a very low glucose utilization rate (Hannigan, Martier, Chugani, & Sokol, 1995a), suggesting decreased functional activity, possibly related to disturbances in fine motor control (Jones et al., 1973), ataxia (Kyllerman et al., 1985; Marcus, 1987), and gait problems (Marcus, 1987).

The cerebellum has received a disproportionate amount of attention from neuroanatomists not only because of its susceptibility to alcohol's neuropathological effects, but also because of its distinctive cytoarchitecture, which enables researchers to observe fine distinctions in the types of cells damaged by alcohol. The two main types of cerebellar cells are the relatively large Purkinje cells and the smaller granule cells. In the rat, Purkinje cells are generated prenatally; granule cells, postnatally. Vulnerability to alcohol's teratogenic effects is greatest if exposure occurs after the cells have passed the formative stage and are in the differentiation stage. In the case of the rat cerebellum, if alcohol exposure occurs prenatally, when Purkinje cells are in their formative stage of neurogenesis, the impact on cell density is minimal. On the other hand, if exposure occurs postnatally, during the brain's growth spurt (corresponding to the third trimester in humans), when the Purkinje cells are undergoing differentiation, dendritic development, and synaptogenesis, they are affected to a much greater extent than the granule cells, which are in their neurogenerative and proliferative stage (Phillips & Cragg, 1982; Pierce, Goodlett, & West, 1989; West et al., 1990).

Alcohol's impact on the most mature cells is also seen in Purkinje cell populations in areas of the cerebellum. Those undergoing dendritic development earliest are affected the most, as reflected by a greater cellular loss, compared with those that develop later (Goodlett et al., 1990; Phillips & Cragg, 1982; Pierce et al., 1989).

The blood alcohol level required to produce cell losses in the cerebellum following a single alcohol treatment in the rat is very high, for example, 360 mg%;

a blood alcohol level of around 150 mg% does not produce significant cell loss, except in one lobule (Goodlett et al., 1990). If exposure occurs over a period of days, the threshold is lower but still relatively high (190 mg%) (Bonthius & West, 1988).

A third structural component of the brain that has received considerable attention in the context of in utero alcohol exposure is the hippocampal formation. Although structural damage to this part of the brain has not been found in FAS, there is considerable evidence of such damage in animals and even evidence of functional damage in humans and animals.

Researchers have been particularly interested in hippocampal damage because of the hippocampus's involvement in memory function, especially long-term potential (LTP). LTP refers to an enhancement of electrical activity in specific neuronal pathways that lasts from several minutes to several days after stimulation. It is widely believed that this prolonged activity is responsible for learning and memory consolidation (Berman & Krahl, 1996). Studies of LTP in animals prenatally exposed to alcohol, however, are inconsistent (Berman & Krahl, 1996).

A practical reason for the interest in the hippocampal formation is that like the cerebellum, it has a relatively distinctive cytoarchitecture. Early-forming, large pyramidal cells are tightly packed together in the hippocampus and spatially isolated from the later-forming, smaller granule cells in the dentate gyrus.

As in the case of the cerebellum, the earlier-forming cells for example, pyramidal cells in the CA_1 region, are significantly reduced in number by high doses of alcohol, whereas cell densities in the CA_3 and CA_4 layers and in the dentate gyrus are not significantly affected (Pierce & West, 1987).

The blood alcohol threshold for such damage is about 150 mg% (West, Hamre, & Pierce, 1984), which is considerably lower than that associated with cerebellar damage in the rat. Although the lower threshold indicates greater susceptibility, the extent of the damage to the hippocampus is less than that to the cerebellum at comparable blood alcohol levels (Pierce et al., 1989).

The optic nerve and the organ of Corti are two additional areas of the brain arising from the ectoderm that undergo damage from alcohol. Although relatively common, these anomalies have received much less attention than those previously mentioned, possibly because sensory function in general has been relatively ignored in fetal alcohol abuse studies (see later).

When specifically looked for, hypoplastic optic nerve heads, either unilateral or bilateral, have been noted in 20% to 50% of FAS cases (Miller et al., 1981; Robinson & Conry, 1986; Stromland, 1985). Optic nerve hypoplasia has also been observed in animals, following the administration of very high doses of alcohol (BALs over 350 mg%) (Clarren et al., 1988).

The organ of Corti is the sensory organ involved in hearing; it is made up of four rows of sensory receptor cells called *hair cells* because of their hairlike appearance. Stimulation of these receptors are converted to nerve impulses by the auditory nerve; they are passed on to the cochlear nucleus in the medulla and then to a series of intermediate nuclei, before they are transmitted to the auditory cortex in the temporal lobe of the brain.

Evidence of hair-cell damage in the organ of Corti in rats prenatally exposed to alcohol is shown in Figure 9.1. As indicated in the figure, punctate loss of hair cells is confined primarily to the three outer hair-cell layers, but damage to the inner hair-cell layer also occurs. Studies in mice and chicks indicate that alcohol also damages cells originating from the ectoderm that give rise to other parts of the auditory system (Church, 1996).

Ultrastructural Damage

In addition to gross anomalies affecting major structures, ultrastructural anomalies due to high levels of alcohol exposure in utero occur throughout the brain. An autopsy of a 4-year-old child with FAS (Ferrer & Galofre, 1987), for example, found that in addition to extensive gross neuroanatomical damage, there were also major decreases in the numbers of dendritic spines and increases in morphologically abnormal spines.

Comparable abnormalities in dendritic spines have also been observed in animals prenatally exposed to alcohol (Abel, Jacobsen, & Sherwin, 1983; Lopez-Tejero et al., 1986; Stoltenburg-Didinger & Spohr, 1983). These clinical and experimental findings are of interest because decreased and abnormal dendritic spines are both compatible with life and have been implicated as the morphological basis for mental retardation (Purpura, 1974). In some cases, however, changes in dendritic arborization and dendritic spines may be ephemeral (Lopez-Tejero et al., 1986) and unrelated to synaptic densities (Druse, Rathbun, McNulty, & Nyquist-Battie, 1986; Hoff, 1988).

Myelination

Experimental studies in animals have generally found that pre- or early postnatal alcohol exposure results in delayed myelination. Decreased myelination has important functional implications because it can result in decreased nerve action potentials and conduction speed. These effects can in turn result in delayed reaction time, as well as motor and sensory impairments and intellectual dysfunction due to "cross talk" between adjacent nerve fibers (Phillips et al., 1991).

Evidence for decreased myelination has been looked for an observed mainly in optic nerve axons (Phillips et al., 1991), but it has also been observed in corticothalamic and callosal axons (Jacobson, Rich, & Tousky, 1979), spinal cord axons (McNeill, Fagan, Harris, & Shew, 1989), and peripheral nerve axons (Baruah & Kinder, 1989).

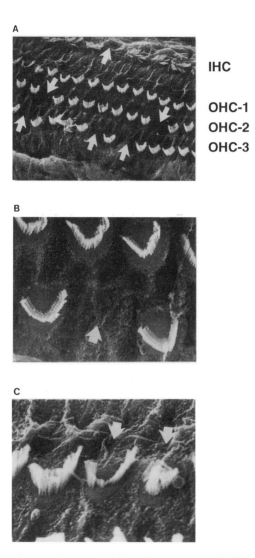

Figure 9.1. Scanning electron micrograph of the auditory sensory epithelium from an untreated control rat and a rat prenatally exposed to alcohol with evidence of hearing loss. Note (in **A**) the single row of inner hair cells (IHC) and three rows of outer hair cells (OHC). Note also the missing or damaged OHCs in the alcohol-exposed animal. (*Source*: M. W. Church, E. L. Abel, J. A. Kaltenbach, & G. W. Overbeck, Effects of prenatal alcohol exposure and aging on auditory function in the rat: Preliminary results. *Alcoholism: Clinical and Experimental Research* (1996), *20*, 172–179. Copyright 1996 by Williams & Wilkins. Reprinted with permission of the publisher.)

A Holoprosencephaly Syndrome?

The fact many of the central nervous system (CNS) anomalies associated with FAS are associated with structures in the midline has been noted by several clinicians who have raised the possibility FAS reflects a mild holoprosencephaly syndrome (Bierich et al., 1976; Bonnemann & Meinecke, 1990; Coulter et al., 1993; Jellinger, Gross, Kaltenbach, & Grisold, 1981; Majewski, 1981; Pfeiffer et al., 1979; Ronen & Andrews, 1991).

Holoprosencephaly is a general term for brain malformations characterized by failures in septation. The condition can range from a very extreme and very rare pathological occurrence called arhinencephaly, in which the early brain fails to separate into two halves, giving rise to such abnormalities as cyclopedia, to less extreme forms in which midline structures like the corpus callosum either do not develop or do not develop to maturity. Problems in septation may also give rise to facial anomalies in the midline, such as an indistinct philtrum. As noted in this and earlier chapters, midline defects, such as missing olfactory bulbs and tracts, absence of optic nerves and chiasma, enlarged dilated lateral ventricles, cleft lip and palate, hippocampal damage, cerebellar damage, and agenesis of the corpus callosum, have also been observed in animals prenatally exposed to alcohol.

However, FAS results in numerous other CNS anomalies, including disordered arrangements and malorientations of nerve cells, cortical heterotopias, ectopic neurons, poor lamination of cerebral cortex, supernumerary mammillary body, and small dysplasias and cortical heterotopies (see Abel, 1990; Mattson & Riley, 1996, for references), that occur at the same time problems relating to septation occur but are not related to them. Furthermore, magnetic resonance imaging has revealed considerable diversity in CNS problems associated with maternal alcohol abuse that go beyond problems attributable to septational anomalies (Gabrielli et al., 1990; Knight et al., 1993; Loock, Conry, Li, & Clark, 1993). Whereas much of the damage associated with prenatal alcohol exposure is located in the midline, the reported diversity means that alcohol's effects are much broader than can be accounted for in terms of a holoprosencephaly syndrome.

Sensory Perceptual Impairments

Sensory processing has been relatively ignored in the context of FAS, although there is consistent evidence that sensory functioning is impaired. In a small pilot study, Morse and Cermak (1994) reported that 12 children with FAS had greater problems with visual and auditory stimuli, and taste and smell, when compared with a control group, although no details were given regarding the control group or the methods used to assess sensory function. Impaired visual and auditory perception, along with form perception, were also reported as being altered in another study evaluating the effects of maternal alcohol abuse during pregnancy (Aronson & Olegard, 1987).

Visual impairment is commonly associated with FAS; it is not uncommon for individuals with FAS to require corrective lenses (see Figure 7.2). In many cases, visual impairment is due to the abnormal curvature of the lens (see Chapter 7).

Visual anomalies appear to be so common that a pediatric ophthalmological examination should be routine for anyone receiving a diagnosis of FAS (Stromland, 1985). Based on the frequency of such FAS-associated disorders, Stromland (1990) was able to identify two additional cases of FAS, attributed to an unknown etiology, in a group of children diagnosed as mildly mentally retarded.

Hearing loss is especially common in FAS and is specifically mentioned by the IOM (1996), in its diagnostic paradigm as evidence of neurodevelopmental disorder. Hearing problems can be subdivided into three main types: conductive, sensorineural, and central hearing loss. Conductive hearing loss typically results from problems affecting the middle ear and occurs in more than 75% of children with FAS. As previously mentioned, recurrent serous otitis media (RSOM) is a leading cause of intermittent conductive hearing loss in children with FAS (Church et al., 1997; Church & Gerkin, 1988; Rossig, Wasser, & Oppermann, 1994). The impediment in sound transmission associated with RSOM results from the buildup of fluid in the middle ear. Hearing losses of 15 db magnitude commonly associated with SOM are clinically significant for young children because this amount of hearing loss can adversely affect school performance and development of speech and language skills (Church, 1996; Rossig et al., 1994; see also Chapter 10).

Sensorineural hearing loss is the result of auditory receptor cell ("hair cell") and/or auditory nerve damage; it is found in 1% to 3% of all children but occurs at a much higher rate in children with Down's syndrome (22%) and submucous cleft palate (22%). It also has been found in as many as 27% to 29% of children with FAS (Church et al., 1997; Church & Gerkin, 1988). Rossig et al. (1994), using a criterion of 20 db for loss, found it in only 6% of their patients with FAS, but they based their findings on brain stem auditory-evoked potentials (BAEPs) (see later), which tests hearing at only 4 kHz. Church and his co-workers (Church et al., 1997) tested hearing at a much broader range of frequencies, using pure-tone audiometry and a criterion of 15 db.

Evoked potentials are electrical responses in the brain that occur in response to various stimuli. Responses are extracted from background EEG activity and can be used to assess neurological function and specific sensory functions. The brain stem auditory-evoked potential, for instance, consists of a series of waves that reflect sequential activation of neuronal nuclei and pathways along the brain stem auditory system. Auditory-evoked potentials may also be abnormal in non-FAS infants whose mothers were alcohol abusers during pregnancy (Pettigrew & Hutchinson, 1984). In Germany, 69% of a group of 29 children whose mothers were alcoholics had abnormal BAEPs (Rossig et al., 1994). Comparable sensori-neural hearing loss has also been found in animals prenatally exposed to alcohol (Church, Abel, Kaltenbach, & Overbeck, 1996).

Prenatal alcohol exposure can also result in damage to auditory nerves in the form of delayed neural transmission (Church et al., 1997; Kaneko, Riley, & Ehlers, 1993). Although the mechanism for this effect has not been determined, decreased myelination or impaired synaptic transmission is possibly responsible.

Church and his co-workers (Church et al., 1997) recently found evidence of central hearing dysfunction as well. Twelve children with FAS were examined using both a dichotic listening task that required them to listen to different "competing" sentences simultaneously presented in each ear, and a task in which they had to pick out words from background noise. All 12 showed clinically significant central hearing impairments on these tests (Kaneko, Ehlers, Phillips, & Riley, 1996; Russell et al., 1991). Studies in animals have likewise found evidence of central hearing impairment following prenatal alcohol exposure (Church et al., 1996).

Prenatal alcohol exposure may also accelerate natural age-related hearing loss. Church et al. (1996) found that most rats prenatally exposed to alcohol that exhibited sensorineural hearing loss at 6 months showed further deterioration in auditory acuity as they aged, and some of the animals with normal hearing at the youngest age developed an exaggerated hearing loss at 12 and 18 months of age. The authors noted that other syndromes associated with sensorineural hearing loss (e.g., Down syndrome) showed progressive age-related hearing loss, and that fetal insults from nicotine and hypoxia likewise were characterized by age-related deterioration of CNS function.

In summary, like sight, hearing is frequently impaired in children with FAS. Given the high rate of hearing problems associated with FAS, it would be worthwhile to test all children with FAS for hearing problems as early as possible.

CHAPTER 10

Neurodevelopmental Abnormalities
Behavioral and Cognitive

The sheer number of behavioral and cognitive abnormalities associated with FAS/ARBE are now so extensive that at least three inferences seem warranted: (a) FAS/ARBE is a very destructive disorder; (b) it has a great many effects; and (c) it is so inscrutable that it has become a magnet attracting every problem for which alternative explanations are not otherwise evident. In this context, greater attention to the syndrome's behavioral and cognitive aspects has meant more studies but not necessarily a better understanding of these problems.

It is worthwhile keeping in mind that although it has been more than 20 years since FAS was brought to light, we still rely on descriptive studies and anecdotes for our impressions about the syndrome. The most haunting and detailed of these is Michael Dorris's biography of his adoptive son, Adam, *The Broken Cord* (Dorris, 1989).

Fueled by gloom-and-doom descriptions of severely affected children like Adam, most people believe FAS/ARBE is inexorably associated with intractable behavioral and cognitive problems. Without the benefit of controlled research studies, however, we cannot assess how typical Adam and the other cases described in the medical literature are. Because all children with FAS/ARBE do not have problems requiring clinical services (Coles et al., 1997), inferences based on such referrals are not necessarily valid for other children with FAS/ARBEs. "It may be that the patients who are referred for evaluation … (in) screening studies and … follow-up projects, are those with the greatest problems" (Morse, 1993; Streissguth & Randels, 1988, p. 149).

Just as we rarely read or hear about everyday occurrences, such as a plane landing on time, baggage uneventfully unloaded, and no traffic jams enroute home, we rarely hear or read about the majority of children with FAS/ARBEs who attend regular classes in public schools, or the young adults with FAS/ARBE who are employed in meaningful jobs or are in college (Kleinfeld & Westcott, 1993; Morse, 1993). As Streissguth (1992) pointed out, "the diagnosis of FAS does not carry with it any particular guarantees or inevitabilities about IQ or about academic achievement levels (and) diagnosis of FAS does not mean that a person cannot graduate from high school or even attend college."

Although we have known for a long time that individuals with FAS/ARBE vary markedly in their abilities and shortcomings, the image of Adam Dorris has become the stereotype for FAS/ARBE. The variant of Gresham's law about money applies to FAS/ARBE—bad news crowds out good—published success stories about people with FAS/ARBE continue to be few and far between because they are far less newsworthy.

Most descriptions of people with FAS/ARBE, including Adam Dorris, are biased in at least two ways: they are typically worst-case scenarios referred for clinical services; with regard to American studies, most are primarily descriptions of Native American children and adolescents with FAS/ARBE (Giunta & Streissguth, 1988; Streissguth, 1994; Streissguth et al., 1985, 1987, 1991). The Streissguth et al. studies, for instance, mainly include adoptees with FAS/ARBE, 50% of whom are Native Americans, as was Adam Dorris.

The fact that so many of these children are Native Americans means that their problems may not be generalizable to African-American or Caucasian children with FAS/ARBE. As will be shown later in this chapter, Native American children, in general, have listening, learning, and behavioral characteristics unique to their cultures. By focusing primarily on these minority children, issues of racial/cultural background have been largely ignored (see chapter "Conclusion"). Because of the inordinate emphasis on minority children, the mistaken inference that these problems are found only in minority children may be drawn.

Inferences based on the study of one minority group are not necessarily generalizable to other minorities or to the wider population. For example, Ernhart's and Cole's reports on African-American children with FAS/ARBE (Coles et al., 1997; Ernhart et al., 1995) do not bear out the twin claims that IQ scores are intractable or that attention deficit disorder/hyperactivity is a general characteristic of FAS/ARBE (see later).

Nevertheless, the common portrayal of FAS/ARBE is disturbing. Adolescents with FAS/ARBE are depicted as mentally incompetent, overly aggressive, and prone to criminal behavior. These depictions, in turn, have generated a deep pessimism about the future of these children, a pessimism many adoptive parents feel incapable of dealing with.

After a typically alarmist program on children with FAS was televised in Boston, the Fetal Alcohol Education Program in the area was inundated with "telephone calls from parents who wished to return their adopted children if this was the future they could look forward to" (Morse, 1993). Adoptive parents who need reassurance that their children with FAS/ARBEs are anything but doomed would be advised to read the upbeat testimonies of parents and care givers of their FAS/ARBE children in *Fantastic Antoine Succeeds* (Kleinfeld & Wescott, 1993).

For the most part, televised programs about FAS/ARBEs offer tabloid entertainment, not fact. There is no scientific evidence that people with FAS are more likely than anyone else to commit criminal acts, or that disproportionate numbers of people with FAS are in prison (Morse, 1993). The best antidote for such misinformation is more and better research and dissemination of the outcomes of this research to the public.

Despite their selectivity, however, studies of children referred for treatment are important. Such studies enable investigators to formulate testable questions concerning the effects of prenatal alcoholism exposure, and they allow for long-term follow-up of these problems. Follow-up studies represent an opportunity to discern what other problems may develop as these children grow older, and whether these problems increase or decrease in severity over time. Without an appropriate control group, however, the extent to which these maladies can be ameliorated or exacerbated by such factors as a child's home environment cannot be adequately assessed. Nor is it possible to determine, on the basis of descriptive studies, if these problems are unique to FAS/ARBE. This is the major failure of the Seattle studies referred to earlier and those discussed below.

These and related issues are examined throughout this chapter in the course of the discussion of the neurodevelopmental consequences of FAS/ARBE. For purposes of presentation, this discussion has been formatted in a developmental framework. This does not mean problems encountered at one age do not occur at another. Categorizing behaviors at various ages is simply one of several ways of integrating a very large and still growing body of information.

Also for purposes of presentation, each developmental period begins with a profile of the behavioral and cognitive problems associated with FAS/ARBE at that age. These profiles are not typical of everyone or anyone with FAS/ARBE. Instead, they are a pastiche derived from descriptive studies of children with behavioral problems. As previously stated, these descriptions are not necessarily characteristic of all children with FAS/ARBE. Instead, they should be regarded only as a starting point for constructing a scientifically based behavioral profile associated with FAS/ARBE. The extent to which these descriptions are supported by scientifically based studies is examined in the controlled studies that follow the descriptive presentations.

Newborns and Infants

Clinical Description

Parents describe caring for newborns and infants with FAS/ARBE as more than exhausting. These children are frequently irritable, hypersensitive to sound, and difficult to console. They do not like to be touched and being touched often makes them cry. They have irregular sleeping habits, are hypotonic ("floppy babies"), hard to feed, and so disinterested in eating that feeding them may take hours. Their mastery of motor milestones, such as speech, grasping, and sitting, is delayed, and they are seemingly unable to bond with caregivers. (Frequent bouts of illness due to infections and failure to thrive were discussed at length earlier in the context of growth and immune function.)

Systematic Studies

Irritability, Hypersensitivity, and Habituation. Neonatal irritability and hypersensitivity have been mentioned in the context of withdrawal from in utero alcohol exposure (see Chapter 4). Indications of irritability are also suggested by a study of increased crying behavior of 3-day-olds whose mothers consumed an average of one to two drinks a day during pregnancy (Nugent, Lester, Greene, Wieczorek-Deering, & O'Mahony, 1996). (Since six of the mothers in this drinking group averaged four drinks per drinking occasion, and some consumed as many as nine drinks per occasion, an association based on "binge" drinking would seem to be more apposite than the "average drinks/day" measure. The authors also failed to take maternal depression into account in their analysis, although maternal depression during pregnancy is correlated with drinking (Bark, 1979) and crying/irritability in newborns [Zuckerman, Baucher, Parker, & Cabral, 1990].) In another study of infant behavior, the association between prenatal alcohol exposure and infant behavior ceased to be statistically significant when maternal depression was taken into account (Jacobson, Jacobson, Sokol, Martier, & Ager, 1993c).

The most commonly used test for systematically detecting subtle differences in neonatal behavior resulting from prenatal exposure to alcohol is the Brazelton test. There are several subcomponents to this test, among them *habituation*, which is evaluated as a response decrement to a rattle and a bell; and *orientation*, which is evaluated as a response to inanimate visual and auditory stimuli. (Results from various studies are summarized in Table 10.1.)

Taken collectively, the results summarized in Table 10.1 indicate that in the absence of FAS/ARBE, prenatal alcohol exposure has no reliable global or specific effect on any of the Brazelton subcomponents.

A mundane reason for the inconsistencies noted in Table 10.1 is that the behavior being scored involves considerable subjectivity (Coles et al., 1985a). However, a more likely explanation is the designated alcohol-exposure groups differed in the number of children with FAS/ARBEs in each study, a problem that befuddles not only these studies but also research evaluating the effects of prenatal alcohol exposure, in general. In many instances, the same children have been extensively studied as part of a longitudinal assessment research program. In the

Table 10.1. Brazelton Test Results Associated
with Prenatal Alcohol Exposure

Subcomponent	Studies reporting a significant effect	Studies reporting no significant effect
Habituation	Streissguth et al., 1983a	Coles et al., 1985a
		Ernhart et al., 1985a
		Fried & Makin, 1987
		Jacobson et al., 1984
		Richardson et al., 1989
		Smith et al., 1986
		Walpole et al., 1991
Lower arousal	Jacobson et al., 1984	Coles et al., 1985a
	Streissguth et al., 1983a	Ernhart et al., 1985a
		Fried & Makin, 1987
		Richardson et al., 1989
		Smith et al., 1986
		Walpole et al., 1991
Orientation	Coles et al., 1985a	Ernhart et al., 1985a
	Richardson et al., 1989	Fried & Makin, 1987
		Jacobson et al., 1984
		Smith et al,. 1986
		Streissguth et al., 1983a
		Walpole et al., 1991

course of describing these studies, added information regarding these children and their mothers indicates that earlier conclusions need reassessment. For instance, in many cases, mothers described as moderate or occasional drinkers when their children were tested as infants on the Brazelton or as toddlers on the Bayley scales (see later) subsequently have been recognized as alcoholics or chronic binge drinkers. It now seems more than likely that there were several children with FAS/ARBE in the studies that found statistically significant associations between maternal drinking during pregnancy and habituation, or orientation. This supposition doesn't invalidate the findings, but it does raise the probability that the significant associations described in these studies are a function of much greater alcohol exposure than is implied by the term *moderate* drinking.

Misclassification of heavy drinkers as moderate or occasional drinkers is common in all alcohol research because people often lie when they are asked how much they drink. If a mother says she has only one drink a day when she actually had seven or eight, perinatal problems that result from that greater level of drinking will be misattributed to the lower consumption. Because "denial" or "underreporting" is most likely for women with a history of alcohol-related problems (Morrow-Tlucak, Ernhart, Sokol, Martier, & Agar, 1989), it is more than likely that perinatal problems attributed to low levels of alcohol consumption are instead due to much higher levels of consumption. Even a single instance of such misclassification may "tilt" an otherwise nonstatistically significant association between occasional or moderate drinking and behavior into statistical significance.

Misclassification still does not explain why only some of the Brazelton components were affected by prenatal alcohol exposure and others were not. Such specificity may have more to do with the time during gestation that the drinking that resulted in FAS/ARBE occurred. As noted later, several studies have found children whose mothers drank throughout pregnancy perform worse on different tasks than children whose mothers discontinued drinking before their third trimester. By analogy, it is conceivable that some children will be differentially affected on the Brazelton and other tests because their mothers drank at times when the brain structures underlying certain behaviors were more susceptible to alcohol's influences. (Examples of such differential susceptibility in parts of the cerebellum were described in Chapter 9.)

Cognitive Processing.   Apical tests like the Brazelton and the Bayley tests (see later) have been widely used to determine if differences between designated groups exist. Beyond this function, however, such tests tell us nothing about the actual cognitive functions (and by inference, the brain structures) that may have been impacted.

In contrast to loosely integrated test paradigms, such as the Brazelton, other studies have attempted to evaluate the behavior of infants by less subjective measures, using more theoretically derived tests of cognitive functioning. One such approach by the Jacobsons recently extended the use of the Fagan Visual Recognition Memory Test to alcohol-exposed infants (Jacobson et al., 1993c).

For this test, infants are seated on their mother's lap and shown two identical stimuli for familiarization. The infant is then shown the same picture along with a novel one. Because infants typically shift their gaze from the familiar to the novel stimulus, the inference is that an infant who shifts to the newer picture or spends more time looking at the new picture is one who is able to recall the original picture and discriminate it from the novel one. Because an infant's eye movements are believed to be independent of sensory and motor activities, this test is assumed to reflect "information-processing" functions, such as encoding, remembering, comparing old information with new, and discriminating the old from the new. *Cognitive processing efficiency* can be defined as the amount of time the infant takes looking at the unfamiliar picture. The shorter the fixation on the previously seen stimulus, the better the information processing. Conceptually, the Fagan test is a counterpart of the Brazelton's habituation component, which likewise requires an infant to encode, remember, compare, and differentiate. The advantage of the Fagan test is that the tracking behavior of the infant's eyes can be assessed more objectively.

Although the Jacobsons reported prenatal alcohol exposure results in slower infant cognitive processing in the Fagan test, the extent of alcohol's impact was no more than 3% of the outcome. Furthermore, although the authors determined that the minimal maternal alcohol consumption that produced this effect was an average of one drink per day during pregnancy, this conclusion is problematic. As with all of the studies attributing significant consequences to minimal levels of consumption, this conclusion is better explained in terms of *abusive* drinking for the following reasons: First, drinking behavior was averaged during different trimesters of pregnancy. Since drinking decreases as pregnancy progresses (see Chapter 11), a finding corroborated in this study, the estimated drinking levels are artifactually lower than they would have been had they been based on the early phases of pregnancy.

Second, as the authors also noted, "few" of the mothers in their study actually drank every day (Jacobson et al., 1993c). Instead, on those days that they did drink, some drank well over 15 drinks that day! After the study was published, the authors learned that at least one of the children in the "average of one drink a day" group had FAS (J. Jacobson, personal communication, 1996). Categorizing drinking behavior in terms of "average drinks per day" when almost none of the mothers drank every day and when many were binge drinkers created an artifact that muddied the association between abusive drinking and infant brain function and overstated the risk of moderate drinking. To further complicate the analysis, the authors found that the significant association between this level of alcohol consumption and infant reaction time ceased to be statistically significant when they included maternal depression as a variable.

Sleep Disorders. Infants whose mothers drank heavily during pregnancy were often described as fitful sleepers (Coles et al., 1985a; Mulder, Kamstra, O'Brien, Visser, & Prechtl, 1986; Rosett et al., 1979; Sander et al., 1977). Their EEG patterns during sleep cycles may exhibit consistent hypersynchrony and delayed maturation of sleep-related EEG. EEG-sleep synchronies for several children with FAS were as much as 200% higher than normal during active REM sleep (Havlicek & Childaeva, 1977). Although sleep disturbances had been reported for infants whose mothers averaged as few as 1.3 drinks a day, this average did not reflect the mother's actual drinking patterns, which in some studies was 12 drinks a day (Scher, Richardson, Coble, Day, & Stoffer, 1988; Stoffer, Sher, & Richardson, 1988)!

Seizures and Convulsions. About 3% of 550 children with FAS surveyed by Abel (1990, appendix L) experienced seizures or convulsions (Azouz et al., 1993; Coulter et al., 1993; Havlicek & Childaeva, 1977). Several reports placed the prevalence of seizures or convulsions in FAS children at considerably higher rates of 6.3% (Iosub et al., 1981), 10% (Spohr & Steinhausen, 1987), and 21% (Majewski & Goeke, 1982). Another study estimated that the prevalence of convulsions among a group of children without a diagnosis of FAS born to alcoholics at about 10% (Olegard et al., 1979). In most of these reports, there was no distinction between seizures and convulsions, and it is possible many of these were febrile convulsions (Marcus, 1987), possibly due to untreated infections (see Chapter 5). Outside of FAS/ARBE, seizures are rarely found in the context of maternal drinking during pregnancy. In her longitudinal studies, Coles has never encountered seizures in any of the children (personal communication, 1996).

Studies of seizure susceptibility in animals exposed prenatally to alcohol have been inconsistent. Although some studies found prenatal alcohol exposure throughout gestation increased susceptibility to audiogenic seizures in mice and shortened seizures onset latencies (Church & Holloway, 1981), most reported prenatal alcohol exposure either had no effect on seizure susceptibility (Kim, Weinberg, & Pinel, 1991), kindled seizures (Savage & Reyes, 1985), or audiogenically primed seizures (Berman, Beare, Church, & Abel, 1992). Another found an attenuated susceptibility to drug-induced seizures (Abel et al., 1993).

Electroencephalogram (EEG). In addition to abnormal electroencephalogram (EEG) patterns during sleep, a few studies have also reported abnormal EEG patterns during awake periods in infants with FAS/ARBEs (Chernick et al., 1983; Havlicek et al., 1977; Majewski, 1981; Mattson et al., 1992; Scher et al., 1988). In contrast to these reports, however, most studies have not reported EEG irregularities, even in cases in which mothers drank 10 drinks or more a day during pregnancy (Mulder et al., 1986). Longitudinal studies indicate in most instances abnormal EEGs due to prenatal alcohol exposure are not increased outside of FAS/ARBE. Although EEG abnormalities have been reported in connection with FAS/ARBE, they often decrease or disappear with aging (see "School Age," this chapter).

The EEG response of fetuses to acute alcohol exposure has been studied in sheep and guinea pigs. At blood alcohol levels of 100 mg%–150 mg%, EEG amplitudes and frequency begin to decrease; above 250 mg%, EEG activity disappears completely in some fetuses (Bergstrom, Sainion, & Taalas, 1967).

Hypotonia and Fine and Gross Motor Dysfunction. Hypotonia may reflect a general muscle weakness exhibited by some infants and newborns with FAS/ARBEs (see Chapter 5, "Myopathy"), but hypotonia itself is not commonly mentioned in the context of FAS/ARBE (Abel, 1984a). Fine motor dysfunction may also underlie feeding difficulties for some infants with FAS/ARBE, including problems defined as abnormal suck, weak suck, and easily tired suck (Ouellette et al., 1977; Van Dyke et al., 1982). In animals, prenatal exposure to blood alcohol levels of around 200 mg% likewise reduces neonatal sucking pressure (Rockwood & Riley, 1986). Attempts to overcome these early feeding problems may create a conditioned emotional response associated with physical contact (see "Preschool

Children," this chapter) and may explain why some children with FAS prefer not to be touched, although, in general, FAS children are very affectionate and enjoy physical contact.

References to gross motor dysfunction in infants and very young children with FAS/ARBE are common in the medical literature. These children are often described as poorly coordinated, ataxic, "clumsy," or developmentally delayed in their motor skills (Aronson, Kyllerman, Sabel, Sandin, & Olegard, 1985; Autti-Ramo & Granstrom, 1991a,b; Marcus, 1987; Steinhausen et al., 1982; Streissguth et al., 1978a). Developmental delays are much greater if mothers continued to drink throughout pregnancy rather than drinking only during the first and second trimesters (Autti-Ramo & Granstrom, 1991a; Coles et al., 1985a). Olegard et al. (1979) considered the combination of small size, poor muscle tone, and incoordination as "quite characteristic" of FAS/ARBE.

In contrast to maternal alcoholism's effects on infant motor development or function, moderate and social drinking (fewer than 2 drinks per drinking occasion) have an ambiguous impact. Though such effects have often been reported (Autti-Ramo et al., 1992; Coles et al., 1987b; Golden, Sokol, & Kuhnert, 1982; Jacobson et al., 1993a; O'Connor, Sigman, & Brill, 1987; Streissguth, Barr, Martin, & Herman, 1980), in several instances, the children being tested had FAS or had mothers who were alcoholics.

A frequently cited study reporting a significant association between poorer performance on the Bayley Scales of Infant Development and maternal consumption of two or more drinks a day (Streissguth et al., 1980) included the children of eight mothers who drank more than 10 drinks a day, and another whose mother consumed 50 drinks a day! Describing this kind of drinking as "two or more drinks a day" distorts the actual relationship with alcohol abuse, as others have previously noted (Rosett & Weiner, 1984).

The inordinate contribution of the children of alcohol abusers to performance on the Bayley test likewise explains the very high 25% decrement in motor scores and the 31% decrement in mental scores attributed to prenatal alcohol exposure in another study. In that instance, however, the authors noted that three of the children included in the prenatally exposed group had FAS, and they specifically examined the role of different levels of drinking (Ioffe & Chernick, 1990). Despite the fact of the obvious confounding—the abstainers were nearly all Caucasian, while the alcohol-consuming mothers were nearly all Native Canadians—the authors found the most important variable was very heavy drinking: "no other factor than a history of excessive alcohol ingestion (binge and frankly alcoholic groups) was a significant contribution to the outcome variables of mental and motor score" (Ioffe & Chernick, 1990, p. 14).

Jacobson and co-workers (1993a) are among the few researchers to acknowledge that even when they place the threshold for alcohol-related effects on psychomotor development at an average daily drinking threshold of four drinks per day, such thresholds are a total artifice "because virtually none of the mothers drank every day" (p. 181). The Jacobsons report that at least one of the women they categorized as a "light" drinker, because her average daily intake was less than 0.5 drinks, consumed 21 drinks on an average drinking day! Another woman in their "very heavy" drinking category consumed almost 50 drinks on an average drinking day. Intuitively, this level of drinking ought to be described as abuse, not "very heavy." Virtually every woman in this group also had an alcoholism-related problem, as reflected in their MAST scores. Because it is obvious that many woman in this and comparable studies have been misclassified, it follows that what passes for moderate drinking, or for an "average of two or four drinks a day" needs to be carefully scrutinized. The deficits are undoubtedly real, their reputed associations with moderate drinking are not.

The same kind of mislabeling artifact precludes a valid assessment of the association between drinking during pregnancy and infant behavior in terms of average drinks per day in other studies. For instance, in their study, Gusella and Fried (1984) calculated their "average drinks" measure by collapsing across the entire pregnancy based on their finding that drinking at each trimester was highly correlated. However, if an association is being sought between average drinks and some outcome, this kind of analysis will underestimate drinking behavior considerably because of the well-known decrease in drinking that occurs as pregnancy progresses (see Chapter 11). The authors noted that 6% of the 84 women categorized as consuming "less than an average of one drink a day" actually drank six to eight drinks during binges. In other words, they were more like alcohol abusers (according to the definition in Chapter 2). The authors argued that this was not an adequate number of subjects to warrant analysis as a separate variable, but instead of removing these cases from their analyses, they "lumped" them together with their much lighter drinking counterparts. This technique likewise created a misleading impression that consumption of one drink a day during pregnancy can result in adverse effects on infant behavior (Gusella & Fried, 1984).

As in the case of the Brazelton studies, the majority of studies using the Bayley test have not found statistically significant decrements attributable to prenatal alcohol exposure (Ernhart, 1991; Forrest, du V. Florey, Taylor, McPherson, & Young, 1991; Fried & Watkinson, 1988; Greene et al., 1991a; Olsen, 1994; Richardson, Day, & Goldschmidt, 1995). On the contrary, since moderate drinking is correlated with higher parental education and many other social advantages (see later), it is not surprising that when middle- and upper-income families are studied, infants whose mothers drink an average of two drinks a day or less perform better on the Bayley compared with those born to abstainers (Forrest et al., 1991; Fried & Watkinson, 1988), although here too the alcohol effect is weak, but nevertheless, statistically significant.

The likely reason why some studies find decrements associated with relatively low levels of maternal drinking when using the Bayley test is that, as in the Brazelton studies, they often include children of alcohol abusers under the guise of moderate or occasional drinkers.

Cerebral Palsy. Cerebral palsy has been mentioned in conjunction with FAS, but supporting evidence is very limited. One Swedish study (Olegard et al., 1979) placed the incidence at 8.3% compared with an overall incidence of 0.02% for Sweden. Another study placed the incidence at 10% (2 cases out of 20) (Lipson, Walsh, & Webster, 1983), In contrast to these two studies, cerebral palsy has rarely been mentioned in the FAS clinical case literature (Abel, 1990).

Preschool Children

Clinical Description

During the preschool years (2½ to 6 years of age), earlier sleep problems, incoordination, and so on continue to exist, and new problems emerge. Some of the more commonly mentioned of these are listed in Table 10.2.

Table 10.2. Frequently Mentioned Behavioral Characteristics of Preschool Children with FAS

Hypersenstivity to touch
Attention Deficit Disorder (ADD)
Hyperactivity ("always on the go," "never sits still," "never seems to listen")
Impulsiveness
Accident prone (possibly a combination of hyperactivity and poor coordination)
Extreme mood changes (laughs or cries too readily)
Heightened anxiety
Constantly demands attention
Low threshold for frustration
Unusual aggressiveness
Frequent temper tantrums over trivial problems
Disobedient in response to requests from parents
Unable to adapt easily to changes in routine activities
Requires more direct supervision than other children
Difficulty forming friendships with other children
Overly friendly and social toward adults
Does not distinguish friends from strangers; has no fear of strangers
Overly talkative; little meaningful content to speech
Talks at inappropriate times

Systematic Studies

Attention Deficit Disorder/Hyperactivity Disorder (ADD/HD). By far the most frequently mentioned and systematically studied of the behaviors listed in Table 10.2 are Attention Deficit Disorder and hyperactivity. These behaviors are so commonly mentioned in the context of FAS/ARBE (Aronson, Kyllerman, Sabel, Sandin, & Olegard, 1985; Iosub et al., 1981; Jones & Smith, 1973; Shaywitz, Cohen, & Shaywitz, 1980; Steinhausen, Godel, & Nestler, 1984; Streissguth & Giunta, 1988) that it is now widely assumed ADD/HD is invariably associated with these conditions (Coles et al., 1997). However, as indicated later (see "School Age"), despite a superficial resemblance, the two conditions are not identical and treatments effective for ADD/HD will likely be ineffective in FAS/ARBE.

In general, about 3% to 5% of all school-age children in the United States are believed to have ADD/HD. These children are a heterogeneous group. They are more likely to be boys than girls, with ratios ranging from 4:1 and 9:1 (American Psychiatric Association, 1994), and there is a marked familial component, with about 30%–50% of affected children having a parent or sibling with the disorder (Woodrich, 1994). Hyperactivity usually becomes apparent in preschool children between the ages of 2 to 5 and continues to occur in school-age children, adolescents, and adults.

Although hyperactivity and Attention Deficit Disorder are considered synonymous, they are clinically distinct (American Psychiatric Association, 1994). Although hyperactivity appears to be common in FAS/ARBE, the association between ADD and FAS/ARBE is more questionable. Two studies of Native American children found considerable similarities between the two conditions (Conry, 1990; Nanson & Hiscock, 1990); however, two studies of African-American children did not (Coles et al., 1996; Morrow-Tlucuk & Ernhart, 1987). (Coles et al.'s [1977] evaluation of school-age children is discussed in detail later, see "School Age.") The other study evaluated 3-year-old African-American children in Cleveland. Although it did not include children with FAS/ARBEs, it cast doubt on an association between ADD and prenatal alcohol exposure. As maternal alcohol consumption during pregnancy increased, signs of ADD, such as emotional reactivity, irritability, and dependence, as well as activity, decreased rather than increased (Morrow-Tlucuk & Ernhart, 1987).

Children with FAS/ARBE diagnosed with ADD/HD have been treated with stimulant drugs such as Ritalin (methylphenidate hydrochloride), Dexedrine (dextroamphetamine sulfate) or Cylert (pemoline) (Coles et al., 1997), but there are no studies directly evaluating their effectiveness for this disorder.

Studies in animals have frequently found that although prenatal alcohol exposure can result in increased activity postnatally, these increases are typically small and transient (Abel, 1984a) and are unresponsive to Ritalin (Ulug & Riley, 1983). Given what we now know about the relationship between FAS/ARBE and

ADD, there is no clinical or preclinical basis for the administration of stimulant drugs to children with FAS/ARBE.

Speech and Communicative Skills. Speech pathology is commonly found in African-American children with FAS (Church et al., 1997; Iosub et al., 1981) and in Native American children with FAS (Becker, Warr-Leeper, & Leeper, 1990). Church and his co-workers (1997) found 21 of their 22 patients with FAS (95%) had clinically significant speech pathology. Because all of these children were seen in a clinic for orofacial problems, this high prevalence is not as surprising as it might otherwise seem.

FAS-related speech pathology is due, in many cases, to articulation problems (Becker et al., 1990; Church et al., 1997; Iosub et al., 1981), arising from physical anomalies in the structure of the jaw, teeth, palate, and gums (see Chapter 4). Alternatively, fine motor dysfunction involving coordination of muscles in the tongue or larynx may be responsible for the inability to articulate vowels and consonants (see earlier). Because speech is also a function of hearing, articulation problems may also be related to alcohol's effects on the auditory system (see Chapter 7).

Linguistic ability was impaired in 82% of the 63 children with FAS studied by Iosub et al. (1981) and 86% of the 12 children with FAS examined by Church et al. (1977) (Becker et al., 1990; Sparks, 1984; Steinhausen et al., 1982). Although these studies involved children from predominantly low SES backgrounds, when children with FAS were compared with children of the same age, sex, and SES background, the same linguistic difficulties were apparent—children with FAS were less advanced in their use of complex grammatical structures, and their short-term memory was not as good as controls (Becker et al., 1990; Hamilton, 1981).

Communication skills are likewise impaired in FAS. In general, these communication disorders and related problems appear to be due to difficulties in cognitive processing rather than speech reception. Morse (1993) has metaphorically described the information-processing problem of the child with FAS as a dysfunctional word processor—full sentences are typed in, but only some of it is saved or stored in an inaccessible area, so only partial sentences can be retrieved. Sometimes the lost material may reappear if a random key is inadvertently hit, or some special cue related to the missing information is accidentally accessed. As a result, the conversation of the child with FAS is often not connected to what is being discussed.

Disturbances in information processing may also be responsible for conduct problems in the classroom. A teacher may believe that these children understand what they have just been told, but when they walk away as if oblivious, the teacher may interpret their behavior as disrespectful rather than as a lack of understanding (Morse, 1993).

Articulation, linguistic, and communication disorders resulting from prenatal alcohol exposure are only encountered in conjunction with FAS/ARBE. At levels that do not cause FAS/ARBE, these skills are not compromised (Fried & Watkinson, 1988; Greene et al., 1991a; Morrow-Tlucuk & Ernhart, 1987; Streissguth et al., 1993; cf., however, Russell et al., 1991).

Mental Retardation/IQ. Whereas children with FAS appear to suffer from problems involving information processing, the association between cognitive function and prenatal alcohol exposure at levels that do not cause FAS are inconsistent. A statistically significant association between maternal drinking of more than an average of three drinks per day during pregnancy and IQ was found in a group of primarily middle-class Caucasian children in Seattle (Streissguth, Brookstein, Sampson, & Barr, 1989b). A comparable association was not found in a group of primarily low SES, African-American children in Cleveland (Morrow-Tlucuk & Ernhart, 1987).

Autism. Autistic behaviors, such as echolalia, indifference to others, frequent temper tantrums, head banging, screaming, "fussy eating," frequent mood changes, fearlessness, inappropriate emotional reactions, difficulty understanding what is said, and perseverative behavior, have been noted in children with FAS (Church et al., 1997; Church & Gerkin, 1988; Harris et al., 1995; Nanson, 1992; Streissguth et al., 1985), but the defining sense of disconnection that characterizes autism is not found in FAS. Coles reflected that unlike autistic children, children with FAS "want to be involved with other people even when they don't know how to do it right" (Coles, personal communication, 1996).

School Age

Clinical Description

It is usually not until children enter school that their FAS/ARBE-related cognitive difficulties and behavioral problems become fully recognized. (School-age here is from 6 years old to adolescence.) Because of their restlessness, distractibility, inability to sit still or focus on their work, and/or comply with the demands placed on them for conformity and adherence to rules, these children quickly come to the attention of their teachers and they are often labeled as ADD or hyperactive.

Academically, children with FAS/ARBEs lag somewhat behind other children their age in arithmetic and reading skills. Although word recognition skills may be somewhat below normal, comprehension of reading passages is considerably delayed, possibly symptomatic of the same impaired information-processing skills that underlies their communication problems. There seems to be a selectivity to some of these impairments. They are found in some study sites and not others, possibly reflecting the ethnic backgrounds of the majority of children being studied; for example, Native American children with FAS have greater problems with arithmetic skills than African-American children with FAS, whereas the opposite is true for reading skills (see earlier). Writing or drawing skills are far below normal, possibly the result of fine motor dysfunction (see "Newborns and Infants," this chapter). Whatever the nature of their cognitive problems, if these children were to be placed in a structured learning environment, they might be able to perform much better, possibly because under such conditions, there would be fewer cognitive demands for processing and responding to new information (Morse, 1993; Morse & Weiner, 1996).

Outside the classroom, children with FAS/ARBE are often described as having poor socialization skills. At playtime, they play alongside, not with, peers; if they do engage in play, it is often with children younger than themselves. Very often they withdraw completely and isolate themselves; they may be teased or bullied or act aggressively (Streissguth, 1992).

At home and at school, children with FAS/ARBEs do not appear to learn from their mistakes as quickly as others. Morse (1993) speculated that this is because they are unable to generalize from one situation to another. Their penchant for repeating the same disapproved behavior, and their need to be taught the same material over and over again may also reflect a short-term memory difficulty; the problem may also be one of not being able to retrieve what has been stored in their memories.

The inability of children with FAS/ARBEs to remember often leads to frustration and temper tantrums; they are also prone to replacing gaps in their memories with inaccurate explanations when they fail to do what is expected of them. Although they believe their explanations to be true, they are typically unrealistic. Instead of being deceitful, Morse (1993) speculated that their prevarications may be an attempt to cope with reality as they perceive it.

Systematic Studies

Attention Deficit Disorder (ADD) and Hyperactivity Disorder (HD). Although FAS has many behavioral characteristics in common with ADD/HD, each of these problems reflects different underlying pathologies. Impulsivity, or lack of self-control, for instance, is a core symptom of ADD/HD (Schweitzer & Sulzer-Azaroff, 1995) but not of FAS/ARBE (Boyd, Ernhart, Greene, Sokol, & Martier, 1991; Coles, Raskind-Hood, Brown, & Sulverstein, 1994, 1997; Kodituwakku, Handmaker, Cutler, & Weatherby, 1995; Nanson & Hiscock, 1990).

Using tests formulated to test attention and information-processing skills, researchers in Albuquerque compared children with FAS/ARBE with age-, sex-

and SES-matched controls. The theory underlying these tests is that self-regulation is a function of two different kinds of attentional systems. One relates to routine performance, such as impulse control, that does not require deliberate attention; the other, called the *supervisory attentional system*, is involved in flexible cognitive activities, such as planning, decision making, and troubleshooting. The Albuquerque study found that children with FAS/ARBEs did not differ in response inhibition (as reflected in tasks requiring impulse control, e.g., delayed responding), but they were less flexible when it came to manipulating information in working memory (i.e., "planning") (Kodituwakku et al., 1995).

Coles and her coworkers (1997) compared four groups of African-American, low SES children: one group was prenatally exposed to alcohol and had dysmorphic signs of FAS/ARBE; another was prenatally exposed to alcohol but was nondysmorphic; a third was clinically diagnosed as ADD/HD; and a fourth was a control group of children with no ADD/HD, whose mothers did not drink during pregnancy. Confirming the Albuquerque findings, Coles and her group found FAS/ARBE and ADD were clinically distinct disorders. Because this is the most thorough of all the studies addressing this issue, a detailed discussion of it is worthwhile.

In the Coles et al. (1997) study, measures of ADD/HD, hyperactivity, and intelligence included standard test batteries and checklists and computerized performance tests for assessing reaction time, vigilance, and impulsivity. Mothers of ADD/HD children were screened for alcohol use by self-report and by measurement of serum gamma glutamyl transpepsidate (GGTP) levels. Only those children in the ADD/HD and control groups whose mothers reported less alcohol consumption and lower GGTP levels than mothers in the other two alcohol groups were included in the ADD/HD group.

Mothers of children in the dysmorphic FAS/ARBE group consumed an average of 25 drinks a week compared with 13 drinks for mothers of nondysmorphic prenatal alcohol-exposed children. Mothers in the other two groups had zero consumption.

When children were compared on the various cognitive measures, dysmorphic children and ADD children had similar global deficits but differed on specific subtests: Children with FAS/ARBE did significantly worse on arithmetic tests, while the ADD/HD group did much worse on reading/decoding tests.

Children with ADD/HD and FAS/ARBE also differed on measures specifically directed at assessing attention. As expected, children with ADD/HD did not perform as well as the normal controls on these measures; alcohol-exposed children, however, did not differ from controls on measures of attention. ADD children also did not perform as well as controls on the computerized attentional measures: Speed and accuracy were both impaired, reaction times on the vigilance test were slower, false alarm rates (indicative of impulsivity) were increased, and they had fewer "hits" and more "misses" on the continuous performance test. In contrast, children with FAS/ARBE did not differ from controls on any of these measures, and in some instances, they actually performed better than controls (Coles et al., 1994).

When the results of this study were subjected to a discriminative analysis, the classification of 85% of the children previously identified as ADD/HD was confirmed as compared with only 44% of the dysmorphic children with FAS/ARBE. Additional analyses suggested that the two groups had unique attentional profiles. While children with ADD/HD suffered from an inability to focus and sustain attention, those with dysmorphic FAS/ARBE suffered from deficits in visual/spatial skills, had information-encoding difficulties, and were more inflexible at problem solving. These latter findings are similar to those reported in the Albuquerque study by Kodituwakku et al. (1995).

In an earlier study, Coles and her co-workers found that teachers were more likely than mothers to label alcohol-exposed children as being hyperactive. When these children were rated by "blind" observers in the laboratory on measures of activity, impulsivity, aggression, or inappropriate mother-child interactions, the blind raters were more likely to agree with the maternal assessments (Brown et al., 1991). The authors suggested that teachers are more likely to label children as hyperactive than are their own mothers because the former need to maintain a learning environment in their classrooms, while parents do not have to maintain the same kind of learning environment in their homes. Put another way, the school environment brings out attention/activity problems that are not seen in the home or the laboratory. The authors also found on a vigilance test used to assess impulsivity that these children were less rather than more impulsive, because they made a greater number of errors of omission rather than commission.

As part of this same study, Coles noted that while children whose mothers drank during pregnancy were more likely to develop "internalized" problems, such as depression, poor self-esteem, and anxiety, these problems were no longer statistically significant when caretaking environment, especially continued maternal alcohol use, was taken into account. The fact that a child's postnatal environment affects his or her behavior is hardly surprising, but it has not received the attention it deserves in the present context. This issue is examined in greater depth later (see "Conclusion").

Because a child's brain is still very plastic for the first two years of life, his or her behavior and cognitive function at school age are products of the pre- and postnatal insults to which it may be exposed. Whatever impact prenatal alcohol exposure may have, that impact cannot be separated from developmental processes that go on prior to or after birth (or from influences that go on prior to and persist into pregnancy). Unless the caretaking conditions to which children are exposed after they are born are taken into account, the relationship between prenatal alcohol exposure and subsequent behavior will continue to be problematic.

Although researchers are well aware of the importance of home environment for a child's development, that influence is typically minimized in FAS/ARBE studies because of the way in which the home environment is assessed. For example, the most widely used test instrument for assessing parent-child interactions in the home is the Home Observation for Measurement of the Environment (HOME). The HOME, however, is sometimes administered in ways for which it was not designed. For example, when African Americans or other low SES groups are being tested, the HOME is often administered not in the home but in the laboratory "due to safety considerations" (Jacobson et al., 1993c). The irony here is that the conditions that make visiting these homes personally dangerous to researchers are considered to have limited impact on the mothers or children who actually live in these homes. Moreover, because the HOME relies for as much as one third of its content on information provided by the mother, it is less than a satisfactory means of assessing actual conditions in a home where there is a drinking problem. If denial is a major problem in obtaining a true drinking history, there is no reason to assume that a mother who denies having a drinking problem would be anymore forthright in describing her home environment.

Mental Retardation/IQ.   Mental retardation has long been considered the most serious persistent consequence of FAS/ARBE (Dehaene et al., 1977; Isoub et al., 1981a; Lemoine, Harousseau, Borteryu, & Menuet, 1968; Majewski, 1981; Olegard et al., 1979; Robinson, Conry, & Conry, 1987; Steinhausen et al., 1982; Streissguth et al., 1978a). FAS/ARBE is now recognized as one of the leading known causes of mental retardation in the industrialized world (Abel & Sokol, 1987). However, mental retardation is not an invariable outcome of FAS/ARBE. The prevalence for mental retardation, as defined by IQ scores below 70, is about 50% in FAS/ARBE (Abel, 1990). Streissguth and her co-workers (1978a) found IQS ranging from 16 to 105 in a group of 20 children with FAS/ARBE. Children with the most severe dysmorphia and growth retardation have the lowest IQ scores (Dehaene et al., 1977; Majewski et al., 1976; Steinhausen et al., 1982; Streissguth et al., 1978a,b).

Five retrospective studies collectively identified 102 probable cases of FAS/ ARBE out of 4,450 mentally retarded individuals living in residential facilities (a rate of 23 per 1,000) (Fryns et al., 1977; Hagberg & Kyllerman, 1983; Mena, Casanueva, Fernandez, Carraso, & Perez, 1986; Shanske & Kazi, 1980; Tanaka, Arima, Ishizuka, Suzuki, & Takashima, 1979). However, none of these studies was very rigorous in design with respect to their criteria for identifying FAS or eliminating other causes. A more thorough analysis using such criteria did not find any FAS/ARBE cases out of the 77 severely retarded and 74 mildly retarded children, 8–9 years of age, systematically examined for causation (Matilainen, Airaksinen, Mononen, Launiala, & Kaarianinen, 1995). In Germany, on the other hand, Spohr and his co-workers (1993) reported 30% of the children with FAS/ ARBE whom they had been following in their longitudinal study were in schools for the mentally handicapped by the time they reached adolescence. The authors suggested that the prevalence would have been higher except that those with the greatest problems had been placed in these schools at an earlier age.

As in the case of ADD/HD, the disturbing high prevalence of mental retardation in the context of FAS/ARBE is based on a select sample of children sent for clinical referral. Shaywitz et al. (1980), for example, reported 15 out of the 87 children born to alcoholic mothers and brought to their attention because of learning problems had normal intelligence but were "hyperactive." Had these children been included in the referrals for mental retardation, the prevalence would have been much lower.

The potential for improvement in intellectual capacity in children with FAS/ARBE is yet to be determined. Several follow-up studies have found IQ scores to be relatively stable (Robinson et al., 1987; Streissguth, Herman, & Smith, 1978b, 1991; Streissguth & Randels, 1988). Some studies also reported that even when children with FAS are raised by adoptive or foster parents who attempt to provide as stimulating an environment for these children as possible, their IQS increase minimally (Janzen et al., 1995; Olegard et al., 1979; Streissguth et al:, 1987).

The possibility of cognitive improvement for any disorder, including FAS/ARBE, however, depends on the extent of the original damage. Individuals with FAS/ARBE whose initial test IQ scores are above 70 appear to have the potential for improvement (Autti-Ramo et al., 1992; Ernhart et al., 1995; Spohr & Steinhausen, 1987), but this possibility has not been systematically evaluated.

It is reasonable to assume that improvement will depend on a combination of the seriousness of the initial brain damage and the home environment in which a child is raised (Sameroff, Seifer, Baldwin, & Baldwin, 1993). To borrow an analogy from the world of horse racing, a good jockey can't get a middling thoroughbred to win the Kentucky Derby, but a poor jockey can cause the best thoroughbred to lose it. A poor jockey aboard a middling horse has no chance whatsoever. Studies in animals suggest that while environmental enrichment may attenuate some FAS/ARBE-related neurodevelopmental effects (Hannigan et al., 1993b), the structural basis for these ameliorative effects may be difficult to identify (Berman & Krahl, 1996).

A stimulating home environment can provide only a modicum of improvement if the brain is incapable of responding to enrichment. Nevertheless, the Hannigan, Berman, & Zajac (1993b) study showed that even affected offspring can benefit from an enriched environment. On the other hand, the combination of brain damage and being raised in a neglectful or cognitively unstimulating environment is unlikely to foster any improvements in intellectual capacity.

Although the association between cognitive problems and FAS/ARBE is generally acknowledged, studies reporting that moderate drinking during pregnancy also adversely impacts on cognitive abilities would be more reasonably attributed to abusive drinking. One such study, for instance, reported moderate drinking tripled the risk in 7-year-olds of having an IQ score lower than 85, and also impaired performance on tests of memory, problem solving, visual/motor performance, and academic skills (Streissguth, Barry, Sampson, & Brookstein, 1989a; Streissguth et al., 1989b). The conclusions from this study are horripilative—if extended to the population as a whole, a decrease in IQ of this magnitude would constitute a major national calamity. However, the methodology on which this worrisome conclusion was based is undermined by the same "lumping" methodology previously shown to distort the relationship between moderate maternal drinking during pregnancy and any outcome being evaluated. In this instance, the leitmotiv resulted in the inclusion among the moderate drinkers of at least three women with major alcohol-related problems. Russell (1991) appropriately pointed out the impropriety of such "lumping" in her discussion of this study and suggested the likelihood that additional children of alcoholic mothers may also have been included in the so-called moderate drinking group.

As frequently mentioned throughout this book, even a single occurrence of misclassification can give an otherwise statistically nonsignificant association between drinking and pregnancy statistical significance. When Greene and his co-workers (1991a,b) excluded the single FAS/ARBE case in their study, the erstwhile statistically significant association between prenatal alcohol exposure and cognitive dysfunction ceased to be significant. Especially noteworthy is the fact that although the child excluded was clearly identifiable as having FAS, his mother's scores on the MAST and her drinking during pregnancy self-report indicated no alcohol-related problems and negligible alcohol consumption. This incongruity reflects the difficulty researchers have avoiding misclassifying alcoholic women as moderate or light drinkers based on self-report. However, when such misclassification is clearly evident, studies should follow the rectitude of Greene and his co-workers in recognizing that children with FAS, by definition, must have had an alcoholic mother and removing them from analyses examining the effects of moderate drinking.

Like Greene et al. (1991b), Russell and her co-workers (Russell, Cowan, & Czarnecki, 1987) found neither intellectual development nor auditory processing were significantly impacted in 6-year-olds by "social" or moderate drinking, while children whose mothers were identified as "problem" drinkers had lower verbal IQ scores, poorer receptive language (contrary to previously discussed studies), and made more errors on a dichotic listening test than did controls.

Beyond the overall cognitive deficits associated with FAS/ARBE, some deficits related to FAS/ARBE have been more difficult to identify consistently. For instance, in a Canadian study, aboriginal children with FAS/ARBE did not differ in math skills compared with normal Native American children (Janzen, Nanson, & Block, 1995), while in Seattle, math skills of children born to binge drinkers were significantly worse than those of controls (Streissguth et al., 1989b). A comparable deficit in math skills was also found by an Atlanta group (Coles et al.,

1991; 1997), but neither the Seattle nor Atlanta studies found significantly poorer verbal skills in their cohorts, while the Canadian study did find such impairment.

Although the difference between the two American studies and the Canadian study may have been related to differences in design or subject populations, these differences do not explain the differential results within each study with respect to mathematical versus reading skills.

One explanation is that the differences between these studies may relate to misdiagnosis. On the basis of the Coles study (Coles et al., 1997), it is possible that the children in the Seattle and Atlanta studies were primarily FAS/ARBE—evidenced by difficulties with math—while those in the Canadian study were primarily ADD/HD, which Coles and her group found to be associated with reading difficulties.

Electroencephalogram (EEG).   Spohr and Steinhausen (1987) examined EEG patterns in a number of children, 8–9 years of age, with FAS and found that their EEGs, though still abnormal, were less pathological than when these same children were examined four years earlier. Two adolescents with FAS examined by Mattson and her co-workers (1992) also had moderately abnormal EEGs (predominantly abnormal neonatal theta activity). In contrast to these reports, most studies have not found abnormal EEGs associated with FAS in school-age children (Abel, 1990).

Adolescence

Clinical Description

There are many anecdotal observations of the behavior of adolescents with FAS, but these are often contradictory in content. As is true for anecdotal evidence at any age, *the plural of anecdote is not data.*

Adolescents with FAS have been described as irresponsible, learning impaired, impulsive, having poor judgment, lacking in inhibition and remorse, and unable to appreciate the consequences of their actions. They are also said to be prone to lying, cheating, and stealing. They continue to be garrulous, socially winsome, and often convincing, insisting that they can control their own lives. However, their conversation is often unresponsive, their winsome behavior may make them easily manipulated and victimized, and they may require constant supervision.

Adolescents with FAS/ARBE are also described as being gullible and having poor problem-solving abilities. Abstract reasoning is difficult for them. Consequently, their mathematical skills are poorly developed. Related problems involve management of time and money. Keeping appointments is difficult because they do not equate clock time with the need to do something or be somewhere. Saving money for a future purchase is too abstract a concept for them to understand it well. Normal functioning is said to be possible for them only in highly structured situations (Morse & Weiner, 1996).

Although there is little doubt that intellectual functioning continues to be impaired in people with FAS, as noted in connection with the Francis case (see Chapter 7), conduct disorders should not be taken for granted as characteristic of in utero alcohol exposure. People with FAS/ARBE are more likely to be victims than victimizers. There is much stronger evidence that conduct disorders are related to early postnatal neglect and abuse rather than prenatal neglect and abuse (see later), and there is still reason to expect that cognitive functioning improves with age, depending on the initial cognitive damage. As mentioned earlier, the chances for improvement depend on a combination of the extent of the neurological damage and home environment. The potential influence of the latter also depends on the age at which a child is placed into an enriching environment (see later).

Systematic Studies

Teachers rated 11-year-old adolescents, whose mothers were binge drinkers during pregnancy, as distractible, lacking in persistence, restless, and reluctant to meet challenges. Their learning problems included difficulties with information processing and reasoning and a "lack of interest in reading." Arithmetic performance was affected most (Carmichael-Olsson, Sampson, Barr, Streissguth, & Brookstein, 1992).

In Germany, Spohr and his co-workers (1994) reported that many of the children with FAS/ARBE whom they had been following in their longitudinal study had a variety of behavioral disorders when they reached adolescence. The prevalence of these problems in 44 children with FAS/ARBE (estimated from the figure presented in their publication) was highest for emotional disorders (50%), followed by speech disorders (38%), hyperkinetic disorders (32%), sleep disorders (24%), conduct disorders (19%), eating disorders (12%), tics (12%), encopresis (8%), and enuresis (5%).

Although earlier studies had not found verbal skills to be significantly decreased in children whose mothers were binge drinkers during pregnancy, arithmetic and verbal skills were decreased by 14 years of age (Sampson et al., 1994; Streissguth et al., 1994b,c). Spatial-visual skills were also impaired (Hunt, Streissguth, Kerr, & Carmichael-Olson, 1995). In the Hunt study, maternal drinking behavior was assessed in terms of the amount consumed during a drinking occasion, rather than average consumption over some period of time, as was done in the earlier studies by this group. The authors indicated that they did not include data from two subjects diagnosed with fetal alcohol syndrome, which apparently they had done in their previous studies.

Even with these refinements, the authors still noted a statistically significant relationship between maternal drinking prior to pregnancy and the speed-accuracy performance of these children. The greater the amount of drinking, the faster and less accurate the behavior, an outcome that the authors interpreted as an indication of increased impulsiveness. Although the authors did not analyze their data with respect to their different drinking categories, the graphic presentation of their data indicated that there was very little difference between their three lowest drinking groups (abstainers, light, and moderate), whereas the heavy drinking group (defined as four or more drinks per occasion) was considerably different from the others.

Adulthood

Clinical Description

There are very few descriptions of adults with FAS and even fewer systematic studies. Many of their problems have been attributed to the persistence of earlier difficulties. Their poor learning abilities mean that they are unable to work steadily; they are unable to live independently and must instead live with family or in group homes. They are unable to manage money, have few friends, and frequently they become withdrawn and isolated. Some have a high incidence of psychosocial problems (LaDue, Streissguth, & Randels, 1992; Streissguth & Randels, 1988).

Systematic Studies

A descriptive study of 92 FAS/ARBE adolescents, 77% of whom were Native Americans, reported IQ scores ranging from 20 to 108, with 46% of the sample scoring 69 or less. Mean verbal IQ was 65 compared to a performance IQ or 79 (LaDue et al., 1992). The authors explained the difference as being due to the fact that the performance subtests require less abstract reasoning (e.g., arithmetic ability) and less short-term memory ability. The authors also noted that arithmetic achievement skills were considerably below what would have been predicted by their IQ scores, while spelling and reading ability were in the predicted ranges. Using the Peabody Picture Vocabulary Test, the authors also found receptive language skills were affected more than general intelligence. Studies of school-age children, however, have found receptive language is not greatly impacted in FAS/ARBE.

On the Vineland Adaptive Behavior Scales, caretakers described children with FAS/ARBEs as having the communication skills of an 8-year-old, although their chronological age was 17 years. Daily living skills and socialization skills were all below normal. Fifty-eight percent of the sample exhibited significant maladaptive behaviors, such as impulsiveness, dependence, stubbornness, defiance, temper tantrums, inappropriate sexual behavior, and physical aggressiveness. Twenty-five percent of the group were drug dependent, and 36% abused alcohol. Legal problems were also common. The rate for petty larceny was 28%; for grand larceny, 4%; the drunk driving rate was 23%. Without a control group of the same racial and socioeconomic background, however, the role of FAS/ARBE in any of these problems continues to remain problematic.

Conclusion

FAS and ARBEs are associated with serious behavioral and cognitive dysfunctions. However, beyond cataloging these dysfunctions, our appreciation and, more importantly, our understanding of FAS/ARBE and its uniqueness has been disappointing. For the most part, this disappointment is due to the apical test strategies, for example, the Brazelton and Bayley tests used routinely to assess behavioral and cognitive dysfunctions associated with FAS/ARBE. Until research progresses beyond simple group comparisons, our understanding of the nature of the cognitive deficits associated with or the uniqueness of FAS/ARBE will never progress beyond superficiality. West and his co-workers (West, Goodlett, Bonthuis, Hamre, & Marcussen, 1990) comments regarding the current status of research involving brain mechanisms and prenatal alcohol exposure in animals applies equally to the behavioral work currently being conducted in human FAS/ARBE studies: "much of the research ... is not only unrelated, it appears to have lost direction and momentum. That is not to say recent results are unimportant, just that currently we are not providing an experimental framework that will generate the needed insight required for continued rapid advancement" (West et al., 1990, p. 684).

Happily, such changes are not occurring. For instance, research in this area has begun to be formulated in terms of theoretical models of cognitive function. Examples include the previously mentioned studies by Jacobson et al. (1993c), Kodituwakku et al. (1995), and Coles and her co-workers (1997). Likewise, whether or not FAS/ARBE is similar to other disorders and therefore can benefit from comparable treatments has begun to be evaluated. One such example of this more progressive approach is the Coles et al. (1997) study, which directly compared FAS/ARBE children with ADD/HD children and found that despite superficialities, the attentional problems underlying these two conditions are not the same. If the underlying anomalies in the brain are not identical, treatments effective for one would not likely be effective for the other. If the behavioral or cognitive anomalies are the final result of different problems in brain function, then a "one size fits all" approach to treatment will be ineffective

A major impediment in furthering our understanding of FAS/ARBE problems overall is the shift in focus from maternal alcoholism or alcohol abuse to the chimerical impact of moderate drinking.

For a birth defect considered to be a leading known cause of mental retardation in the industrialized world (Abel & Sokol, 1987), the fact that prenatal alcohol exposure accounts for no more than 5% of any behavioral or cognitive outcome when this relation is examined systematically means that the research strategies for examining cognitive function in the context of prenatal alcohol exposure need to be revised. The incongruity between the clinical descriptions of FAS/ARBE and the trivial impact alcohol has when its in utero effects are examined systematically cannot be glossed over. As Coles pointed out in her assessment of such studies, "had these individuals not been participating in research studies, their behavioral differences would usually not have been noted, or, if noted, would not have been associated with exposure to alcohol" (Coles, 1992, p. 21). Andersen and Olsen (1996) made a similar point: "many researchers have looked for all kinds of effects of a low to moderate alcohol consumption in pregnancy without reporting any significant findings.... No data point toward low or moderate alcohol consumption during pregnancy as a potential cause of birth or developmental defects" (p. 294). This statement is incorrect insofar as some researchers have reported significant findings associated with low or moderate drinking. What the authors undoubtedly intended to say was that these findings are essentially nugatory.

The obdurate fact, as Coles pointed out, is that the overwhelming majority of children whose behavior or cognitive function has been evaluated in terms of their prenatal exposure are normal. The reason alcohol's impact is so small despite being statistically significant is that moderate drinking has a trivial effect on the embryo/fetus. Based on the analyses presented in this chapter, all of the previously mentioned studies attributing effects to maternal "moderate," "social," or "light" drinking should be reassessed, addressing the question of whether those effects were instead attributable to a few cases of children whose mothers were alcohol abusers during pregnancy. Because the dangers from drinking during pregnancy appear to arise from "heavy" or binge drinkers, we should focus much more closely on these children than on the overwhelming majority of children whose mothers rarely consumed more than two drinks per drinking occasion. One is hard put to justify the time and effort that continues to be spent uncovering associations that account for less than 5% of an outcome, when other conditions account for a much greater effect.

Furthermore, unless cause and effect can be clearly articulated and reliably demonstrated in children, FAS/ARBE cannot be properly understood or prevented. Lumping children with FAS/ARBE together with children whose mothers are "light" or "moderate" drinkers deflects the impact of alcoholism and minimizes its important effects.

A particularly obfuscating issue that has thus far escaped scrutiny concerns the subject populations that are being examined for FAS/ARBE. As mentioned in the beginning of this chapter, most of the descriptive studies of children and young adults with FAS/ARBE are vignettes of Native Americans with FAS/ARBE. Despite attempts to be neutral, such studies are invariably culturally and socioeconomically biased because normality is determined by comparability with the dominant culture. In only a few instances have these cultural biases been acknowledged. One such instance is a study that tested several Native American children with FAS—all of whom fell below the normal range on a number of tests, such as the Bayley or Infant Development. In discussing their findings the authors commented, "No Native American children were included in the normative samples for any of these tests" (Harris et al., 1993, p. 616). Unless matched controls are used, these studies are too confounded to make them interpretable.

One of the reasons Native American children, especially those living in remote parts of Canada, do poorly on language tests is they "do not learn English until they are into middle school, as they receive all their early education in their native languages. This makes psychological assessment in the children extremely challenging" (Nanson, personal communication, 1996). The biases associated with such measurement tools may explain, in part, why aboriginal children are reported to have the highest rates of FAS/ARBE in the world (see Chapter 11).

Because Native Americans have been so frequently studied in the context of FAS/ARBE, researchers conducting such studies should at the very least be familiar with some of the basic differences between indigenous and nonindigenous peoples in brain lateralization and information processing. For instance, while Navajo children favor the left ear for processing auditory information, Caucasians favor the right (Hynd & Scott, 1980). This basic difference reflects different linguistic predispositions, which are apparently culturally learned, because Navajos who go on to college train themselves toward the same hemispheric specialization as Caucasians (Hynd, Teeter, & Stewart, 1980).

In the classroom, Native American children speak less and are more observant than Caucasian children (Guilmet, 1981). Their laconic behavior reflects what Guilmet (1981) calls their tendency to be less "oral-linguistic," for example, less laughing and crying. Native American children also tend to avoid direct eye contact; instead, they spend more time looking at teachers from a distance (McShane & Plas, 1984). These are cultural differences, not "behavioral anomalies," but they may be regarded as anomalies when there are no cultural standards against which to evaluate them, and when the teachers doing the rating are from a different culture than those whom they are rating. Whenever studies rely on teachers' ratings of children, those ratings should be analyzed with respect to the child's cultural background, as well as his or her possible prenatal alcohol exposure. Similarly, Native American children who are diagnosed with FAS and who are adopted into Caucasian homes may appear to their new parents to be unresponsive and passive because of FAS, but their behavioral pattern may instead reflect their cultural heritage.

Another factor that has not received the scrutiny it deserves is the home environment. Confounding of pre- and postnatal factors is especially likely for children with FAS/ARBE who are raised by their biological mothers. As Andersen and Olsen (1996) pointed out, "the damage caused by growing up in an alcohol-abusing family is probably not of lesser consequence than the damage that occurs during fetal development, and it is a far more widespread problem" (p. 289). Although continuity of environment is important for most children (Streissguth & Giunta, 1988), the kind of continuity that a child with FAS can expect from a biological mother whose alcoholism is unarrested is often nightmarish. Child neglect or abuse is common. Streissguth described the home environments of these children as "tumultuous" (Streissguth et al., 1985, 1991).

The idea that FAS/ARBE is entirely preventable if an alcoholic does not drink during pregnancy is simplistic and naive; it implies that after she gives birth, a woman's alcoholism has inconsequential effects on her child. Mothers who give birth to children with FAS do not stop drinking after they give birth, nor do they stop having more children with FAS (Abel, 1988). Children with FAS who remain with their biological mothers are burdened with the "double whammy" or pre- and postnatal alcoholism. Being raised in such an environment can only exacerbate underlying biological problems. "Continuity" under these conditions is hardly to a child's benefit.

Based on studies of children with low birth weight and various other perinatal problems (Sameroff et al., 1993), on the other hand, it is likely that being adopted into a "good" environment may attenuate many of the developmental problems associated with FAS/ARBE (unless the uniqueness of this disorder does not preclude such improvement). But if placement in foster or adoptive homes does not occur until children are one or two years of age, neglect or abuse may already have occurred, and the time during which environmental enrichment may compensate for prenatal damage may have long since passed. In Adam Dorris's case, for instance, he was not adopted until he was three years old. Prior to that he was malnourished, tied to his crib, and chronically ill. Adam's problems may have been due to his FAS, but given his deplorable infancy, who is to say his problems were solely the result of FAS?

When FAS is described in the medical literature or portrayed in the media, what is often lost sight of is not only are those the worst-case scenarios, these are also the stories of children whose earliest years were also their most traumatic. Yet neither Dorris's book nor the television movie about Adam gave anything but a passing nod to the damage Adam suffered after he was born. Instead, attention was focused almost exclusively on the single issue of prenatal alcohol exposure. Little time has been spent exploring the potential harm associated with being raised in a home where children are neglected and possibly physically abused by their alcoholic parent(s). The impact of being raised in such an environment can be just as devastating as that from in utero alcohol exposure. Adoption, itself, is a risk factor for many behavioral problems. Although adopted children are usually raised in families with higher socioeconomic status and better parental relations than their biological families, children, especially boys, adopted in the first year of life are much more likely to exhibit attentional deficit disorder, conduct disorders, and general behavioral problems (Sullivan, Wells, & Bushnell, 1995).

Because the cognitive and behavioral problems associated with poverty are the same kinds of cognitive and behavioral problems one encounters with FAS/ARBE, it is understandable why children with FAS/ARBE from different homes vary so much in their intelligence or their behavior. FAS/ARBE is not simply the result of being born to an alcoholic mother. It is also the result of being raised by an alcoholic mother; and it is especially the result of being born and raised by a poverty-stricken alcoholic mother (see Chapter 11).

Closely related to the problem of maternal alcoholism is the perennial but scarcely investigated question of the impact of a "significant other." Female alcoholics are disproportionately likely to be married to other alcoholics (McLeod, 1993), and the fathers of children with FAS are almost always alcoholics (Abel, 1983). There is now a small but growing body of literature that indicates that many of the preclinical effects of in utero alcohol exposure, including the occurrence of physical abnormalities, can also result from paternal alcoholic exposure prior to conception (Abel, 1989b; Bielawski & Abel, 1997). There is also a large body of literature on the children of alcoholics that documents the adverse impact of living with an alcoholic father.

Growing up in an alcoholic environment in which a child has no opportunity to become socialized results in many of the same conduct disorders currently associated with FAS/ARBE. Such children do not form intimate lasting relationships and do not develop a sense of remorse. In their behavioral profiles, these children bear a striking similarity to those with FAS. Both have been described as impulsive, hyperactive, aggressive, disobedient, antisocial, insecure, emotionally disabled, academically delayed, and so on (Steinhausen et al., 1984). However, when assessing the home environment, the father's role is typically ignored in FAS/ARBE studies, especially when instruments such as the HOME are used. If a father's alcoholism is ignored, the validity of the results provided for the potential impact of the home environment by these instruments is meaningless. In the context of alcoholism, this is especially so when the home itself is not observed.

CHAPTER 11

The American Paradox

The ability to recognize something out of the ordinary is the hallmark of the dysmorphologist or the medical geneticist, but recognizing the abnormality and determining its cause are not one and the same.

The frequency of occurrence of a birth defect like FAS is described in terms of incidence and prevalence. *Incidence* refers to the number of new cases of an anomaly entering a population at a particular time; *prevalence* refers to either the frequency of a condition among identified cases regardless of when they entered, or the frequency of a condition in a population at a particular time.

For example, if 10 cases of FAS are born for every 10,000 births, the incidence would be 1 per 1,000; if 20, the incidence would be 2 per 1,000. This increase, however, would not affect the prevalence of any FAS-related disorder. If the prevalence rate of cleft palate in FAS is 10%, it doesn't matter if 10 or 20 cases of FAS are born. A 10% rate means there will only be one case of cleft palate for every 10 FAS cases, no matter how many total cases of FAS there are.

For structural birth defects like atrial septal defect, prevalence rates are lower in older children than at birth or in utero for a number of reasons: the child may have died in early infancy; surgery may have been performed to correct the problem; or the defect may have healed on its own. The prevalence of congenital functional anomalies, such as hearing impairment or cognitive disturbances, on the other hand, is generally higher for older versus younger children because the disorder is not life threatening and usually not recognized until several years after birth.

Prevalence rates for various disorders were examined in earlier chapters of this book. This chapter focuses exclusively on the incidence of FAS in populations. Why such a narrow focus? Because fetal alcohol abuse syndrome is a diagnosable clinical disorder, whereas individual alcohol abuse-related birth defects are not pathognomonic, that is, exclusively the result of in utero alcohol exposure.

On the basis of what has already been presented, it should be clear to the reader that FAS is not the result of one or two drinks a day. Instead, it is the result of maternal alcohol abuse, the lower level of which is close to five drinks per drinking occasion, on two or more occasions a week. The incidence of FAS in a given population will therefore depend on the number of alcohol-abusing mothers in that population. However, although alcohol abuse is a sine qua non for FAS, FAS is not an inexorable consequence of maternal alcohol abuse during pregnancy. Instead, FAS occurs selectively for reasons we do not fully understand. This same selectivity is also found in conjunction with other conditions associated with alcohol abuse, such as cirrhosis (Mezzich, Arria, Tarter, Moss, & Van Theil, 1991).

Disparities in the occurrence of FAS can be a source of frustration for individuals who think of FAS in terms of an overly simplistic, reductionistic framework. These disparities, however, are valuable clues to the puzzle of why FAS occurs selectively. Once we recognize the reasons for this selectivity, we will be better able to make inferences about potential predisposing sociobehavioral risk factors that contribute to alcohol's teratogenic effects.

Strategies for Estimating FAS

The main epidemiological procedures for estimating the frequency of occurrence for FAS are retrospective studies, population-based prevalence studies, passive surveillance programs, and prospective/active surveillance studies. Each of these procedures has intrinsic biases that preclude consistency with one another. In other words, depending on the methods epidemiologists use, they will arrive at a relatively high or low estimate of the frequency of occurrence of a disorder like FAS in any population.

Retrospective Studies

Following the report of a birth defect, one of the most common analytical procedures for determining its frequency is the retrospective study, an "after-the-fact" strategy in which pregnancy and birth records or birth-defect registries are scoured, and the frequency of an anomaly is determined relative to the number of cases that are examined.

Retrospective studies typically result in inflated estimates for many medical disorders. In some instances, these estimates are the result of mundane factors, such as medical reimbursements. Because the diagnostic code associated with a particular case is the basis for payment by health insurers, there may be a not-so-subtle pressure to record the presence of a disorder, even though a physician may not have specifically noted its existence, because it results in greater remuneration (Hexter et al., 1990). For example, out of the 43 cases of FAS listed in discharge records at Hutzel Hospital in Detroit for the years 1988 to 1989, only 8 cases had a physician's diagnosis of FAS. If the coder saw maternal drinking in the patient's file, a code for FAS was introduced into the reporting record. Based solely on these hospital records, the incidence of FAS at this hospital was 17.7 per 1,000 (43 out of a total of 24,261 live births). Based on physician diagnosis and inclusion of three additional cases with features compatible with FAS, the incidence was 0.45 per 1,000 (Abel & Sokol, 1991).

A similar result was found in a study conducted in South Dakota, involving Native American children from birth to 14 years of age. Out of the 205 cases coded as FAS, only 7 were considered valid by a pediatric dysmorphologist who examined the case notes. The rate of occurrence for FAS based on the original data was 0.87 per 1,000; the revised rate was 0.3 per 1,000 (Canfield & Selva, 1993).

A study conducted in Atlanta provides another example. Potential FAS cases identified from birth certificates were considered true positives if they were also registered as FAS in the Metropolitan Atlanta Congenital Defects Program, a population-based birth-defects registry. FAS entries in the birth certificate that were not recorded in the registry were considered false positive. In this study, false positives accounted for 71% of the cases (11 out of 14) reported on birth certificates. yet another Centers for Disease Control (CDC) study found a false positive rate of 76% in the medical records for Native Americans (CDC, 1995b).

Birth certificate and medical record data, which are often used in retrospective studies, can be highly inaccurate sources of information regarding FAS for many reasons.

Just as estimates may be inflated for remunerative reasons, they can also be deflated due to physician bias. A study comparing death records and records of lifetime drinking histories, for example, found for certain patients, cirrhosis was rarely attributed to alcoholism, even when the drinking history would warrant such an inference (Dufour & FeCaces, 1993). The reason physicians may not record a particular condition for some patients is a reluctance to stigmatize them or their families as "alcoholic."

Population-Based Prevalence Studies

A variant of the retrospective study is the population-based prevalence study. These studies are often conducted in Native American communities and typically result in the highest of all prevalence estimates.

In a typical study, children are referred to a center because of some problem or characteristic, and then they are examined for evidence of FAS. Using the minimal criteria paradigm (see Table 2.1, p. 25). Asante and Nelms-Matzke (1985) found out that of the 586 children referred to them in the Yukon and Northwestern British Columbia areas in Canada, 82 had FAS and 94 had FAE. Based on the total population of children in these areas, they estimated the prevalence rate for FAS plus FAE among Native children at 46 per 1,000 compared with 0.4 per 1,000 for non-Native children.

There are many problems associated with relying on referrals for estimating the prevalence of a disorder in the larger population, especially where minorities are concerned. For one thing, Native American children may be referred to a center because of a "language problem." The problem, however, may be a result of the environment in which the children were raised; for example, a child may have a hearing impairment that resulted from a mother's ignoring or being unable to attend to an inner ear infection (see Chapter 5), or being forced to conform to behavioral standards that are unusual in a child's normal environment.

Nevertheless, the 100-fold difference between Native and non-Native populations in the Asante and Nelms-Matzke (1985) study is startling. Unfortunately, the authors were unable to obtain information concerning drinking histories of the mothers of these children, nor were they able to provide sociodemographic information for their subjects other than race.

One of the highest prevalence rates ever reported is associated with a small Native community in British Columbia (Robinson et al., 1987). All children under the age of 19 were examined. Diagnosis of FAS was based on the minimal criteria paradigm, coupled with a history of maternal alcohol abuse or FAS in a sibling. Fourteen of the 116 children examined for FAS received a positive diagnosis; another 8 were given a diagnosis of FAE, resulting in an estimated prevalence of 120 per 1,000 for FAS, and a prevalence of 190 per 1,000 for FAS/ARBE combined (22 out of 116).

Although these estimates are very high, it is worth noting that five mothers accounted for 12 (54%) of the affected children. Because population-based studies often count each sibling as a single case, they tend to give undue influence to what may be a relatively small proportion of mothers. Prevalence rates tend to presume a mother-child ratio of one to one, whereas in fact, one mother may give birth to five FAS children.

Similarly, high prevalence rates for FAS have been reported for Native populations in South Dakota, 39 per 1,000 (Duimstra et al., 1993); Alaska, 14 to 29 per 1,000 (CDC, 1993a); 31 to 38 per 1,000 (Egeland, Perham-Hester, & Hook, 1995); and the southwestern United States, 313 per 1,000 (May, Hymbaugh, Aase, & Samet, 1983). The last study noted important tribal differences: Navajo and Pueblo tribes had the lowest prevalences (1.3 and 2.2 per 1,000, respectively), while the Plains tribes (Apache and Ute) had a rate of 103 per 1,000. As in the Robinson et al. (1987) study, several mothers accounted for more than one FAS child.

Population-based prevalence studies all suggest very high rates of FAS among some tribes of indigenous people. Although rates may indeed be much higher in these populations than in Caucasian populations, the way in which the data are gathered introduces biases that preclude accuracy. Subjects are typically preselected for examination because of some departure from a subjective or objective norm, and this in itself may bias evaluations because examiners may be more likely to make the diagnosis due to the referral. Comparisons with non-Native populations in the same area and same level of poverty would indicate whether these rates are specific to indigenous peoples.

The large differences in prevalence rates among different tribes suggests that either they differ in the amount and pattern of their drinking or the kind of alcohol they consume. Alcohol-related health problems may be more prevalent among Native Americans in general because they tend to be binge drinkers (May et al., 1983), and they are more likely to rely on Lysol, Aqua Net, and other forms of "mountain gin" (Burd, Shea, & Khull, 1987). These commercial products contain up to 90% alcohol, along with various solvents. The hazards of these ersatz alcohol sources for fetal development has never been examined.

Cultural bias may also account for the relatively large numbers of FAS cases reported by German clinicians (Majewski, 1993). Germany, for example, has the highest number of medical diagnoses per capita in the western world (Payer, 1988), with *harzinsuffizien* one of the most commonly diagnosed disorders. In one study, 40% of a normal population were considered to have an abnormal electro-cardiogram using German criteria for abnormality compared with only 5% when American criteria were used (Payer, 1988). The tendency to overdiagnose cardiac problems may explain the very high rates of "congenital heart defect" in patients with alcohol embryopathy I and II (9%–19%) and alcohol embryopathy III (63%) (Majewski, 1993).

This cultural tendency to overdiagnose problems may also account for the greater number of anomalies reported in Berlin compared with other European cities participating in the multisite European Concerted Action Study (EURO-MAC). Over 8,000 pregnancies were prospectively followed, and anomalies were examined and coded according to a standardized EUROCAT code, an abbreviated version of the ICD code. In addition to Berlin, data were collected from Odense, Denmark; Roubaix, France; The Netherlands; Porto, Portugal; Valencia, Spain; Vizcaya and Guipuzcoa, the Basque country, Spain; and Dundee, the United Kingdom. Some centers recorded anomalies in greater detail than others. The anomalies count in Berlin was considerably higher than those from many other sites.

Population-based studies rarely include information about possible confounding factors. Accepting the estimates from these studies without critical appraisal would lead to a conclusion that FAS is occurring at epidemic proportions among the indigenous peoples of North America (Bray & Anderson, 1989).

Although this may be true, these studies should only be considered a starting point for further study; not the basis for hastily implemented programs that are wasteful and misguided (Bray & Anderson, 1989).

Passive Surveillance Studies

Passive surveillance studies involve collecting data from birth records or pediatric records at institutions that agree to participate in a monitoring program.

The largest birth-defects passive surveillance program in the United States is the Birth Defects Monitoring Program (BDMP) directed by the Centers for Disease Control (CDC). This nationwide program collates data from hospital discharge diagnoses for newborns from over 1,200 hospitals with obstetrical services.

In 1988, the CDC's passive surveillance program estimated the overall incidence rate for birth defects in the United States for the years 1981–1986 at about 0.1 case per 1,000. Differences between racial groups were relatively high, but compared with the population-based rates mentioned earlier, they were very low. The rate among Native Americans, for instance, was 2.99 compared to 0.6 for African Americans, 0.09 for Caucasians, 0.08 for Hispanics, and 0.03 per 1,000 for Asians.

Although the rate among Native Americans in these studies is far greater than among other groups, the prevalence rate for FAS among Native Americans is nevertheless about ten times lower than the rate derived from population-based studies.

Rater bias may be one reason FAS rates are so much higher on reservations and at inner-city hospitals compared with suburban hospitals. A CDC study comparing FAS rates in and around Atlanta, for instance, found 88 FAS cases out of 98,000 births in the city's hospitals compared with only 3 FAS cases out of 72,000 births in one of its large suburban hospitals. Although the difference in rates between the inner-city and suburban hospitals may be real, the authors suggested that selective case finding, in other words, a "bias in suspecting diagnosis," may otherwise be a "potential reason for the difference" (Cordero, Floyd, Martin, Davis, & Hymbaugh, 1994, p. 83).

Biased rates can also arise from a reliance on coding paradigms, such as the International Classification of Diseases, Ninth Revision (ICD-9), which, as the CDC itself recognizes, is not specific for FAS because it includes drinking during pregnancy ("noxious influences affecting fetus via placenta or breast milk, specifically alcohol) as a criterion for FAS. If this were true, however, every child born to a woman whose drinking is considered "noxious" would have FAS. Using this criterion, the infant's condition is irrelevant; all that is needed is a notation in the mother's medical history of drinking. Even so, estimated rates for FAS based on surveillance studies are very similar to retrospective studies in North America:

Retrospective studies suggest rates of 0.3 to 0.45 cases per 1,000 (Abel & Sokol, 1991; Canfield & Selva, 1993), which are similar to the CDC's estimates of 0.1 per 1,000 (CDC, 1995a), 0.37 per 1,000 (CDC, 1993b), and 0.67 per 1,000 (CDC, 1995a). Population-based studies, by contrast, suggest rates of 14 to 313 per 1,000 (see earlier).

Passive surveillance studies are valuable for tracking changes in relative rates of major defects over time, but they were not designed for identifying or tracking syndromes like FAS, which have relatively few structural defects (Cordero et al., 1994). This may be one of the reasons why the estimated incidences of FAS are very low in passive surveillance studies. Because the syndrome is subtle, divergences from the norm can easily escape detection, unless clinicians are specifically trained to recognize the syndrome; clinicians who are less knowledgeable can be expected to be more uncertain.

Prospective Studies/Active Surveillance

Prospective studies employ an active surveillance strategy for identifying cases and are generally considered to yield the best estimates for the incidence of an anomaly. In contrast to the outcome-to-antecedent strategy of the retrospective study, prospective studies proceed in an antecedent-to-outcome direction. Such studies follow a case from some predetermined starting point to a predetermined end point.

For an FAS study, the starting point is typically a woman's first prenatal care visit, and the end point is the examination of her child at birth. In between, her pregnancy is continually monitored while a thorough history of her health, family background, eating and drinking habits, and so on are obtained, using a standardized questionnaire. Because information is collected on a reliable basis prior to birth, memory loss or deliberate falsification is less likely to occur than might otherwise be the case if the same information were collected after birth, especially if a child were born with a birth defect, and a mother was defensive or felt guilty about its cause.

Prospective strategies are also more likely to result in valid and reliable case findings compared with other methodologies because every newborn is examined. This means that there is minimal bias due to selective evaluation of children, especially if those evaluations are conducted by an examiner who is "blind" to the child's prenatal alcohol exposure.

Prospective/active surveillance studies are not without their own inherent problems, however. If women most at risk of having a child with FAS refuse to participate or do not attend prenatal care clinics, their pregnancies and children will not be included in the study. In an otherwise prospective study in France, for example, Larroque and her co-workers included a number of women who were examined retrospectively because they had received no prenatal care. As stated by the authors, "this latter group, although interviewed retrospectively, was entered in the study because mothers with no hospital prenatal care usually include a high proportion of heavy drinkers" (Larroque et al., 1995, p. 1655).

If women who are the least likely to seek prenatal care and therefore least likely to participate in a prospective study are at the greatest risk for giving birth to a child with FAS, the exclusion of one or two cases may thus have a relatively large impact on the estimated incidence. Likewise, women who seek prenatal care may be at the lowest risk for giving birth to a child with FAS because of their demonstrated concern for their own health and the health of their unborn child. Their inclusion would inflate the number of negative cases, resulting in an artifactually low estimate.

Another source of bias associated with prospective studies involves the sites where they are generally conducted, which are invariably large inner-city hospitals where large academic programs are located. The patient populations in these studies are overwhelmingly of very low socioeconomic status and likely to suffer from many risk factors that affect the well-being of the unborn child (see Chapter 12). As such, they may not reflect patient populations at large.

Worldwide Estimated Incidence of FAS

Because prospective/active surveillance studies provide the most accurate estimates for the incidence of a disorder, the following analyses and inferences are based on results obtained from that experimental strategy.

As of 1995, 29 prospective studies had been conducted relating to the incidence of FAS (see Table 11.1). Based on these studies, the overall worldwide incidence for FAS in the industrialized world is 0.97 cases per 1,000 live born children. This estimate was arrived at by adding all the cases of FAS (95) and dividing that number by the total number of cases (97,576).

If, however, the incidence data from each study are averaged, the overall incidence is a much lower 0.50 cases per 1,000, which, incidentally, is much closer to estimates based on retrospective and surveillance methods. In neither instance, however, is the mean very representative because in most studies, the modal incidence was zero cases. When distributions of numbers are as skewed as those in Table 11.1, the median, representing the point where the entire group is divided into halves, one greater and one smaller, may be the more appropriate statistic for representing the population. In this instance, the median, like the mode, is zero per 1,000 cases. The discrepancy between the mean and the median reflects the fact that FAS has not been uniformly encountered in the various studies that contributed to the overall estimates of its incidence. In other words, FAS appears to occur more often (or less often) at some sites than others.

Table 11.1. Per Capita Alcohol Consumption and Estimated Incidence
of FAS per 1,000 Births Based on Prospective Studies

Study site (source)	Per capita consumption (liters)	Race and socioeconomic status	Sample size	Number of FAS cases	Estimated incidence per 1,000
Australia					
Bell & Lumley, 1989	10	Caucasian/middle class	8,884	0	0.00
Gibson et al., 1983		Caucasian/middle class	7,301	0[b]	0.00
Lumley et al., 1985		Cross-sectional	14,923	0	0.00
Walpole et al., 1990		Caucasian/middle class	605	0	0.00
Canada					
Fried & O'Connell, 1987	7.8	Caucasian/middle class	600	0	0.00
Denmark					
Ogston & Parry, 1992	9.6	Caucasian/cross-sectional	286	0	0.00
France					
Rostand et al., 1990	13.0	—	684	2	2.92
Germany					
Ogston & Parry, 1992	10.5	Caucasian/cross-sectional	999	0	0.00
Italy					
Primatesta et al., 1993	10.0	Cross-sectional	1,516	0	0.00
Netherlands					
Verkerk et al., 1993	8.3	—	3,447	0[c]	0.00
Portugal					
Ogston & Parry, 1992	10.5	Caucasian/cross-sectional	430	0	0.00

(continued)

Table 11.1. (*Continued*)

Study site (source)	Per capita consumption (liters)	Race and socioeconomic status	Sample size	Number of FAS cases	Estimated incidence per 1,000
Spain					
Bolumar et al., 1994	13.0	Caucasian/cross-sectional	1,004	0	0.00
Ogston & Parry, 1992		Caucasian/cross-sectional	866	0	0.00
Ogston & Parry, 1992		Caucasian/cross-sectional	793	0	0.00
Sweden					
Larsson, 1983	5.4	Caucasian/Low SES	464	1	1.43
Larsson et al., 1983		Caucasian	669	1	2.20
Switzerland					
Fricker et al., 1985	11.0	Caucasian	996	0	0.00
Halperin et al., 1985		Caucasian	541	0[d]	0.00
United Kingdom					
Wright et al., 1983	7.3	Caucasian/middle class	900	0[a]	0.00
Plant, 1985		Caucasian/low SES	1,008	0[e]	0.00
Waterson & Murray-Lyon, 1989		Cross-sectional	2,266	0[f]	0.00
Primatesta et al., 1993		Cross-sectional	996	0	0.00
Sulaiman et al., 1988		Cross-sectional	901	0[g]	0.00

United States

Boston					
Hingson et al., 1982	7.3	Low/African American (inner city)	1,690	1	0.59
Ouellette et al., 1977		Low/African American (inner city)	633	1*	1.58
Rosett et al., 1978		Low	322	0	0.00
Cleveland					
Sokol et al., 1980		Low/African American (inner city)	12,127	5	0.41
Sokol et al., 1986		Low/African American (inner city)	8,331	25	3.00
Denver					
Tennes & Blackard, 1980		Caucasian/middle class	278	0	0.00
Detroit					
Sokol et al., 1993		Low/African American (inner city)	14,707	57	3.90
Loma Linda					
Kuzma & Sokol, 1982		Caucasian/middle class	5,093	0[i]	0.00
Pittsburgh					
Day et al., 1989		Low SES (50% African American)	595	0[i]	0.00
Cornelius et al., 1994		Low SES	391	0[i]	0.00
Seattle					
Hanson et al., 1978**		Caucasian/middle class	1,529	2	1.31
Little, 1977		Causcasian/middle class	801	0	0.00

Number of FAS cases Totals:	95.00
Rate per 1,000	0.97
Average rate per study (based on estimated incidence per 1,000)	0.50
Median rate per study (based on estimated incidence per 1,000)	0.00
Modal rate per study	0.00

[a]Barrison et al., Adverse effects of alcohol in pregnancy. *British Journal of Addiction*, 80, 11–22, 1985.
[b-j]Personal communications: [b]Gibson; [c]Verkerk; [d]Halperin; [e]Plant; [f]Waterson; [g]Florey; [h]Marier; [i]Sokol; [j]Cornelius.
*Both cases African American and on welfare.
**Source: E. L. Abel, An update on incidence of FAS: FAS is not an equal opportunity birth defect, *Neurotoxicology and Teratology* (1995), 17, 438. Copyright 1995 by Elsevier Science Ltd. By permission of the publisher.

Per Capita Consumption

One of the possible explanations for the disparity in incidence among the various studies in Table 11.1 is a difference in the number of people drinking or the number of alcohol-abusing drinkers at a particular study site.

Whereas countries that have the highest rates of per capita alcohol consumption might be expected to have the highest rates of alcohol-related problems, researchers are confronted with what has come to be called the "French paradox" (Criqui & Ringel, 1994). The essence of this paradox is that France, which has the highest per capita alcohol consumption rate in the world, and a very high rate of liver cirrhosis, nevertheless has a very low rate of cardiovascular disease, compared with countries with much lower per capita consumption rates.

Although France has a relatively high rate of FAS, many countries with relatively high per capita rates of alcohol consumption have very low FAS rates. For example, Spain, Switzerland, Germany, Italy, and Australia have relatively high rates of consumption but have 0 FAS cases per 1,000. The United Kingdom, which has an annual per capita consumption very similar to that of the United States, likewise has 0 cases per 1,000 births. Drawing an analogy to the "French paradox," just as the inverse correlation between alcohol consumption and cardiovascular disease in France has been called the French paradox, the inverse relationship between the relatively low per capita alcohol-consumption rate and the very high rate of FAS in the United States can be called the "American paradox." Because 91 out of the 95 cases of FAS observed in worldwide prospective studies were diagnosed in the United States, the "American paradox" seems to account for the entire worldwide incidence of FAS!

Data regarding drinking during pregnancy, like per capita data, do not reflect the type of alcoholic beverages consumed in a particular country or the context of their consumption. For instance, the main alcoholic beverage consumed in Mediterranean countries (Italy, France, Spain, and Portugal) is wine, while in northern European countries like Germany, Denmark, and the United Kingdom, as well as the United States, the main alcoholic beverage is beer (Pyorala, 1990). Many studies have found alcohol-related reproductive problems occur primarily among women who drink beer (Dehaene et al., 1977; Kaminski et al., 1976, 1981; Kline et al., 1987; Kuzma & Sokol, 1982; McDonald et al., 1992; Walpole et al., 1989). Because beer is consumed by a small minority of women, many of whom are characterized by low SES, it is possible that it is not so much the amount of alcohol they consume, but the combination of alcohol consumption and low SES that is the important etiological factor in FAS.

Patterns of consumption in these countries also differ. In Mediterranean countries, alcohol consumption is characterized by daily wine drinking that occurs primarily at meals, and intoxication is rare. In Northern Europe, drinking occurs mainly on weekends, typically involves beer, usually occurs outside meals, and drunkenness is socially tolerated to a much greater extent than in Mediterranean countries (Bennett & Ames, 1986). In Scandinavian countries, drinking is typically excessive when it occurs, and it is also concentrated during the weekends, resulting in a binge pattern of consumption (Zeeman-Polderman, 1994). Likewise, in the United States, which has the highest rate of FAS in the world, alcohol is commonly consumed on weekends (Abel & Kruger, 1995), and there is a relatively high social tolerance for drunkenness. Since binge patterns of consumption have been found to be more frequently associated with FAS than patterns of regular consumption (see later), not only the amount, but also the frequency and pattern of drinking is undoubtedly a factor influencing whether FAS does or does not occur.

As indicated in Table 11.1, although there were far more studies conducted in the United States, fewer children were examined (46,497) than the number examined in other countries (51,079). In other words, although fewer children were examined in the United States, the incidence of FAS in the United States is about 20 times higher than it is for the rest of the world.

Prevalence of Drinking during Pregnancy

Per capita consumption data do not differentiate between men and women. Comparisons of the incidence of FAS and per capita consumption data may be misleading if the proportion of male to female drinkers is not the same in each country. The "American paradox" may not be a paradox at all if rates of drinking among women in various countries, and especially the number of women in different countries who drink during pregnancy, differ with regard to the amount they drink. Estimating rates and levels of drinking during pregnancy, however, is befuddling because drinking tends to decrease as pregnancy progresses (Little, 1977; Little et al., 1976; Sokol et al., 1980). However, the decrease in consumption is usually proportional to prepregnancy levels (Little et al., 1976). Because drinking levels during pregnancy are closely related to drinking levels prior to pregnancy, international comparisons relating to drinking during pregnancy may be more valid if based on prepregnancy drinking behavior. However, as Tables 11.2 and 11.3 indicate, the rates of drinking before and during pregnancy among European/Australian and American/Canadian women are almost identical. This means that differences in the overall rates of drinking while pregnant cannot account for the American paradox.

Incidence among Heavy Alcohol Users

Because FAS is associated with chronic alcoholism, one might expect greater concordance between alcohol consumption data and FAS if alcohol consumption data were narrowed to include only women identified as alcoholics. However,

Table 11.2. Percentage of Pregnant Women Who Drink Prior to or during Early Pregnancy in Countries Other Than the United States and Canada

City/Country	Prepregnancy %	During pregnancy %	Reference
Netherlands	77.2	51.9	Ogston & Parry, 1992
Netherlands	78.0		Verkerk et al., 1993
Roubaix (France)	61.1	48.5	Ogston & Parry, 1992
Valencia (Spain)	72.7	52.8	Bolumar et al., 1994
Vizcaya	60.0	35.3	Ogston & Parry, 1992
Guipuzoa	72.0	42.1	Ogston & Parry, 1992
Odessa	71.0	68.0	Ogston & Parry, 1992
Berlin (Germany)	37.6	61.6	Ogston & Parry, 1992
Porto	59.7	53.5	Ogston & Parry, 1992
London (UK)	81.0	55.0	Griso et al., 1984
European	90.0	58.0	Waterson & Murray-Lyon, 1989
Afr-Caribbean	75.0	31.0	
Oriental	56.0	29.0	
Asian	47.0	18.0	
Dundee (UK)	90.0	55.0	Sulaiman et al., 1988
London (UK)		49.0	Peacock et al., 1990
London (UK)		50.0	Brooke et al., 1989
London (UK)	88.0	56.0	Waterson & Murray-Lyon, 1989
Edinburgh (UK)	92.0		Plant, 1984
Southampton (UK)	80.0	54.0	Primatesta et al., 1993
Adelaide (Australia)	74.5		Gibson et al., 1983
Italy	37.0		Lazzaroni et al., 1993
Italy	35.0	29.4	Bonati & Fellin, 1991
Melbourne (Australia)		36.2	Bell & Lumley, 1989
Sydney (Australia)	79.0	43.0	Kesby et al., 1991
Dunedin (New Zealand)		41.6	Counsell et al., 1994 (R)
Milan (Italy)	79.0	78.0	Primatesta et al., 1993
Tasmania (Australia)		57.0	Lumley et al., 1985
Copenhagen (Denmark)	70.0		Rubin et al., 1988 (R)
Belgium	52.0		Lodewijckx & DeGroof, 1990 (R)
Average	69.0	49.0	

Table 11.3. Prevalence of Drinking Prior to or during Pregnancy
in the United States and Canada

Study site	Prepregnancy %	During pregnancy %	Reference
Northern California[P]		47.0	Mills & Graubard, 1987[a]
		48.0	
Southern California[R]		51.0	Kuzma & Kissinger, 1981
Canada, Ontario[P] (Ottawa)	95	82.0	Fried et al., 1980
	97	83.0	Fried et al., 1984
Colorado[P] (Denver)		61.0	Tennes & Blackard, 1980
Maryland[P] (Baltimore)	45	29.0	Fox et al., 1987
Michigan[P] (Detriot)		91.2	Sokol et al., 1989
Massachusetts (Boston)		48.0	Ouellette et al., 1977
			Weiner et al., 1983
Massachusetts[R] (Boston)		35.0	Hingson et al., 1982
		23.0	Marbury et al., 1983
Mississippi (Jackson)	53	28.0	Stephens, 1985 '
Missouri (Calaway County)[R]	49	23.0	Kruse et al., 1986
New York			Kline et al., 1980
New York (New York City)		72.0	Kline et al., 1987
New York (Buffalo)			Russell & Bigler, 1979
Ohio[P] (Cleveland)			Sokol et al., 1986
Ohio (Cleveland)			Sokol et al., 1980
Pennsylvania[P] (Philadelphia)		13.0	Brooten et al., 1987
Pennsylvania (Pittsburgh)	86	60.0	Cornelius et al., 1994
Washington (Seattle)			Little, 1977
	80	81.0	Streissguth et al., 1977
Washington[P] (Seattle)	65	42.0	Streissguth et al., 1983b
USA[P]		25.1	Serdula et al., 1991
USA[R]	53		Bruce et al., 1993
	55	39.2	Praeger et al., 1983
Average	68	49	

P = Prospective
R = Retrospective

alcoholism (as noted in Chapter 2) has not been operationally defined in terms of levels of consumption. Instead, the overriding concept is one emphasizing obsessive-compulsive use of alcohol. Although "heavy" drinking is an inadequate surrogate for alcoholism—or alcohol abuse—it has been widely used as such for the purposes of estimating the incidence of FAS among a group of women whose drinking is characterized as being greater than the general population's. These comparisons are shown in Table 11.4.

**Table 11.4. Estimated Incidence of FAS
per 1,000 Live Births among "Heavy" Drinking Women***

Study site (source)	Heavy drinkers (%)	Number of heavy drinkers	Number of FAS cases	Estimated incidence per 1,000
Australia				
Bell & Lumley, 1989	0.4	38	0	0
Gibson et al., 1983	10.8	79	0	0
Lumley et al., 1985	13.0	79	0	0
Walpole et al., 1990	1.0	44	0	0
Canada				
Fried & O'Connell, 1987	3.1	21	0	0
Denmark				
Ogston & Parry, 1992	3.1		0	0
Finland				
Autti-Ramo et al., 1992		85	20	235
Halmesmaki, 1988		82	10	122
France				
Rostand et al., 1990	7.6	52	2	38
Germany				
Ogston & Parry, 1992	0.6		0	0
Hungary				
Vitéz et al., 1984		301	25	83
Italy				
Primatesta et al., 1993	7.0	257	0	0
Netherlands				
Verkerk et al., 1993	9.0	274	0	0
Portugal				
Ogston & Parry, 1992	5.1		0	0
Spain				
Bolumar et al., 1994			0	0
Ogston & Parry, 1992	0.2		0	0
Ogston & Parry, 1992	0.5		0	0
Sweden				
Aronson, 1984		26	5	192
Larsson, 1983	3.0	17	1	59
Larsson et al., 1983	4.0	21	1	48
Olegard et al., 1979		21	7	333
Switzerland				
Fricker et al., 1985			0	0
Halperin et al., 1985			0	0

Table 11.4. (*Continued*)

Study site (source)	Heavy drinkers (%)	Number of heavy drinkers	Number of FAS cases	Estimated incidence per 1,000
United Kingdom				
Plant, 1985	35.6	281	0	0
Primatesta et al., 1993	1.0	81	0	0
Suliaman et al., 1988	0.4	8	0[f]	0
Waterson & Murray-Lyon, 1989	4.1	22	0	0
Wright et al., 1983	1.0		0	0
United States				
Boston				
Hingson et al., 1982	2.7	45	1	22
Ouelette et al., 1977	9.0	42	1	24
Rosett et al., 1978	13.0		0	0
Cleveland				
Sokol et al., 1980	1.7	204	5	25
Sokol et al., 1986	7.2	600	25	42
Denver				
Tennes & Blackard, 1980	2.0		0	0
Detroit				
Sokol et al., 1993	6.0	882[a]	57[a]	65
Loma Linda				
Kuzma & Sokol, 1982			0	0
Pittsburgh				
Day et al., 1989**	24.0	64[a]	0	0
Cornelius et al., 1994	13.0–19.0	16	0	0
Seattle				
Hanson et al., 1978	7.0	70	2	29
Little, 1977	9.0		0	0
TOTAL		3761	162	
Rate per 1,000	43.1			
Average rate per study	47.0			
Median rate per study	11.0			
Modal rate per study	0.0			

*Defined as average of 2 or more drinks per day, or 5–6 per occasion, or positive MAST, or clinical diagnosis, except as noted elsewhere.
**Heavy* defined as average ≥ 0.89 drinks/day.
[a]Martier, personal communication.
[b]Waterson, personal communication.
Source: Modified from E. L. Abel, An update on incidence of FAS: FAS is not an equal opportunity birth defect, *Neurotoxicology and Teratology*, (1995) 17, 439. Copyright 1995 by Elsevier Science Ltd. By permission of the publisher.

The rate of FAS among heavy drinkers is 4.3% (162 cases out of 3,761). The average incidence rate for FAS per study is 4.7%, which is very close to that estimate. Because the distribution of FAS cases is highly skewed in these studies, the median rate of 1.1% may be more representative.

In the context of the American paradox, Table 11.4 indicates that the twenty-fold difference in incidence between the United States and other countries cannot be attributed to differences in the number of heavy drinkers at different sites. For example, the rate of heavy drinking in Cleveland, a city with one of the highest rates of FAS, was 1.7%; whereas Boston, with a rate ranging from 2.7% to 13.0%, had only one case of FAS; Australia, with a rate of 0.4% to 13.0%, and Scotland, with an even higher rate of 35.6%, reported no cases. Women in Little's (1977) study of mainly middle- and upper-SES women from Seattle had the same 9% prevalence rate of "heavy" drinking as the low-SES, mainly inner-city African-Americans studied by Ouellette et al. (1977). Alpert and co-worker's (Alpert et al., 1981) study of the same inner-city population as studied by Ouellette et al. (1977), however, found a prevalence rate for "heavy" drinking during pregnancy of only 2%. Likewise, when Streissguth examined drinking behavior in the same population studied by Little (1977), she and her co-workers reported a prevalence rate of 0.8% in one study (Streissguth, Martin, & Buffington, 1977) and 2.9% in another (Streissguth, Darby, Barr, Smith, & Martin, 1983b).

Nevertheless, Table 11.4 indicates that the incidence of FAS increases when we focus on women who are selected on the basis of their drinking. The incidence of FAS among these pregnant heavy drinkers, however, is only about 4%. This relatively low incidence is likely the result of setting the criterion for heavy drinking too low to isolate those women who put their children at risk for FAS.

Misclassification of drinking amounts has a minor impact on incidence rate compared with the impact of criteria used to define heavy drinking. For example, if 10% of the women drinking five or more drinks per day claim to be drinking only an average of two drinks a day, then the total number of heavy drinkers in the five-or-more-drinks-per-day category would be 45, and the number of children with FAS in this group would be the same (6% of 5 is less than 1). The incidence of FAS among heavy drinkers, however, would now be 6.6% (3 out of 45). Inclusion of the five women in the two-or-more-drinkers-per-day category would result in the same incidence of 0.46% (3 out of 655), as if they were not included. If 20% of the women consuming five or more drinks are placed in the two-or-more-drinks category, then the higher incidence remains relatively unchanged at 6.5% (2 out of 40, since one of the children with FAS is removed from this group), while the lower incidence decreases to 0.45% (3 out of 660).

Denial is a perennial problem in accurately estimating prevalence and amount of substance abuse, including drinking. By way of illustration, a study of Zuckerman et al. (1989) showed that 16% of the 202 pregnant women who denied using marijuana had positive urine samples for it, and 24% of the 114 denying cocaine use had positive urine tests for that drug.

Similar underreporting is widely suspected for alcohol use during pregnancy. Researchers sometimes use a deception called the "bogus pipeline," telling patients that their verbal or written responses regarding alcohol use may be independently checked by laboratory tests of their blood or urine. In one such study, 14% of a group of pregnant patients responding to a questionnaire only said that they drank compared with 27% when the respondents were told that lab tests also would be conducted to verify their responses (Lowe, Windsor, Adams, Morris, & Reese, 1986).

There are also several other possible reasons for discrepancies in incidence rates of FAS among heavy drinkers. As noted earlier, studies comparing different countries face the formidable problem of discussing a drink as if it contained a standardized amount of alcohol. A "drink" in the United States, however, contains about 13g of alcohol compared with 8g in the United Kingdom. This means a standard drink in the United States contains the equivalent of about 1.6 standard drinks in the United Kingdom. This may be the reason the percentage of heavy drinkers is so high in Scotland (Plant, 1985; see Table 11.4), while the incidence of FAS is so low. Even at a consumption rate of seven drinks per occasion, the total amount of alcohol consumed in Scotland would be 56g, far short of the 65g (5 drinks × 13g per drink) needed to meet the criterion for heavy drinking in the United States. Thus, differences in the alcohol content of a drink make international comparisons as to the relationship between the amount of drinking and FAS, or the comparable relationship between heavy drinking and FAS, very tentative.

The inference drawn from a relatively low occurrence rate of FAS, even among heavy drinkers (4.3%), is that alcohol is a necessary, but not sufficient, cause of FAS. Factors in addition to alcohol consumption during pregnancy must clearly affect the expression of FAS.

CHAPTER 12

Permissive and Provocative Factors in FAS

The relatively low rate of occurrence of FAS among heavy drinkers means alcohol is a necessary, but not sufficient, cause of FAS. The fact that individuals differ in their responses to alcohol implies that they have inherent physiological susceptibilities to its effects. Unlike the simple concept of *response* which carries with it the expectation of a single causal agent, acknowledging that alcohol is not a sufficient cause for FAS implies that the concept of *responsiveness*—in the sense of a differential level of susceptibility and biological defense (Hart & Frame, 1996)—is much more apt.

The model presented in this chapter develops this theme by identifying predisposing behavioral, social, or environmental factors, called *permissive conditions*, that create the differential reaction to alcohol responsible for the occurrence/ nonoccurrence of FAS/ARBE. These permissive conditions are then related to physiological changes in the internal milieu, called *provocative conditions*, that increase vulnerability to alcohol's toxic effects. Without an explanation as to how permissive factors create a biological environment that increases or decreases the susceptibility to alcohol's effects, identifying such factors would mean little more than acknowledging the fact the alcohol abuser does not live in a vacuum. By characterizing these personal and environmental conditions in terms of their biological consequences, a model such as the one proposed here offers a heuristic explanation as to how these factors produce the sufficient conditions that act in conjunction with alcohol to produce FAS.

Permissive Factors

Alcohol Intake Pattern

Fetal alcohol abuse syndrome and fetal alcohol abuse effects only occur in the children of alcohol-abusing mothers (see Chapter 2). Although alcohol abuse or alcoholism is not generally defined in terms of a number of drinks or a drinking pattern, there is widespread agreement that it is characterized by consumption of large amounts of alcohol either periodically or chronically. When consumed periodically, such drinking is often described as bingeing or a "bender." When consumed on a regular basis, it is often described as alcoholism.

In general, the minimum number of drinks per occasion in a binge is five (this is related to how alcohol abuse was operationally defined in Chapter 2). Estimated blood alcohol levels associated with consumption of 9 to 20 drinks over a 5-hour period for a 60-kg man are listed in Table 1.2. Making allowance for male–female differences (see Chapter 2), Table 12.1 illustrates some estimated peak blood alcohol levels associated with a binge of five drinks for women of varying body weights. Blood alcohol levels for binges involving more drinks would, of course, be considerably higher.

It is now very clear that bingeing, especially chronic bingeing, is more dangerous for the unborn child than consumption of the same amount of alcohol over an extended period. Newborns whose mothers are binge drinkers have more serious facial anomalies (Clarren et al., 1988), greater EEG hypersynchrony (Ioffe & Chernick, 1988), and greater cognitive impairment (Streissguth et al., 1989b) than newborns whose mothers consume the same amount of alcohol on a regular,

**Table 12.1. Peak Blood Alcohol Levels Following
a "Binge" of Five Drinks*
as a Function of Maternal Body Weight
and Time Spent Drinking**

Body weight (lb)	Time spent drinking (hr)	BAL
100	1	.16
	2	.15
	3	.13
120	1	.13
	2	.12
	3	.10
140	1	.11
	2	.10
	3	.08

*A drink is 12 oz. of beer or 1 oz. of 86-proof alcohol.

but not bingelike, basis. The more chronic the bingeing, the greater the damage, because chronic bingeing extends the period of alcohol toxicity over a longer duration of pregnancy. As a result, exposure is more likely to occur during critical periods of development (see Chapter 2). Differences in times and frequency of exposure are among the reasons that some alcohol-abusing women have children with FAS, others have children with FAE, and still others have apparently normal children (Abel, 1995; Streissguth & Martin, 1983). If bingeing is more common in America than in countries with higher per capita consumption, this would be a likely explanation for the higher rate of FAS in the United States (see Chapter 11). Evidence that this is so will be presented shortly.

Because the potential for damage is related to bingeing, there is little point in describing drinking in terms of "average drinks per day" because that statistic tells us virtually nothing about bingelike patterns of consumption and therefore very little about risk. To be biologically relevant, researchers would be well advised to abandon the average-drinks-per-day measure in favor of one that reflects maximal drinking per occasion and its frequency.

Health Status

Majewski has often made the point that a mother's health status with respect to her alcoholism is a key factor determining ultimate embryonic toxicity (Majewski, 1993; Majewski, Fishback, Pfeiffer, & Bierich, 1978; Seidenberg & Majewski, 1978). Using Jellinek's three stages of alcoholism paradigm, Majewski found no cases of FAS among women in the beginning stage of alcoholism, a frequency of 20% among those in the critical stage (psychologically and physically dependent), and 43% for those in the chronic stages (compulsive drinking). Majewski's results implied that how long a woman has been an alcoholic is less important than the severity of her alcohol-related pathology (e.g., alcoholic liver disease, DTs).

Table 12.2, which lists some of the more common problems of mothers with children with FAS, supports Majewski's findings. As indicated by the table, there is little doubt that women who give birth to children with FAS have severe alcohol-related pathology (Coles et al., 1985a). As many as three quarters of these women will die within five years of giving birth to their children with FAS (Clarren, 1981; Olegard & Sabel, 1979; Streissguth et al., 1987).

Not surprisingly, cirrhosis is the most common ailment in this patient population. Because cirrhosis, regardless of its etiology, is associated with increased rates of spontaneous abortion and preterm birth (see Chapters 4 and 6), and detectable levels of acetaldehyde in the blood are more likely to be produced by alcoholics with cirrhosis than by those with nonalcoholic liver disease (see later), many of the effects directly attributed to alcohol exposure in utero may instead be due to the combined effects of maternal cirrhosis and alcohol consumption.

In addition to their disease states, alcoholic women are typically emaciated.

**Table 12.2. Heatlh Problems Commonly
Encountered in Mothers
of Children with FAS**

Disorder	%
Cirrhosis (and liver dysfunction)	29.5
DTs	18.0
Psychiatric hospitalizations	16.0
Anemia, poor nutrition, emaciation	15.0
Tremors	9.0
Gastrointestinal bleeding, etc., due to alcohol	8.0
Epilepsy, seizure disorders	7.0
Diabetes, pancreatitis, obesity	4.0
Various infections during pregnancy	4.0
Korsakoff's syndrome	3.0
Preeclampsi	4.0
Neuropathy	2.0
Polyhydramnios	2.0
Polyneuritis	2.0
Pyelonephritis	2.0
Edema	1.0

$N = 122$.

Although weight gain during pregnancy is rarely reported in most case or epidemiological studies involving FAS, a survey of the available literature, scant as it was, found a prepregnancy weight of 98.6 lb ($SD = 6.7$), with a range of from 94.6 to 110 lb. During pregnancy, average weight gain was 14 lb ($SD = 12.4$); four mothers actually lost weight during their pregnancies (average $= -6.5$ lb) (Abel, 1982).

Prepregnancy weight and weight gain during pregnancy far outweigh any effect of moderate or occasional alcohol consumption on pregnancy outcomes. In one study of women whose alcohol consumption was relatively low (Kuzma & Sokol, 1982), alcohol consumption during pregnancy accounted for only 0.1% of the decrease in birth weight associated with maternal drinking compared with 3.5% for prepregnancy weight and 5.3% for weight gain. Another study found no effect of alcohol consumption, while prepregnancy weight accounted for 6% and weight gain during pregnancy accounted for 3% of the effect (Hingson et al., 1982).

Maternal Age/Parity

Case reports and epidemiological studies clearly indicate the prevalence of FAS increases as maternal age and parity increase (Abel, 1988; Jacobson, Jacobson, & Sokol, 1996; May, 1991; Sokol et al., 1986). The effect of maternal age is illustrated by a study comparing the birth weights of rats prenatally exposed to alcohol whose mothers differed in age. Dams were 2, 4, or about 6 months of age at time of alcohol treatment. (The results are shown in Figure 12.1.)

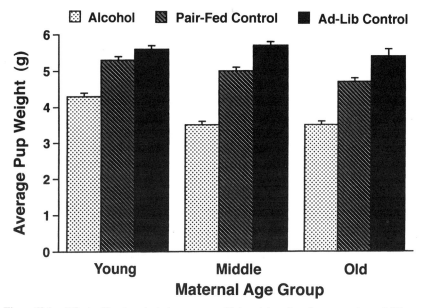

Figure 12.1. Effects of in utero alcohol exposure on birth weights of rats born to mothers of different ages. (Modified from Abel and Dintcheff, 1985).

As is evident in Figure 12.1, prenatal alcohol exposure had a greater impact on birth weights of offspring born to "older" and "middle-aged" mothers than on those born to younger mothers (Abel & Dintcheff, 1985).

Tables 12.3 and 12.4 illustrate the frequency of FAS among sibs of patients with FAS. The risk for FAS in the general population is 0.97 per 1,000 (see Chapter 11). Tables 12.3 and 12.4 clearly show the very high risk of a sib having FAS when there is another case in the family.

The fact that each child born to alcohol abusers is typically more impaired than older siblings has been frequently noted (Abel, 1988; Majewski, 1993; May,

Table 12.3. Increased Probability of a Previous Child with Fetal Alcohol Syndrome

Total number of live births prior to birth of FAS child	Number of children with FAS in prior births	Estimated incidence of FAS per 1,000 live births	Incidence of FAS in previous births per 1,000 live births	Risk increased by
135	23	0.97	170.4	172×

Source: E. L. Abel, Fetal alcohol syndrome in families, *Neurotoxicology and Teratology* (1988), *10*, pp. 1–2. Copyright 1988 by Elsevier Science. Adapted with permission of the publisher.

**Table 12.4. Increased Risk of Having a Second Child
with Fetal Alcohol Syndrome**

Total number of live births after birth of FAS child	Number of children with FAS in subsequent births	Estimated incidence of FAS per 1,000 live births	Incidence of FAS in subsequent births per 1,000 live births	Risk increased by
35	27	0.97	771	795×

Source: E. L. Abel, Fetal alcohol syndrome in families, *Neurotoxicology and Teratology* (1988), 10, pp. 1–2. Copyright 1988 by Elsevier Science. Adapted with permission of the publisher.

1991). Although the probability of a second child with FAS in a family increases dramatically if there is a previously affected child, researchers have not been able to determine if the more important risk factor is increased maternal age or increased parity. Studies in animals, however, suggest maternal age as the greater risk factor (Abel & Dintcheff, 1984, 1985; Vorhees, Rauch, & Hitzermaun, 1988). In pregnant primiparous rats, for instance, the same amount of alcohol has a greater impact, in terms of pregnancy loss and lower birth weight, on older compared with younger mothers (Abel & Dintcheff, 1984). When pregnant mothers of different parities but the same age are treated with the same amount of alcohol, parity does not affect the outcome (Abel & Dintcheff, 1985). This implies the important factor is age, not parity.

One possible explanation for the augmented effect of maternal age in alcohol's toxicity is illustrated in Figure 12.2. In this study (Church, Abel, Dintcheff, & Matyjasik, 1990), pregnant rats 2¼, 3¾ or 5¼ months of age were intubated with 3.5 g/kg of alcohol twice daily at 6-hour intervals on gestation days 11 to 19 inclusive. Blood alcohol levels were determined on gestation day 19. As indicated by the figure, there was a progressively greater blood alcohol level associated with increasing age, even though animals received the same amount of alcohol on the basis of body weight. In fact, the body weights of animals in the "middle" and "old" age groups were almost identical, indicating that the older animals did not achieve high BALs because they received more alcohol than the middle-aged animals.

Another interesting aspect of this study was the high incidence of toxicity in the older animals compared with those of the two younger groups. For instance, 33% of the older females died from the alcohol doses they received, whereas there were no deaths due to alcohol in the two younger age groups.

A subsequent study (Church et al., 1990) found that although differences in body water were correlated with age, when alcohol was administered on the basis of body-water content, differences in blood alcohol levels could not be accounted for solely in terms of that variable. The authors speculated that age-related

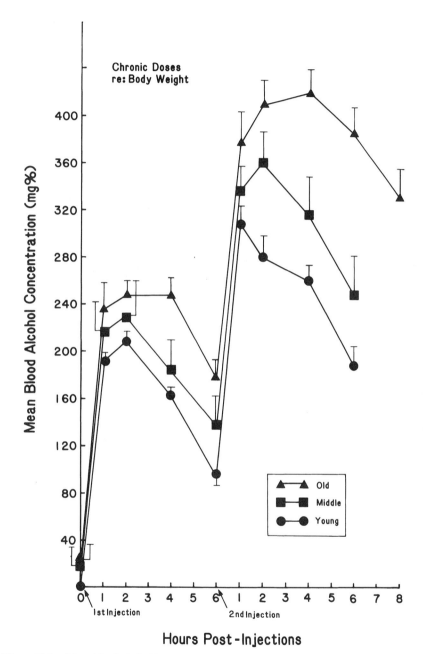

Figure 12.2. Mean blood alcohol levels on gestation day 19 in " young," "middle," and "old" pregnant rats following two intubations of alcohol (3.5 g/kg). *Source*: M. W. Church, E. L. Abel, B. A. Dintcheff, and C. Matyjasik, Maternal age and blood alcohol concentration in the pregnant Long-Evans rat, *Journal of Pharmacology and Experimental Therapeutics* (1990), *253*, p. 1991. Copyright 1990 by American Society for Pharmacology and Experimental Therapeutics. By permission.

differences in absorption may also have contributed to the different blood alcohol levels and toxicities.

Teenage Pregnancies

The age factor raises an interesting question that has largely been ignored in FAS research, namely, whether pregnant teenagers are less likely to give birth to children with FAS/ARBEs than are older women.

Relatively high rates of drinking are not uncommon among teenage girls. About 27% of female high school seniors in the United States self-report consuming five or more drinks on occasion (Johnston, O'Malley, & Bachman, 1989). Teenagers who drink during pregnancy are also not uncommon: Prevalence rates range from a high of 70% for mainly Caucasian, low SES teenagers in Seattle (Lohr, Gillmore, Gilchrist, & Butler, 1992) to 54% for a group of primarily African-American, low SES teenagers in Pittsburgh (Cornelius, Day, Cornelius, Geva, & Taylor, 1993) and 24.8% among a group of predominantly Caucasian adolescents in Madison, Wisconsin (Kokotailo, Langhough, Cox, & Davidson, 1994). The lowest reported rate is 3.3% for a group of pregnant, mainly African-American, low SES teenagers in Baltimore (Kokotailo, Adger, Duggan, Repke, & Joffe, 1992). In Pittsburgh, 3.4% of the teenagers reported being intoxicated at least once a month while pregnant, and though pregnant teenagers drank less on a daily basis than pregnant adults, their rate of binge drinking was higher (Cornelius et al., 1993, 1994).

If alcohol ingestion, especially bingeing, were the only factor in the etiology of FAS, then the number of drinking years should not be an important factor; as far as the fetus is concerned, it would not matter whether a mother drank for 2 years or 12 years before becoming pregnant—the only important factor would be the amount of alcohol exposure during pregnancy. As of yet, there are no clinical or epidemiological studies addressing this question with respect to teenagers, but as noted earlier, older women are at greater risk for FAS than younger women. Whether this higher risk factor is because of a longer history of drinking, higher blood alcohol levels associated with the same amount of drinking, development of alcohol-related such as cirrhosis (Majewski, 1981), or other factors has not been determined.

Alcohol Metabolism

Although alcohol is capable of reducing fetal growth and inducing malformations in vitro without being metabolized (Brown, Goulding, & Fabro, 1979), its metabolite acetaldehyde is more than a thousandfold more embryotoxic than ethanol (Campbell & Fantel, 1983; Higuchi & Matsumoto, 1984) and may affect fetuses directly or augment ethanol's fetotoxicity.

Acetaldehyde's role as a mediator of fetal alcohol abuse effects, however, is indeterminate. Although relatively high blood acetaldehyde levels have been found in some studies of pregnant women (Veghelyi & Osztovics, 1978), these findings are suspect due to the likelihood of artifactual ex vivo formations of acetaldehyde (Fukumaga et al., 1993).

Nevertheless, it is possible that some alcoholic women are at higher risk for giving birth to a child with FAS because they produce a higher-than-normal amount of acetaldehyde when they drink (Majewski, 1981; Veghelyi & Osztovics, 1978). There are at least two ways this could occur. One is if they are in an advanced stage of alcoholism. After drinking, acetaldehyde can be detected in the blood of alcoholics with cirrhosis, but it is not detectable in individuals with nonalcoholic liver disease (Panes et al., 1993). This finding supports Majewski's argument that women in advanced stages of alcoholism pose a greater danger to their unborn children than those in an incipient phase, despite equal amounts of alcohol intake (see earlier).

A second way is if someone has a unique enzyme system that is more likely to produce acetaldehyde than other enzyme systems.

One of the main enzymes involved in alcohol's metabolism to acetaldehyde is alcohol dehydrogenase (ADH). Because there are several variants of this enzyme (Thomasson, Crabb, Edenberg, & Li, 1993), some alcoholics may develop higher levels of acetaldehyde than others. Although acetaldehyde is aversive and generally regarded as a deterrent to developing alcoholism, its aversiveness is less than absolute (see later). There are also several variants of aldehyde dehydrogenase (ALDH), the enzyme that converts acetaldehyde to acetate. An inactive form of this enzyme, ALDH (ALDH2+2), leads to the buildup of acetaldehyde following alcohol consumption and an accompanying characteristic cutaneous vasodilatory "flush," tachycardia, and nausea. This inactive form is present in Asians and not in African Americans, Native Americans or Caucasians (Thomasson et al., 1993).

To an important extent, the rapid buildup of acetaldehyde in Asians is believed to be responsible for the lower prevalence of alcoholism in this population (Higuchi, Maramatsu, Matsushita, Murayama, & Hayashida, 1996). However, individuals with the enzyme variants that result in high levels of acetaldehyde do become alcoholics and, in fact, studies from Japan found a higher prevalence of these inactive enzymes in the general population than in Japanese alcoholics (Higuchi et al., 1996). These and other related observations indicated that although genetic variations in alcohol-oxidizing systems may be involved in developing alcoholism, these systems are not the main factor in their etiology (Higuchi et al., 1996).

Alternatively, a non-ADH pathway for metabolizing alcohol, such as the microsomal enzyme oxidizing system (MEOS) located in the endoplasmic reticulum (Lieber, 1991), may be involved. A functional component of the MEOS system, called cytochrome P450 IIE1 (P450 2E1), is of particular interest because it is highly inducible. The proliferation of the endoplasmic reticulum, which is associated with chronic drinking, is in large part due to induction of this enzyme, and, in alcoholics, this is the primary means by which alcohol's metabolism occurs (Lieber, 1991).

If vulnerability to FAS is related to variations in acetaldehyde production, that vulnerability is much more likely to be related to individual, rather than racial, variations, because FAS occurs in all races. Although alcoholics continue to drink despite developing high acetaldehyde levels, variations in metabolism due to the presence of a particular variant of maternal ADH, ALDH, or MEOS enzymes could result in greater fetal exposure. If differential maternal enzymes are involved, an equally important issue awaiting clarification is whether acetaldehyde crosses the placenta and, if so, at what levels of exposure.

Studies in animals have been inconsistent with respect to detecting acetaldehyde in fetal blood. Some studies have found very low levels (Gordon et al., 1985); others have not been able to detect it at all (Kesaniemi & Sippel, 1975). As in the case of studies in humans, technical problems in measuring acetaldehyde cannot be ignored when assessing these findings.

It is also possible that enzyme variants in the embryo, rather than in the mother, may be a source of acetaldehyde. If so, this would depend on the activity of these enzymes during the time of organogenesis. Alcohol dehydrogenase and aldehyde dehydrogenase are both present in mouse embryos (Deltour, Ang, & Duester, 1996; McCaffery & Drager, 1994), but the amount of acetaldehyde they produce or metabolize is unknown.

One small study published in abstract form reported that five African-American children with FAS had a higher than expected frequency of a rare ADH form, but the study did not include a comparable control group (Sokol et al., 1989). Another abstract found no association between the occurrence of "atypical ADH and ALDH genotypes" and the clinical features of FAS (Faustman, Streissguth, Stevenson, Ouenne, & Yoshida, 1992). Because both studies examined children, neither addressed the question of enzyme activity during organogenesis.

As noted earlier, alcohol is capable of affecting fetal growth under conditions that do not involve its metabolism. It is not only toxic to embryos in vitro (see earlier), but it also causes malformations in the wings and legs of fruit flies, a species that does not convert alcohol to acetaldehyde (Ranganathan, Davis, & Hood, 1987), and it produces teratogenic effects when administered along with pyrazole, which inhibits its conversion to acetaldehyde. Until shown otherwise, the possibility that acetaldehyde is responsible for or contributes to alcohol's teratogenic effects on the fetus has yet to be proven.

Race/Socioeconomic Status

Within the United States, incidence rates for FAS are clearly related to socioeconomic status. Inner-city hospitals, where the populations are predominantly African American whose SES is characterized by poverty, have much higher rates of FAS than do sites where the populations are primarily Caucasian or middle class. The same is true for population-based studies, which are primarily studies of Native Americans (see Chapter 11). Despite the fact African-American and Native American populations are disproportionately poor, the focus of attention with respect to alcohol's effects whenever minorities are studied has typically been on race, rather than income.

Tables 12.5 and 12.6 provide separate estimates from the standpoint of racial demographics and socioeconomic status, of the number of women who give birth to children with FAS each year.

As Tables 12.5 and 12.6 indicate, the incidence of FAS at sites serving primarily Caucasian/middle-socioeconomic-status patient populations is about 10 times lower than the rate at sites where the majority of patients are primarily African American/low SES (0.26 vs. 2.29 per 1,000).

Table 12.6, which estimates the number of women who gave birth to children with FAS on the basis of maternal socioeconomic status, using incomes of $10,000 or less as the criterion for a family of three (U.S. Department of Commerce, 1993), projects almost the same number of FAS cases as were projected on the basis of racial demographics.

As Tables 12.5 and 12.6 clearly indicate, FAS does not discriminate on the basis of race, but it is by no means an equal opportunity birth defect because it occurs predominantly in low SES populations. Race and socioeconomic status are confounded in these studies, but descriptions of the patient populations in these studies and elsewhere indicate that poverty, not race, is the handmaiden of FAS. This is clearly suggested by the case report literature.

The first FAS case reports by Jones and Smith (1973), for example, included Caucasian, African-American, and Native American children. All of these children were seen at Harborview Medical Center in Seattle, which served "a low

Table 12.5. Number of Women (15–44 Years Old) Giving Birth to Children with FAS in the United States in 1992 Based on Racial Demographics

Racial background	Estimated incidence per 1,000	Number of deliveries	Number of FAS births
Caucasian*	0.26	2,985,734	776
African American*	2.29	553,173	1,267
Native American†	?	39,000	?
Total			2,043

Source: E. L. Abel, An update on incidence of FAS: FAS is not an equal opportunity birth defect, *Neurobehavioral Toxicology* (1995), *17*, 440. Copyright 1995 by Elsevier Science Ltd. Reprinted with permission of the publisher.

**Table 12.6. Number of Women (15–44 Years Old)
Giving Birth to Children with FAS in the United States in
1992 Based on Socioeconomic Status**

Socioeconomic status	Estimated incidence per 1,000	Number of deliveries	Number of FAS births
Low*	2.29	712,500	1,632
Middle-High	0.26	2,823,145	734
Total			2,366

*<10,000 per year.
Source: E. L. Abel, An update on incidence of FAS: FAS is not an equal opportunity birth defect, *Neurotoxicology and Teratology* (1995), *17*, 440. Copyright 1995 by Elsevier Science Ltd. Reprinted by permission of the publisher.

socioeconomic urban population" (Ulleland, 1972). Streissguth and Martin (1983) likewise commented that "centers reporting high proportions of Indian children with fetal alcohol (Seattle; Vancouver, British Columbia; New Mexico) are from areas where race and socioeconomic factors are confounded ... the preponderance of cases from the lower social classes has led some authors ... to suggest some of the risk factors may be associated with socioeconomic status" (pp. 553–554).

In Boston, Rosett et al. (1978) reported that "most of the women (they) interviewed were poorly nourished." Morse and Weiner (1996) found the children with FAS enrolled for services in Massachusetts came from families that "differed significantly from other families with at-risk children" on several demographic variables, especially "annual income below $10,000 [and] unemployed parents."

In New York, Bingol et al. (1987) found that only one case of FAS out of 109 children born to 36 Caucasian, upper-middle-class alcoholics (1%) compared with 54 cases out of 133 children (40.5%) for African-American and Hispanic, lower SES alcoholics. All of Iosub's et al.'s (1981a,b) clinical patients were on public assistance and were either African American or Hispanic (Iosub, personal communication). In another study from New York, an alcohol-related increase in spontaneous abortions among women on public assistance could not be replicated when the same investigators studied patients not on public assistance (Kline et al., 1980; Kolata, 1981).

In Cleveland, the African-American and Caucasian children with FAS identified by Sokol et al. (1980, 1986) were characterized by low SES. All of the more than 14,000 patients in Sokol's Detroit sample were African American and low SES.

Of the 207 FAS cases seen at the Kinsmen Children's Centre in Saskatchewan, Canada (up to 1994), 178 were Native Americans or Metis (mixed heritage), 20 were Caucasian, and the remainder were of unknown background, and "the large majority have biological parents with a low SES" (Nanson, personal communication, 1996).

In other countries, where the populations are more racially homogenous and predominantly Caucasian, children with FAS are nearly always characterized by low SES.

Lemoine's 127 French children born with what is now recognized as FAS (Lemoine et al., 1968) were the progeny of "mostly poor" women, all of whom smoked one to two packages of cigarettes per day (Lemoine, personal communication, 1995). Similarly, Dehaene et al. (1981) noted that all of the 45 French FAS cases they observed were born to women of "low socioeconomic status."

All of the mothers studied by Manzke and Spreter von Kreudenstein (1979) in Germany were Caucasian; 14 of these 17 mothers were low SES, and all smoked, as did the two middle SES and one upper SES mothers (Manzke, personal communication, 1995)—in the few cases women from middle- or upper-class backgrounds gave birth to children with FAS, they were invariably smokers. (As explained later in this chapter, smoking results in "provocative" factors very similar to those associated with poverty.)

All of the 151 FAS cases studied by Steinhausen in Switzerland were Caucasian, but the overwhelming majority had less than a high school education (45 out of 63 known cases) (Steinhausen, personal communication, 1995).

Nine of the 10 Caucasian children with FAS studied by Autti-Rämö et al. in Finland (1992) were born to mothers characterized by low SES and/or smoking; the mothers of the five children with FAS studied by Aronson (1984) in Göteborg, Sweden, were all smokers.

Of the 147 cases studied by Lesure in Reunion (1988), "most of the mothers … are unusual smokers, most of them all lower social class and very rarely middle social class" (Lesure, personal communication, 1995).

The mothers of 34 children with FAS studied by Mena and her co-workers in Chile (1986) had unbalanced diets and, partly because of their low socioeconomic status, their diets were deficient in calories and proteins.

In Cape Town, South Africa, all of the 14 FAS cases were observed at Somerset Hospital, which serves a population of low socioeconomic background (Palmer, 1985).

Studies looking for evidence that so-called moderate, social, or occasional drinking affects children have likewise almost exclusively relied on minority/low socioeconomic populations. In Detroit, for example, 83% of the mothers studied by Jacobson and co-workers were on welfare (Jacobson et al., 1994). In Atlanta, infants were recruited, "at a large university teaching hospital that serves a predominantly black, low socioeconomic status population" (Brown et al., 1991). In Pittsburgh, mothers were "of low socioeconomic status," three quarters of whom earned less than $400 a month (Day et al., 1989). In France, mothers were seen at a hospital "located in an area of low socioeconomic status" (Larroque et al., 1995).

Although race and SES are inextricably confounded in the United States, as mentioned earlier, most studies of FAS-related risk factors have focused on race and have largely ignored SES. Other studies, however, have found racial differences in poor perinatal outcome, mortality, and developmental disabilities frequently disappear when SES is taken into account (Cooper, 1993; Polednak, 1991). In other words, as differences between social classes narrow, racial differences in prenatal problems decrease.

Studies based on racial susceptibility to various health-related disorders, including FAS, are fundamentally flawed because they rest on a misconception that race reflects biological homogeneity, and the genes determining race are linked to those affecting health (Williams, Lavizzi-Mourey, & Warren, 1994). A variety of genetic studies, including DNA analyses, indicates *intragroup* genetic variability among African Americans is greater than *intergroup* genetic variability between African Americans and Caucasians (Cooper, 1993; Williams et al., 1994). Even a recognized single-gene disorder, such as sickle-cell anemia, which is frequently cited as evidence of a racially homogeneous disorder, is not unique to Africans or African Americans. Although certainly more common among African Americans, the genetic trait also occurs among Caucasians of a Mediterranean background, but is almost nonexistent among blacks in South Africa (Viljoen, personal communication, 1997). Occurrence of the sickle-cell trait is dependent not on race, but on geographical origin—people whose ancestry is traceable to areas where malaria is common have a higher prevalence of the trait (Williams et al., 1994).

Collectively, these considerations clearly point to socioeconomic status, rather than biological factors related to race, as the major permissive factor for FAS. Genes, however, are easier to characterize and study than SES, and, because race is highly related to SES (Cooper, 1993), investigators have largely ignored SES as a factor in FAS research in favor of race-related genetic susceptibilities.

Genetic Susceptibilities

The current research focus on genetic differences between populations based on race has diverted attention from socioeconomic or environmental contributions to disease in general and to poor infant outcome in the case of FAS in particular. The biological unimportance of race in FAS, however, does not imply genetic factors are not involved. Reports in which one twin has FAS and the other only partial effects, or one twin has more severe partial effects (Figure 7.1A; see also Crain, Fitzmaurice, & Mondrey, 1983; Lesure, 1988; Miller et al., 1981; Streissguth et al., 1993) indicate genetic susceptibilities to alcohol's toxic effects.

Discordance, however, could also be due to other factors, such as different placental vasculatures (Fogel et al., 1965), different rates by which each fetus metabolizes alcohol (unlikely for reasons mentioned earlier), and differences in fetal position. In the twin study illustrated in Figure 7.1A,B and Table 12.7, for instance, the twin most affected at birth was lying in the breech position in utero. As noted earlier, this is a risk factor for many of the characteristics associated with FAS (see Chapter 4).

A noteworthy feature relating to the twins described in Figure 7.1A,B and Table 12.7 is that the affected twin exhibited considerable postnatal catch-up growth. If these twins had only been observed at 17 months of age, instead of at birth, a diagnosis of FAS would not have been warranted using the minimal criteria paradigm (see Chapter 2) because there were no differences relating to body weight or height, one of the paradigm's main diagnostic features.

A high concordance for FAS/ARBEs among monozygotic twins (Harris et al., 1993; Streissguth et al., 1993) and differential sensitivities to in utero alcohol exposure (Gilliam et al., 1989) indicate that genotype is a factor affecting alcohol's toxicity.

Culture/Ethnicity

Although a lower threshold for FAS has been reported for African Americans compared with Caucasians (4 versus 6 drinks per day, respectively) (Sokol et al., 1986), for several reasons, this apparent differential susceptibility does not necessarily relate to different genotypes among racial groups. First, as noted earlier, threshold estimates based on self-reported drinking are unreliable, especially

**Table 12.7. Comparison of Physical Features
in Dizygotic Twins Whose Mother Drank 10 Bottles
of Beer a Day during Pregnancy**

Physical characteristics	Unaffected twin	Twin with FAS
Birth weight (g)	3,480	2,400
Height at birth (cm)	47	44
Head circumference (cm)	34	33
Palpebral fissure size (cm)	2.5	1.9
Philtrum length (cm)	1.2	1.5
Interpupillary distance (cm)	5.0	5.5
Weight at 17 mo. (g)	10,075	11,380
Height at 17 mo. (cm)	79.5	81.5
Head circumference (cm)	47.5	47

Source: Modified from R. S. Riikonen, Differences in susceptibility to teratogenic effects of alcohol in discordant twins exposed to alcohol during the second half of gestation, *Pediatric Neurology* (1994), *11*, pp. 334.

when obtained from problem drinkers. We do not know if people from different racial or SES backgrounds, pregnant or otherwise, differ in denial or distortion of self-reported drinking behavior. We do know, however, that as a group, African-American women are more likely to be abstainers than are Caucasian women (Caetano, 1984). If drinking is a greater stigma among African-American women, they may be more likely to deny their drinking, or if they do admit drinking, they may underestimate the amount of drinking to a greater extent.

Like SES, *ethnicity*, defined by Warren, Hahn, Bristow, & Yu (1994) as "self-perceived membership in populations defined by diverse criteria, including common ancestry, nationality, culture, language, and physical appearance," has been virtually ignored in favor of race. Differences among ethnic groups and cultures with respect to social or behavioral characteristics, however, may increase the risk of FAS for one group as compared with another. African-American and Native American alcoholic women, for example, tend to drink in prolonged binges, while Caucasian alcoholic women are more likely to engage in short, frequent binges (Dawkins & Harper, 1983; May, Hymbaugh, Aase, & Samet, 1983).

Cultural factors in drinking patterns are a major permissive influence on the incidence of FAS and are analogous to the drinking behavior associated with increased risks for FAS in different countries. For example, FAS appears to be much more common in Germany and the United States than in Italy or Great Britain, even though total per capita alcohol consumption is similar for these countries (see Chapter 11).

Cultural differences in diet may also be a factor in FAS/ARBE (see later), although it has not received much attention as such.

Smoking

The final major permissive factor for FAS that requires mention is smoking. Smoking is a permissive factor because it causes the products of tobacco smoke to be taken into the body. There is no doubt that these products themselves contribute to adverse pregnancy outcome, especially decreased birth weight (Abel, 1984b). Because alcohol consumption is highly correlated with smoking (Brooke et al., 1989; Ernhart et al., 1988; Olsen et al., 1991; Sokol et al., 1980; Wright et al., 1983), assignment of subjects with different smoking histories to different alcohol-consuming groups in clinical or epidemiological studies is problematic for reasons discussed at length in Chapter 6. Although the concurrent influences of alcohol and smoking can be examined statistically to assess the independent effects of each alone, statistically significant interactions between the two are very hard to demonstrate, other than by stratification, because there are usually too few subjects in any study who are heavy drinkers and light smokers, or light drinkers and heavy smokers.

Smoking cigarettes is not only an important permissive factor in FAS, it may be the reason FAS occurs in the rare occasions when it is not associated with poverty. The common link between poverty and smoking is that each provokes a common biological milieu that increases susceptibility to alcohol's teratogenic action.

Provocative Factors

Epidemiological studies typically focus on identifying the *permissive* factors associated with a particular condition. More often than not, however, these "black box" epidemiological studies to not explain how these conditions relate to the problem being examined. Unless these conditions can be associated with a biological milieu that affects the occurrence of that condition, they cannot lead to any meaningful inferences about the condition itself.

Once we understand how permissive factors lead to changes in the biological milieu, we will be better able to suggest possible reasons for the selective occurrence of FAS and its prevention. This section considers some of the ways the permissive factors identified previously "provoke" these changes in the body.

Alcohol Intake Pattern and Blood Alcohol Levels (BALs)

Studies in animals clearly indicate that blood alcohol level (BAL) is a critical variable affecting development, especially the developing brain. Given the same amount of alcohol—the shorter the time period over which it is consumed, the higher the resulting BAL, and the higher the BAL, the greater the reduction in brain growth and amount of brain damage (Bonthius & West, 1988; Webster et al., 1983).

The reason bingeing is a potential hazard for a mother and her unborn child is the accompanying high BAL is more likely to exceed a biological threshold for perturbation of cellular function. In the rat, the blood alcohol threshold for perturbing brain growth is a relatively high 150 mg/dl (Samson & Grant, 1984)—much higher than the legal level of intoxication in humans (100 mg/dl) and the level associated with moderate drinking.

All teratogens, including alcohol, produce their effects within a range of alcohol exposures. Below one level, they are harmless; above another level, any of the various anomalies described throughout this book may occur. At very high levels, a teratogen may be embryo- or fetotoxic, thereby providing an upper limit on the number of potential live births associated with exposure to that teratogen. In nonhuman primates, following exposures of about 200 mg/dl, abortions from alcohol begin to occur in the first trimester of the 164-day gestation period (see Chapter 3), corresponding to consumption of about 8.5 drinks within a 4-hour period (1 drink per half hour) for a 55-kg (120-lb) woman. Drinking patterns such as bingeing are permissive because they produce high peak BALs. High peak BALs are provocative because they exceed toxicity thresholds and thereby induce biological changes at the cellular level that result in FAS.

Low SES and Alcohol-Related Health Problems

Although FAS occurs in all races, poverty-stricken alcoholics are far more likely (one is tempted to say "almost exclusively") to have children with FAS than affluent alcoholics.

Environmental and social correlates of poverty that are directly provocative or exacerbate other provocative factors for FAS include inadequate diet or poor nutrition, inner-city residency, psychological stress, high parity, smoking, and abuse of other drugs.

Undernutrition

The embryo and fetus are totally dependent on the mother for their nutrients ("building blocks") and fuel supply. Maternal diet is therefore the most critical factor affecting growth and development in utero.

Although it has always been assumed that all alcoholics are undernourished, this assumption is overly broad but appears to apply to alcoholics in the lower socioeconomic groups (Salaspuro, 1993), who, as previously noted, are characterized by low prepregnancy weight or poor maternal weight gain during pregnancy and/or by smoking. Mothers do not become alcoholics when they become pregnant, so the influence of alcoholism-related nutritional factors begins long before pregnancy (Crawford et al., 1993).

Suboptimal maternal nutrition is a provocative factor for FAS because when it occurs, the nutrient pool necessary for supporting fetal growth and maintaining maternal health is reduced. Nutrition is compromised in alcoholism because alcohol has a high energy content and replaces other energy sources in the diet. While nutritional factors alone cannot give rise to FAS, alcohol consumption alone cannot account for its occurrence (see Chapter 11). The two almost invariably go together.

Although rarely appreciated, research studies that use animal models of FAS reliably indicate that alcohol's teratogenic actions are related to nutritional status; alcohol exposure is typically accompanied by decreased food and water intake and decreased weight gain during pregnancy. As shown in Figure 12.3, all three parameters decrease as alcohol exposure increases. In such cases, the interaction between nutritional status and alcohol exposure cause adverse outcomes in offspring.

Techniques such as pair-feeding, whereby one group of control animals receives the same amount of food and water consumed on the previous day by

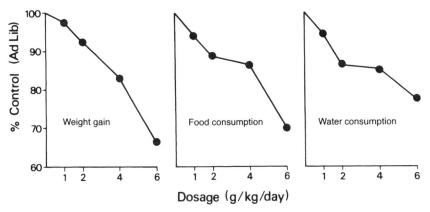

Figure 12.3.   Weight gain and food and water consumption of pregnant rats intubated with different amounts of alcohol each day of pregnancy, relative to nontreated females.

alcohol-treated animals, have already been mentioned in the context of growth retardation (see Chapter 6).

The shortcoming of this procedure is that it only controls for the influence of undernutrition per se. Pair-feeding provides equivalent caloric or sometimes equivalent specific nutrients for alcohol and control groups, but the alcohol-treated groups under such conditions are always both alcohol-treated and undernourished (Khera, 1987).

In addition to reducing food consumption, alcohol also can reduce nutrient absorption, so that even if nutrient intake were the same, the concentration of nutrients absorbed into the mother's blood and potentially available to cross the placenta could be reduced. Because alcohol can also prompt vomiting and diarrhea in humans, with concomitant loss of fluids and absorption of water (Lieber, 1991), there are those problems to consider as well. Thus, any differences between alcohol-treated groups and nonalcohol-treated controls is likely due to the interactive effects of alcohol plus undernutrition. The fact that anomalies occur to a greater extent in alcohol-exposed animals than in pair-fed controls does *not* eliminate the likelihood of a nutritional contribution but only indicates undernutrition per se cannot account for these anomalies.

In vitro studies, likewise, do not eliminate the potential role of nutritional factors because the artificial media may not contain dietary substances, for example, vitamins, whose effects may attenutate alcohol's biological effects on embryos (Davis et al., 1990). The same potential for interactions between alcohol and nutrients exists in cultured cells from whole animals. Disproving the provocative influences of undernutrition in FAS/ARBE would require demonstrating specific FAEs when alcohol-treated dams maintain the same body weight and the same functional nutrient status as untreated animals given ad libitum access to food. This has never been and probably cannot be shown.

Environmental Pollutants

Low SES is associated with living in the inner-city (Polednak, 1991), which can increase exposure to environmental pollutants. Although the effects of many of these pollutants could be mentioned (Longo, 1980), only lead from industry and paint is considered here because more is known about the effects of lead exposure on development.

The threshold level for CNS damage from lead for children was recently lowered to 10 μg/dl with increasing damage associated with increased exposures (Ernhart, 1992; Ernhart et al., 1985b). Many of the effects of prenatal alcohol exposure, for example, intrauterine growth retardation (IUGR) and CNS dysfunction, are also associated with prenatal lead exposure (Ernhart, 1992). Because alcohol consumption can increase blood lead levels (Ernhart et al., 1985b), the likelihood of fetal damage from a synergism between alcohol and lead exposure is increased for infants born to alcoholics living in the inner-city.

Age/Parity

Advanced age/high parity, another correlate of poverty (Polednak, 1991), can be a provocative factor for FAS/ARBE because of the obvious relationships between age and history of alcoholism. The longer a woman drinks heavily, the more severe her potential medical complications (Ashley et al., 1977). Later born children may thus be more prone to FAS because they are exposed to higher BALs in utero than their older siblings. This higher exposure may, in turn, be due to lower body water (Church et al., 1990), tolerance-related increases in maternal alcohol intake, a greater severity of maternal alcohol-related medical problems, and so on, interacting with continued alcohol exposure (Khera, 1987; Majewski, 1981; Sanchis, Sancho-Tello, Chirivella, & Guerri, 1987). Increased parity is also associated with increased uterine collagen and elastin content. This condition can have the effect of decreasing blood flow to the conceptus, contributing to fetal hypoxia (Robertson & Manning, 1974; Woessner, 1963), and thereby further exacerbating the impact of alcohol. However, as noted previously, increased age appears to be the greater risk factor.

Psychological/Physical Stress

Maternal stress (marital discord, overcrowding, negative attitudes about pregnancy, etc.) and physical abuse are prominent correlates of poverty (Amaro, Fried, Cabral, & Zuckerman, 1990; Polednak, 1991). Stress can impair maternal physiology and health and contribute to increased rates of spontaneous abortions (Scarpellini, Sbracia, & Scarpellini, 1994), obstetric complications (Laukaran & VandenBerg, 1980), and low birth weight (Edwards et al., 1994). Stress can also potentiate alcohol's toxicity and may initiate or encourage continued alcohol abuse (Bresnahan, Zuckerman, & Cabral, 1992). Whether by cause or effect, victims of violence during pregnancy are also more likely to be "heavy" drinkers (Amaro et al., 1990).

Childhood disorders, such as bed-wetting, distractibility, sleep disturbances, disorders in reading ability, and cognitive impairment, have also been attributed to the effects of maternal stress during pregnancy (Pasamanick & Lilienfield, 1955), but such associations in humans are equivocal because of the confounding of pre- and postnatal conditions. However, such relationships have been amply documented in animal studies (see Table 12.8). Interestingly, all of the effects listed in Table 12.8 are also encountered in conjunction with in utero alcohol exposure. (Readers interested in the references associated with Table 12.8 can obtain them by request from the author.)

Further evidence that adrenal stress-related hormones, such as corticosterone, may also be involved in some ARBEs is present in studies that report attenuation of the effects of prenatal alcohol exposure on growth retardation and immunosuppression by maternal adrenalectomy (Redei, Halasz, Li, Prystowsky, & Aird, 1993; Tritt, Tio, Brammer, & Taylor, 1993).

Ethnicity

Ethnicity and culture are influenced by SES and, in turn, can influence patterns of alcohol consumption and diet. In cultures in which alcohol is consumed regularly at meals, infants are found to be at less risk for FAS than those whose culture encourages periodic drinking behavior (e.g., concentrated on weekends), or where alcohol abuse is characterized by bingeing (see Chapter 11). Differences in diet can also influence the risk for FAS/ARBE when particular diets

Table 12.8. Effects of Prenatal Stress on Offspring

Low birth weight	Altered male sexual behavior
Prematurity	Decreased sexually dismorphic nucleus
Increased postnatal mortality	Decreased hippocampal size
Postnatal growth retardation	Altered play behavior
Developmental delays in maturation	Hyperactivity
Congenital malformations	Altered plasma testosterone levels
Increased distractibility	Increased corticosterone response to stress
Low muscle tone	Decreased immunocompetence
Poor coordination	Decreased learning ability
Altered maternal behavior	Impaired reversal learning

provide (or do not provide) nutrients (e.g., saturated fats, vitamins) capable of exacerbating (or attenuating) alcohol's effects. (Examples are presented in Chapter 13.)

Tobacco and Other Drugs

Alcohol's toxic effects on the developing human fetus are augmented substantially among women who inhale tobacco smoke. Smoking is a "permissive factor" (see early) because it is highly correlated with poverty (Hogue, Buehler, Strauss, & Smith, 1987; Nordstom, Cnattinguis, & Haglund, 1993; Polednak, 1991) and alcohol consumption. The ingredients in tobacco smoke are what makes smoking a provocative factor for FAS because, like alcohol, some of these ingredients, for example, nicotine and carbon monoxide, directly reduce blood flow and oxygen content, respectively; can cause ischemia and fetal hypoxemia; decrease nutrient availability to the fetus (Abel, 1984a); and promote teratogenesis through free radical formation (see Chapter 13). Smoking also increases blood lead levels (Ernhart et al., 1985b), creating an additional risk factor from that element.

Other drugs associated with alcohol abuse are potential risk factors and contribute to alcohol's impact on the fetus. Consumption of marijuana, cocaine, and caffeine are significantly correlated with alcohol consumption during pregnancy (Brooke et al., 1989; Coles et al., 1992; Jacobson et al., 1991). Like tobacco smoke, marijuana smoke can also increase maternal blood levels of carbon monoxide. Increased blood levels of carbon monoxide or exposure to the many ingredients in marijuana smoke, for example, tetrahydrocannabinols, may negatively affect fetal outcome (Abel, 1985; Day et al., 1992; Fried & Watkinsson, 1988; Jacobson et al., 1994a;b) or may interact with alcohol to potentiate its effects on the fetus (Abel, 1985).

Caffeine use is also commonly associated with alcohol intake (Brooke et al., 1989; Coles et al., 1992; Jacobson et al., 1991). Epidemiological studies have linked caffeine to lower birth weight in humans (Dlugosy & Bracken, 1992), and caffeine has an additive effect with prenatal alcohol in reducing birth weight in rats (Hannigan, 1995). Caffeine may exacerbate alcohol's effects on the fetus (Hannigan, 1995) by reducing folate and/or zinc levels (Yazdani et al., 1992).

Among the other drugs associated with alcohol abuse, most of the attention has been focused on cocaine. However, reports of the impact of prenatal cocaine exposure in humans and animals are inconsistent (Hutchings, 1993). Likewise, studies examining interactions between prenatal alcohol and cocaine (Church et al., 1991; Coles et al., 1992) are also inconsistent. Yet, there are aspects of cocaine pharmacology that are potentially important for mechanisms of alcohol teratogenesis (Hutchings, 1993). For example, cocaine-related anorexia could compromise maternal nutrition (Hutchings, 1993). Cocaine also causes uterine artery

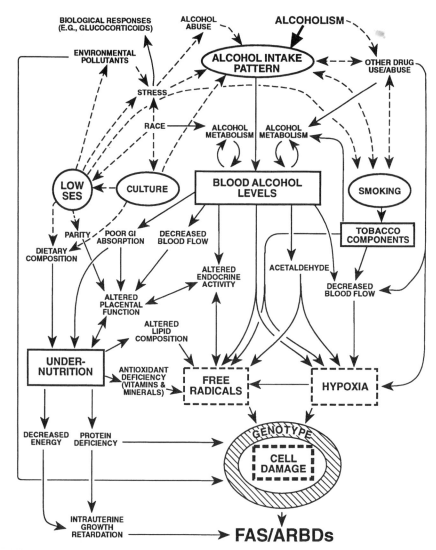

Figure 12.4. Schematic summary of relationships among permissive and provocative maternal risk factors underlying FAS/ARBEs. *Source*: E. L. Abel, & J. H. Hannigan, Maternal risk factors in Fetal Alcohol Syndrome: Provocative and permissive influences, *Neurotoxicology and Teratology* (1995), *17*, 445–462. Copyright 1995 by Elsevier Science, Ltd. Reprinted with permission of the publisher.

vasoconstriction, decreases oxyhemoglobin saturation, and exacerbates underlying hypoxic conditions (Hutchings, 1993).

Conclusion

The relationships between the various permissive and provocative factors and the proposed mechanisms involved in FAS/ARBEs are summarized in Figure 12.4.

To summarize Figure 12.4: Sociobehavioral *permissive factors* (inside the circles), such as alcohol intake patterns, low socioeconomic status (low SES), particular aspects of culture, and smoking behavior, are highly correlated among themselves and constitute an increased risk for FAS/ARBDs by provoking, that is, establishing an environment for and/or predisposing fetuses to, alcohol's direct, cellular teratogenic effects. The key biological *provocative factors* (inside the rectangles) are peak blood alcohol levels (BALs), undernutrition, and tobacco smoke components. Similar to the relationship between alcohol drinking pattern (permissive factor) and BALs (provocative factor), smoking is essentially a permissive and a provocative risk factor because (a) cigarette smoking is highly correlated with alcohol abuse and poor nutrition (permissive factor), and (b) because tobacco smoke exacerbates the effects of alcohol and directly impacts fetal development.

The various pathways by which the permissive and provocative risk factors act on the maternal/placental/fetal unit are indicated by the dotted-line arrows ($- - - \blacktriangleright$), which show recognized, sometimes bidirectional, associations among various environmental, demographic, and behavioral variables. For example, low SES is highly correlated with parity, smoking, and stress. The solid-line arrows ($\longrightarrow$) indicate biological relationships and physiological pathways. For example, binge drinking (alcohol intake pattern) increases peak BALs, which, in turn, leads to decreased placental blood flow, altered placental function, undernutrition, and so on.

Key teratogenic mechanisms are examined in depth in Chapter 13. Hypoxia and free-radical damage (broken rectangles), the two main mechanisms shown here, converge on the necessary proximal cause of FAS, cell damage, which leads to FAS/ARBE. The shaded circle ("genotype") around "cell damage" indicates that vulnerability to all of these factors is affected by individual genetically related susceptibilities to cellular perturbation.

CHAPTER 13

Mechanisms

In keeping with its characterization as a pattern of defects, FAS must be the result of alcohol abuse during more than one day or one period of pregnancy. This means in producing FAS, alcohol exposure must occur repeatedly throughout pregnancy, that is, during critical periods of organogenesis, as well as during periods of maturation and functional organization. Partial FAS, ARMs, or ARNDs, on the other hand, may occur as a result of isolated episodes of alcohol abuse, that is, bingeing. The one common thread linking all of these effects—the anatomical pathology as well as the growth retardation—is a reduction in cell populations. Although many substances have the potential for reducing cell populations, there are relatively few ways these reductions can occur during development. One way is cell death. Another is decreased cellular proliferation.

There is little doubt alcohol can cause cell death in the developing embryo/ fetus by either necrosis or aberrant apoptosis (Renau-Piqueras, Minagali, Guerri, & Baguena-Cervellera, 1987; Sancho-Tello, Renau-Piqueras, Baguena-Cervellera, & Guerri, 1987; Sulik et al., 1981). Necrotic cell death can occur at any age. Apoptotic cell death, on the other hand, is a naturally occurring phenomenon that is part of normal development. The constant renewal of skin cells is an example of apoptosis: Cells that migrate from deeper layers to the surface die naturally on the way, and the dead cells form the body's protective layer before sloughing away. In the case of menstruation, cells migrating to the uterine wall undergo apoptosis and are sloughed away in menstruation. In the developing nervous system, between 40% and 85% of the neurons produced during neurogenesis die prior to an individual's birth (Schwartz, 1991). The death of these cells provides our nervous system with considerable plasticity because the neuronal connection and pathways for every neuron are not necessarily predetermined. However, if apoptosis is accelerated or retarded, and repair does not spontaneously occur, aberrations in cell populations may occur. Premature apoptosis could result in clefts because when target cells are eliminated the pathways for migrating cells are disrupted (West et al., 1981); failure of the neural tube to close, for instance, may arise from the death of cells that normally migrate to the rim of the neural fold, thereby preventing them from fusing and closing the tube (Kotch & Sulik, 1992a).

Excessive cell death in the midline may be the reason FAS abnormalities take the form of short palpebral fissures, an indistinct philtrum, cleft lip and cleft palate, left-right asymmetries, and behavioral anomalies that involve the hippo-campus and corpus callosum. The kind of midline damage will depend on time and duration of toxicity. Genotypic predispositions, which increase vulnerabilities for alcohol-induced anomalies in certain areas, for example, microphthalmia in $C_{57}B1$ mice, are also involved. Whether it causes necrosis or premature apoptosis, alcohol's developmental effects are in large part traceable to local cell death. Localized cell death, in turn, interferes with the normal cascade of cellular events and results in abnormalities.

Morphologically, apoptotic cell death differs from necrosis. Apoptotic cell death is reflected in cellular shrinkage and a separation from neighboring cells. Internally, the cell seems to be boiling: blebs form briefly on the surface, dis-appear, and new blebs form shortly afterward. Organelles retain their structure, but the chromatin mixture of DNA and protein in the nucleus condenses at the internal surface of the nucleus. Subsequently, the nucleus breaks apart and the cell disinte-grates.

Necrosis, in contrast to apoptosis, is reflected in swelling and often results from oxygen deprivation. Oxygen deprivation shuts down the cell's ability to make energy; without energy cells are unable to maintain their integrity. Under extreme conditions, the neuronal cell's energy-driven ion channels become in-operative, pores open, and sodium ions rush into the neuron. The increased cellular levels of sodium alter osmotic gradients across the cell membrane, and water moves into the cell. Organelles within the cell, such as the mitochondria, Golgi apparatus, and lysosomes, swell and rupture, and the otherwise organized stacking of the cisternae of the rough endoplasmic reticulum becomes disorgan-ized. Other vacuoles are emptied of their contents, and only fragments remain visible. All of these signs of cell death have been observed in conjunction with prenatal alcohol exposure (Renau-Piqueras et al., 1987; Sancho-Tello et al., 1987; Sulik et al., 1981).

One reason damage to the hippocampus is such a common ARBE may be that excessive amounts of glutamate are released within the cell. Glutamate is the brain's major excitatory neurotransmitter and is especially concentrated in hippo-campal neurons (Collingridge & Lester, 1989). When released from its vesicles, it crosses the synaptic cleft and acts on the same receptors that it would if its release were due to ordinary neuronal stimulation. But, whereas the amount of glutamate that is normally released is carefully regulated, membrane disintegration results when relatively large quantities of the cell's glutamate is released into synapses.

The fact that glutamate receptors are densely located on the dendrites of hippocampal CA_1 pyramidal cells (Greenamyre, Olson, Penney, & Young, 1985) is another likely explanation for the selective vulnerability of the CA_1 area to alcohol-induced brain damage and the attendant memory dysfunction associated with prenatal alcohol exposure (see Chapter 10).

The neuronal response to glutamate is mediated by several different receptors described in terms of their reactions. Two of these receptors activate sodium and potassium channels; the third controls the calcium channel. The last is called the N-methyl-D-aspartate (NMDA) receptor, and it has been the focus of considerable research in recent years, especially with respect to "long-term potentiation," a phenomenon believed to underlie the cellular changes responsible for memory (see Chapter 10).

Glutamate receptors do not necessarily respond independently. Ordinarily, calcium is prevented from entering the cell by magnesium ions that fit into the channels used by calcium. The entry of sodium into the cell, however, causes neurons to become partially depolarized. In turn, partial depolarization reduces magnesium's blocking influence at calcium channels, and calcium then enters the neuron. Glutamate thus increases calcium entry into the cell by binding to the NMDA receptor or through depolarization.

Ordinarily, calcium acts as a "second messenger" by activating a number of cellular proteins, such as calmodulin, which amplifies calcium's signal. One such amplification effect is believed to be mediated by nitric oxide, which in turn also activates a number of protein kinases that control the cell cycle and influence protein synthesis. In cells involved in memory, nitric oxide may also act as a retrograde messenger, diffusing back to the presynaptic neuron and causing it to release more glutamate to prolong the activity that presumably involves consolidation of memory

Ordinarily, activation of NMDA receptors is a controlled process. At high levels of alcohol exposure, however, a much greater amount of calcium enters the cell because of the breakdown in ionic pumps. Following this increased calcium entry, calmodulin's effects may be greatly amplified and nitric oxide, which acts as a gaseous second messenger at low concentrations, may form the potent and relatively long-lived free radical, perosynitrite anion, in the presence of another free radical, superoxide (see later).

One way that the fetal brain protects itself from alcohol-induced glutamate damage is *down regulation*, a phenomenon through which the density of glutamate sensitive NMDA receptors are reduced in areas where they are highly concentrated, such as the hippocampus (Savage et al., 1991). This down regulation reduces the possibility that excitotoxicity will follow large increases in intracellular calcium. Such down regulation, however, is seen only when alcohol exposure occurs during the last part of gestation (Abdollah & Brien, 1995; Savage et al., 1991), protecting cells from necrotic cell death.

Although one study associated this down regulation with relatively low blood alcohol levels (39 mg%), sampling occurred as long as 9 hours after alcohol diets were offered, and therefore assessments did not reflect peak blood alcohol levels. Although the authors indulged in speculating on the significance of these changes in the context of "relatively low blood ethanol concentrations," these values do not reflect peak levels. As the authors themselves admitted, their blood alcohol data are at variance with virtually every other study in this or related areas (Savage et al., 1991).

Alcohol-related premature apoptosis is less readily demonstrable than necrosis, but it is suggested by enhanced death of neural crest cells in mice and chicks when exposure occurs during gastrulation (Cartwright & Smith, 1995a, b; Kotch & Sulik, 1992b; Sulik, Cook, & Webster, 1988; Webster et al., 1983), a developmental period corresponding to the third week of gestation in humans. Studies in chicks differ from those using mammalian animal models, however, in that alcohol only reduces populations of cranial neural crest cells but does not alter the migration of those cells that survive treatment (Cartwright & Smith, 1995a,b). Altered cell migration is characteristic of prenatal alcohol exposure in mammalian animal models (see Chapter 10).

Although apoptosis may underlie many ARBEs, this still does not explain how such death is initiated. One possibility is that the trophic growth factors that influence cellular development become unavailable or become overabundant. Alcohol's effects on one of these target-derived tropic factors, nerve growth factor (NGF), are too diverse to derive any consistent role for its involvement in ARBEs. For instance, alcohol has been found to both increase and decrease NGF activity (Heaton, Swanson, Paiva, & Walker, 1992; Walker, Lee, Heaton, Kuig, & Hunter, 1992) and to alter a cell's response to NGF (Heaton et al., 1992), resulting in inhibition (Dow & Riopelle, 1985) or stimulation of neurite outgrowth (Wooten & Ewald, 1991).

An alternative target-derived trophic factor with a possible involvement in ARBEs is glutamate (Reynolds & Brien, 1994), which, as noted earlier, is also believed to be intimately involved in cell necrosis. In addition to its role as the brain's main excitatory neurotransmitter, glutamate's neurotrophic role in the developing brain is related to its involvement in the regulation of dendritic growth, axonal growth, and synaptogenesis (McDonald & Johnston, 1990). Although these events occur considerably later in brain development, overstimulation of glutamate's receptors—the NMDA complex—during early development could result in apoptosis and necrosis. Even if glutamate proved to be a mediating factor, however, this still does not explain how alcohol initiates its release from its vacuoles.

In the remainder of this chapter, I attribute the initiation of the mechanisms that ultimately mediate event(s) in necrosis or apoptosis to two conditions: free radical formation and decreased cellular oxygenation. The assumption is that these conditions "provoke" more specific mechanisms, depending on the developmental stage at which such "provocation" occurs. In other words, a dynamic relationship between general mechanism and developmental susceptibility is presumed to account for the various phenotypic outcomes associated with maternal alcohol abuse during pregnancy.

The reason for the emphasis on decreased cellular oxygenation and free radical formation is that their involvement in cellular function is indisputable. These are general biological influences. As such, their influence extends beyond embryonic or fetal development. Hypothesizing their involvement in ARBEs not only allows for a biologically parsimonious explanation of ARBEs, but also enables us to relate information from other biological studies to those involving embryonic and fetal development. Proposing two mechanisms, however, is not meant to imply an either-or dichotomy in which only one mechanism is involved in cell damage at a particular time. In most cases, it is difficult to determine whether cell damage is precipitated by changes in cellular oxygenation by excessive free radical generation, or, most likely, by both because reperfusion of previously oxygen starved cells typically results in a large increase in free radical production, so a certain redundancy is to be expected.

Cellular Metabolism

Before discussing the involvement of altered oxygenation or oxygen free radical formation in ARBEs, a review of some fundamentals of cell metabolism is worthwhile to place these mechanisms in their normal biological context.

Respiration, through which oxygen is taken into the body and carbon dioxide is given off in exchange, is a normal everyday occurrence. Physiologically, respiration is the process by which the oxygen that is taken into the body is used by every cell to generate the metabolic energy from organic fuels that it needs to carry out its activities.

The conversion of organic fuels to energy takes place in the mitochondria, where electrons in a very high energy state are generated from organic fuels, such as carbohydrates and fatty acids, as part of an intricate metabolic process called the Krebs, or citric acid, cycle. In the course of this reaction, hydrogen atoms are removed from these substrates. These hydrogen atoms lose electrons, which are passed along a chain of electron carriers called cytochromes. The final step in this chain involves the transfer of these electrons to molecular oxygen, resulting in the formation of water and carbon dioxide. During this transport process, the electrons impart some of their energy to adenosine diphosphate (ADP), enabling it to take up a phosphate molecule to form adenosine triphosphate (ATP) in a process called oxidative phosphorylation. In the course of glucose's combustion each glucose molecule produces 38 high-energy ATP molecules. The energy stored in these

ATP molecules is then used to fuel the cell's internal activities. If this fueling system is impaired, the cell will be unable to function in the same way that an automobile will become nonfunctional if it runs out of gas or if its internal combustion engine becomes dysfunctional.

The reason oxygen is so critical in this process is that it acts as the "magnet" that attracts electrons through the various cytochromes as they impart energy to ADP. If there were no oxygen in the cell, the electron train would not be able to run because the electrons would not be funneled along a common pathway. Anaerobic pathways would then have to be found for creating energy. This sometimes happens, but these alternative sources are soon used up, the cell quickly loses its ability to function, and destabilizing forces that destroy it are set in motion.

Decreased Oxygenation

The standard clinical marker for anaerobic metabolism is lactic acid in the blood. This condition is a common occurrence in alcoholism (Cate, Hedrick, & Morin, 1983). It is not necessarily present in every mother who gives birth to a child with FAS, but it has been noted in some. Lactic acidosis is also found in maternal blood in newborn primates, sheep, and rats (Abel, 1996a; Mukherjee & Hodgen, 1982; Reynolds et al., 1996a) following maternal alcohol administration, so it is not a unique or uncommon occurrence in the context of maternal alcohol exposure.

Because the embryo/fetus is entirely dependent on the mother's blood for its oxygen, any conditions that impair that blood supply, reduces its oxygen content, or decreases its ability to give up that oxygen have the potential for reducing the oxygen a fetus needs to carry out its vital functions.

Decreased blood flow to the uterus or interruption of umbilical blood flow are an unlikely cause of ARBEs. For one thing, alcohol increases blood flow to the uterus rather than reducing it (Reynolds et al., 1996). Decreased fetal oxygenation due to interrupted umbilical blood flow is also unlikely. Although infusion of a very high dose of alcohol (3 g/kg) over a 2-minute period precipitates a very marked collapse of the umbilical vasculature and subsequent acidosis and hypoxemia (Mukherjee & Hodgen, 1982), such a sudden massive infusion of alcohol is unrealistic (Reynolds & Brien, 1995). Even binge drinking over a short period of time would result in a much more gradual exposure to alcohol. For example, exposure to an equivalent amount of alcohol (3 g/kg) for a 60-kg (120-lb) woman would involve an unrealistic consumption of about 14 drinks—in less than a 1-hour period.

Although human umbilical cord arteries can be constricted in vitro by relatively low concentrations of alcohol—equivalent to BALs of 10 mg/dl (Altura et al., 1983; Savoy-Moore, Dobrowski, Cheng, Abel, & Sokol, 1989)—measurements of umbilical blood flow in pregnant women, using Doppler ultrasound, indicated that at blood alcohol levels of around 40 mg%, umbilical blood flow is not compromised in humans (Erskine & Ritchie, 1986). Administration of the same amount of alcohol as that used to produce collapse of umbilical vessels, but given as six doses of 0.5 g/kg rather than as a single bolus over an 8-hour period, produced minimal changes in fetal arterial blood gases or acid-base status (Patrick et al., 1988; Richardson, Patric, Bosquet, Homan, & Brien, 1985; Smith, Coles, Lancaster, Fernhoff, & Falek, 1989).

Whereas alcohol does not appear to interfere with blood supply to the embryo/fetus, blood flow within the embryo/fetus itself, especially in the brain, does occur. A dose of 1 g/kg (equivalent to about five drinks for a 60-kg woman) infused over a 1-hour period, for example, produced a decrease of 41% in cerebral blood flow in term sheep fetuses (Richardson et al., 1985). Four doses of 0.5 g/kg administered over a 5-hour period also significantly reduced blood flow to the fetal brain (Richardson, Patrick, Homan, Carmichael, & Brien, 1987). This decrease in brain blood flow resulted in a net reduction in cerebral oxygen delivery (Richardson et al., 1987) and decreased fetal EEG activity (Patrick et al., 1985). Petechial hemorrhages similar to those observed in human fetuses following hypoxia have also been observed within the lateral ventricles of alcohol-exposed mouse fetuses (Kotkoskie & Norton, 1990).

Although blood flow to the fetus is not compromised, the embryo/fetus could still experience decreased cellular oxygenation if considerable oxygen is removed from the mother's blood during hepatic metabolism of alcohol (Lieber, 1991). Although lactic acidosis is a byproduct of anaerobic metabolism, the increase in blood acidity that it produces increases the readiness with which oxygen is dissociated from blood, thereby counteracting the condition that gave rise to it. To further increase oxygen availability, a metabolic acidosis also triggers hyperventilation, which increases the amount of carbon dioxide removed from the blood relative to that normally produced by the cell. The loss of carbon dioxide lowers plasma arterial PCO_2, disturbing the equilibrium between carbonic acid and formation of hydrogen and bicarbonate ions. As the hydrogen ion content is lowered, the acidity is decreased and blood pH is raised. These kinds of changes (illustrated in Figure 13.1) have been seen in pregnant rats and sheep following alcohol administration (Abel, 1996a; Urfer, Fouron, Bard, & DeMuylder, 1984).

If hyperventilation is persistent, the increase in blood pH it produces can overcompensate for the conditions it is intended to stabilize. Instead of being slightly less acidic, the blood becomes alkaline, a condition called *respiratory alkalosis*. The consequence of this alkalosis is a shift in the oxygen dissociation curve to the left, a phenomenon called the Bohr effect. As a result of the Bohr effect, hemoglobin has an increased affinity for oxygen, which results in less oxygen unloading and additional cellular hypoxia, even if blood oxygen content or saturation were normal. The respiratory alkalosis resulting from hyperventilation

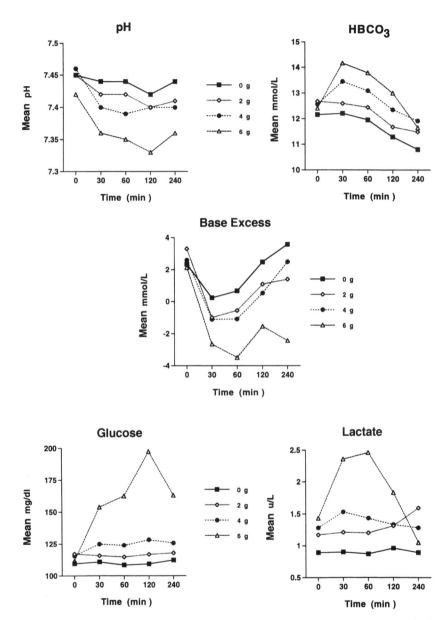

Figure 13.1. Effects of alcohol on blood pH, HCO_3, base excess, glucose, and lactate concentration in female rats. Results for pregnant and nonpregnant rats were not different and were therefore combined. *Source*: E. L. Abel, Alcohol-induced changes in blood gases, glucose, and lactate in pregnant and nonpregnant rats. Alcohol (1996), *14* p. 27. Copyright 1996 by Elsevier Science Ltd. Reprinted with permission of the publisher.

can also have a vasoconstrictive effect on arterioles, causing the decrease in cerebral blood flow and cerebral oxygen tension previously mentioned.

Hyperventilation also occurs as a response to stress, anxiety, tension, anger, or restlessness (Magarian, 1982). The condition is prevalent in about 27% of the general female population and is most common during the peak reproductive years (Magarian, 1982). In chronic hyperventilators, respiratory alkalosis is maintained by subtle and persistent increases in the respiratory rate or occasional deep breathing (Magarian, 1982). Persistent hyperventilation is also associated with certain organic conditions, such as cirrhosis (Magarian, 1982). Maintenance of a alkalotic state associated with hyperventilation would itself have the effect of decreasing oxygen release in blood. If chronic alcohol consumption exacerbated this condition, even in the absence of cirrhosis, it might constitute an additional factor contributing to ARBEs.

While any of these effects would result in a global impairment in cellular oxygenation, each would have a much greater impact on organs with very high metabolic rates, like the brain. Specific areas within the brain, such as the hippocampus and cerebellum, which have especially high metabolic rates, would experience greater damage from alcohol than cells in other areas of the brain (Jorgensen & Diemer, 1982). Likewise, cell populations within these areas, such as the pyramidal and Purkinje cells in the hippocampus and cerebellum, respectively, would be more susceptible to alcohol-related hypoxic episodes compared with metabolically less active cells, such as those in the dentate gyrus or cerebellum. In other words, while all cells are vulnerable to alcohol's toxicity, some are more vulnerable than others.

Another of the mechanisms the body uses to deal with alcohol-related changes in cellular oxygenation is the release of a subfamily of prostaglandins (PGs) from the placenta.

Prostaglandins are long-chain, fatty acid metabolites of arachidonic acid. PGs and, in particular, levels of the PGE_2 subfamily of PGs, are increased in the fetal brain, cerebrospinal fluid, and blood following maternal alcohol administration (Phillips, Henderson, & Schenker, 1989).

Since alcohol does not increase synthesis or release of PGE_2 or alter its catabolism in the fetal brain in vitro (Sinervo, Smith, Bocking, Pachick, & Brien, 1992), the increase in fetal PGE_2 in the brain following alcohol exposure or hypoxia is most likely due to its release from the placenta, the major source of PGs during pregnancy (Bocking, Carmichael, Abdollah, Simenvo, & Smith, 1994), and its subsequent transfer across the blood–brain barrier (Reynolds & Brien, 1995).

Although PGs can cause fetal anomalies (Persaud, 1978), they only do so when they are administered in doses up to 1 million times normal serum levels. Sodium chloride and water are also teratogenic when administered in unrealistic amounts, but, like prostaglandins, they are essential for normal bodily functioning. The fact that PGEs may be teratogenic at unrealistically high physiological levels is therefore irrelevant. At normal physiological concentrations, PGs clearly have an essential role in normal fetal development, because drugs such as indomethacin, aspirin, and ibuprofen, which inhibit cyclo-oxygenase, can be teratogenic (Klein, Scott, Clark, & Wilson, 1981; Peterson, 1985). The fact that PGE_2 levels are elevated in response to alcohol exposure and hypoxia suggests that PGE_2 has a cytoprotective effect with respect to attenuating damage due to these insults. The protective effect may arise from its vasodilatory activity. PGE_2 levels, for example, are elevated during ischemia to restore the blood flow reduced by the actions of peroxide-stimulated thromboxanes (Sardesai, 1992). PGE_2 also attenuates the fetal acidemia that occurs during hypoxia, thereby reducing the potential liberation of iron from organelles and free radical formation.

Consequences of Impaired Oxygenation

Embryological and fetal growth and development are dependent on cellular proliferation and differentiation. Because these processes are in turn dependent on protein synthesis, protein synthesis has been a major focus of alcohol's effects on the fetus.

Protein synthesis is a multistage process, which involves the incorporation of amino acids into the endoplasmic reticulum, their synthesis into protein, transport to the Golgi apparatus, glycosylation, and transport to their final destinations. The net result of these various processes is fetal protein synthesis. All of these steps in protein synthesis require energy. Regardless of how oxygen supply to cells is impaired, any such impairment will result in a decrease in ATP, the cell's primary source of energy, and therefore a decrease in protein synthesis. As long as the oxygen supply is reduced, rather than cut off, the reduction process involved in generating ATP will continue, albeit at a less than optimal rate.

Amino acid deficiencies are common in alcoholics (Lieber, 1991), although such generalizations may pertain primarily to low SES alcoholics, because they are as a group the most widely studied. If alcohol-abusing mothers consume less than optimal amounts of the amino acids required to support optimal fetal protein synthesis, this could be one way alcohol abuse indirectly contributes to fetal growth retardation. Another possibility is that maternal diet is adequate, but active amino acid transport across the placenta and into cerebral, cardiac, and hepatic ribosomes is less affected due to decreased ATP synthesis.

Although amino acid uptake and transport by human placental cotyledons in culture is not inhibited by alcohol (Fisher & Karl, 1996; Schenker, Dicke, Johnson, Hays, & Henderson, 1989) transport of certain amino acids in rats and nonhuman primates is reduced (Fisher et al., 1983, 1985; Henderson et al., 1981, 1982) due to decreased placental blood flow (Falconer, 1990) or decreased efficiency of energy-dependent Na-K-ATPase membrane-transport processes (Fisher, Duffy, & Atkinson, 1986).

Alcohol also reduces incorporation of amino acids into cerebral, cardiac, and hepatic ribosomes, and their subsequent transcription into protein in animals (Dreosti et al., 1981; Henderson, Hoyumpa, Rothschild, & Schenker, 1980; Rawat, 1979), and it interferes with their glycosylation (Renau-Piqueras, Sancho-Tello, Cervellera, & Guerri, 1989). Animal models that circumvent placental transport, for example, chicks and embryos grown in culture, likewise point to the direct effects of alcohol on protein synthesis at the embryo/fetal level (Brown, Goulding, & Fabro, 1979; Pennington, Boyd, Kalmus, & Wilson, 1983).

Concomitant alcohol-related inhibition in DNA synthesis, as reflected in decreased ^{3}H-thymidine incorporation into fetal rat DNA (Dreosti et al., 1981; Henderson et al., 1980) and/or an increase in the length of the mitotic cycle, may also result in delayed transcription and translational processes (Rawat, 1975, 1985). Decreased DNA synthesis is a well-known cause of cell death (Langman & Cardell, 1978), and altered DNA synthesis during active periods of cellular development could explain selective cell death (Kotkoskie & Norton, 1990; Miller, 1986; Miller & Muller, 1989). Because only cells undergoing DNA synthesis would be affected by alcohol, a minority of cells might die. Alcohol's selective effects on brain cells would thus depend on when during their neurogenesis alcohol exposure occurred (O'Shea & Kaufman, 1981).

Effects on gene function and activity might likewise arise from interference with the methylation process that activates or suppresses DNA-protein binding, thereby altering gene expression (Holliday, 1987). Because embryonic DNA is highly methylated, substances that inhibit the methylation process have the potential to alter gene expression and development. Alcohol alters the activity of enzymes involved in DNA methylation (Espina, Lima, Lieber, & Garro, 1988), and prenatal alcohol exposure can result in hypomethylation of fetal DNA (Garro, McBeth, & Lima, 1991). However, altered DNA methylation has not as yet been shown to be a causal factor in alcohol's teratogenicity.

Free-Radical Damage

Free radicals are molecules with one or more unpaired electrons. Because of their unpaired electron configurations, these molecules are highly unstable and reactive, becoming more stable by either removing an electron from, or donating an unpaired electron to, other molecules. This action, in turn, generates a chain of similar responses, as each newly formed radical attempts to satisfy its thirst for an electron, until these radical species are neutralized. The substrates for this disruptive chain reaction include lipids, proteins, receptors, DNA, and so on.

Neural crest cells—those from which craniofacial features and CNS structures are derived—are particularly sensitive to alcohol exposure (Davis et al., 1990). As shown in Figure 13.2, alcohol is capable of inducing reactive oxygen radicals in these cells.

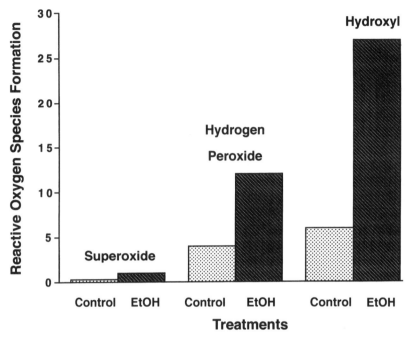

Figure 13.2. Effects of 12-hour exposure (in vitro) to EtOH (0.2%) on production of superoxide (nmol/min/2 × 10⁴ cells), hydrogen peroxide (pmol × 10²/min/2 × 10⁴ cells), and hydroxyl radicals (pmol × 10²/min/2 × 10⁴ cells) by chick neural crest cells treated for 12 hrs. (Modified from Davis et al., 1990, pp. 277–293.)

Figure 13.3 shows that alcohol-induced oxygen radicals are a likely cause of cell death in the neural crest because the toxicity of these radicals is attenuated when superoxide dismutase is added to the medium and, by implication, malformations.

Cotreatment with superoxide dismutase (300 units/ml) is also able to reduce the incidence of alcohol-induced (0.5 g%) neural-tube closure failures in mouse embryos in vitro by 35% (Kotch, Chen, & Sulik, 1995).

Whereas oxygen is essential for normal metabolic cell function, the same oxygenated free radicals produced in neural crest cells by alcohol are constantly being produced in the course of normal metabolism as electrons shuttling along the metabolic chain in mitochondria and are taken up by molecular oxygen in the intermediatory phase prior to conversion to water (see earlier).

The first of the free radicals formed as a byproduct of cellular metabolism is the superoxide radical. In aqueous environments, superoxide may then be converted by superoxide dismutase into hydrogen peroxide and oxygen. The more

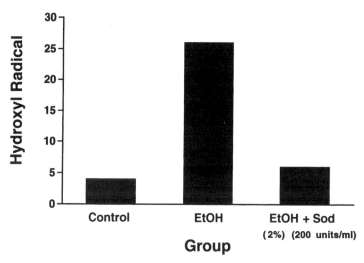

Figure 13.3. Effects of alcohol (0.2%) and alcohol plus superoxide (200 units/ml) on hydroxyl radical formation. (Modified from Davis et al., 1990, p. 286.)

acidic the cell's pH, the more rapidly that this change occurs (Hooper, Harding, Deaton, & Thorburn, 1992). This relationship assumes a new importance in light of previous remarks concerning the formation of lactic acid in the cell during periods of anaerobic metabolism and the role of PGE_2 in attenuating such activity.

The formation of hydrogen peroxide does not itself result in further toxicity because it has no unpaired electrons. But hydrogen peroxide is very water soluble, a condition that enables it to cross membranes very easily. As a result, it can diffuse throughout the cell. If unbound transition metal ions, such as ferrous iron, are present in the cell, they will remove a single electron from hydrogen peroxide to create their more stable ferric form. In so doing, hydrogen peroxide will be converted into the hydroxyl radical, one of the most reactive of all the radicals formed in the body. The hydroxyl radical will strip an electron from any bio-molecule in its vicinity, setting a chain reaction of molecular destruction in motion unless it is stopped.

Because of the potential for ferrous iron to generate hydroxyl radicals, iron's availability to cells is highly restricted in the body. The duodenal and jejunal mucosa, for instance, restrict its absorption into the circulatory system. The freedom of whatever is absorbed into the circulation is further restricted by virtue of its being bound to a considerable extent by protein. About two-thirds of absorbed iron is present in hemoglobin and another 10% in myoglobin (Spatz, 1992). Transferrin, the plasma transport protein, tightly binds ferric iron at neutral pH. Because it is only partially saturated, virtually all of the iron in plasma is bound and is in the unreactive ferric state.

Decreased iron binding will result in altered levels of carbohydrate-deficient transferrin and will elevate levels of free iron in the blood. Within the cell, ferric iron is bound by the related protein, ferritin. However, when protein consumption is very low, cells are damaged, or iron is released from hemoglobin, transferrin, or ferritin in response to lowered tissue pH, free iron will be liberated.

Cirrhosis is associated with marked disturbances in iron homeostasis, resulting in high serum levels in the liver (Sanchez, Casas & Rama, 1988), which may be one of the reasons cirrhosis is associated with a large number of perinatal problems, including FAS (see earlier). High levels of free iron are potentially damaging because, as previously noted, in its free state, iron can catalyze the generation of the highly damaging hydroxyl radical. One way in which iron's damaging effects may be minimized, however, is if the alcoholic also takes aspirin or indomethacin regularly, because both are iron-chelating agents (De Groot & Littauer, 1989). Organs such as the brain are especially vulnerable because extracellular cerebrospinal fluid has no iron-binding capacity (Spatz, 1992), rendering neurons and glia more vulnerable to an iron-catalyzed attack from free radicals, such as the hydroxyl radical.

How alcohol produces increases in free radical formation is still unclear. Alcohol does not generate free radicals in the course of its own metabolism via cystolic alcohol dehydrogenase or aldehyde dehydrogenase (Dianzani, 1988). Although the microsomal enzyme-oxidizing system (MEOS) is also involved in the metabolism of alcohol in adults and is a major source for producing reactive oxygen radicals (Lieber, 1991), the P_{450} 2E1 gene responsible for alcohol's metabolism in this system is not expressed in the human fetus (Hakkola et al., 1994) and cannot be detected in either the rat (Song, Gelboin, Park, Yang, & Gonzalez, 1986) or mouse fetus (Deltour et al., 1996). The absence of this gene means that the source of oxygen free radicals likely involved in producing ARBEs in the embryo must also involve some mechanism other than the MEOS system.

One such alternative may involve the peroxynitrite anion, formed when excessive nitric oxide is produced as part of the cell's second messenger system (see earlier), reacting with the superoxide radical or other radicals to produce the hydroxyl radical or other secondary oxidants. The conversion of nitric oxide to a radical or secondary radical involves excessive stimulation of NMDA receptors by glutamate (see earlier); areas with high levels of nitric oxide synthase suffer greater damage than others because of the formation of these nitric acid radicals.

The blood alcohol levels required to bring about a marked increase in free radicals are very high. In the study describing alcohol's effects on neural crest cells (see earlier), concentrations of 200 mg% were employed. A similar study employed alcohol concentrations of 500 mg% (Kotch et al., 1995). A study demonstrating in vivo alcohol-induced oxidative stress in rat embryos had blood alcohol levels over 0.3g% (Henderson, Devi, Perez, & Schenker, 1995). In virtually every in vitro as well as in vivo study, concentrations exceed 0.1g%, and exposure occurs for about the equivalent of 1½ days in the human (Kotch & Sulik, 1992a). These very high concentrations are typically associated with chronic bingelike patterns of consumption (permissive factor), and, as previously indicated, the concentrations are provocative of free oxygen radical formation resulting in lipid peroxidation.

Antioxidant Defense Mechanisms

Usually there is a balance between the free radicals produced through normal metabolism and the body's antioxidant defenses. However, if the cell is called on to deal with increased production of oxygen free radicals resulting from alcohol exposure, the balance will be shifted in favor of the radicals, and cell damage will be more likely to occur.

The cell's protective mechanisms take the form of nonenzymatic antioxidants that act as free radical "scavengers" and endogenous antioxidative enzymes, such as superoxide dismutase and catalase. Antioxidants, such as ascorbic acid (Vitamin C), α-tocopherol (Vitamin E), and β-carotene, quench or trap radicals. Vitamin C, for instance, is located in the cytosol and quenches radicals, thereby keeping them from reaching the cell's membranes. Vitamin E, located in the cell membrane, prevents or markedly attenuates lipid peroxidation by acting as an electron donor, thereby transforming free radicals into more stable materials. Deficiencies in antioxidant nutrients, especially vitamin E and vitamin C, can therefore potentiate alcohol's toxic effects throughout the body.

One condition associated with decreases in reserves of antioxidant nutrients is smoking, which increases maternal and fetal concentrations of free radicals (Niki, Minamisawa, Oikawa, & Komuro, 1993; Pryor & Stone, 1993). These concentrations have the effect of depleting antioxidants, such as vitamins A, C, and E, and antioxidant enzymes that scavenge these tobacco-related free radicals (Haste et al., 1990). Smoking also contributes to free radical formation by inhibiting absorption of antioxidant vitamins (Norkus, Hsu, & Cehelsky, 1987).

As a result of the depleted antioxidant reserves and reduced intake of antioxidants related to smoking, the potential for scavenging alcohol-generated radicals is greatly compromised in smokers. This may account for the additivity or synergism between alcohol and smoking in producing FAS/ARBDs (Abel & Hannigan, 1995b).

Dietary deficiencies can also affect antioxidant enzymes because they rely on essential nutrients, such as zinc and manganese (superoxide dismutase), selenium (glutathione peroxidase), riboflavin (glutathione reductase), and niacin (NADH/NADPH), for their activation. As a result, the normally short intracellular life of radicals is prolonged, and this increases the likelihood of extensive cell death.

Experiments attempting to verify the role of dietary factors in ARBEs have been only marginally successful. The reason, in many cases, is an artifactual methodology that assumes dietary changes can produce immediate effects.

Although vitamin E has been shown to provide some measure of protection against alcohol-related lipid peroxidation (Davis et al., 1990), increases in membrane levels of vitamin E in the adult require considerable time for accrual. Therefore, it is unlikely that supplementation beginning in pregnancy will have much of a protective effect with respect to alcohol-induced radicals. Nor is it surprising that vitamin E supplementation does not attenuate alcohol's in utero effects under adequately nourished conditions (Tanaka et al., 1988) because the cell membrane is already saturated with vitamin E. The fact that vitamin E levels in cell membranes are not immediately responsive to dietary changes means that decreased vitamin E in the diet also has less of an exacerbating effect on alcohol-related free radical damage if it also begins with pregnancy. The fact that nearly all animal models begin treatments at pregnancy means that they are basically artifactual—they do not model conditions in the human that exist prior to pregnancy.

Experimental diets commonly used for administering alcohol to animals may also obscure the search for mechanisms of action. The Lieber-DiCarli liquid diet contains five times more vitamin E than what is recommended for growth of mice. This diet also contains 45 times more vitamin A, and 10 times more vitamin D (Watzl et al., 1993). Although chronic alcohol abuse in humans would deplete tissue reserves of these vitamins, this would not happen in animal models using these and other diets because they overcompensate for various nutrients.

By far, most of the attention relating to dietary substances in the context of modifying alcohol's in utero effects has been directed at zinc. Because zinc transport is not significantly reduced in human placental cotyledons by alcohol even at very high concentrations (Beer et al., 1992), and zinc levels in fetal brain tissue in nonhuman primates are not affected by maternal alcohol treatment (Fisher et al., 1988), deficiencies in fetal zinc levels associated with maternal alcohol consumption are unlikely to be due to any effects of alcohol on placental zinc transport (Fisher & Karl, 1996). This means that any role zinc may have in influencing ARBEs must be the result of preexisting zinc status. The corollary to this conclusion is that any zinc deficiency related to FAS/ARBE is probably of long standing duration rather than suddenly coincident with pregnancy. An underlying zinc deficiency coupled with heavy alcohol consumption is a much more likely clinical scenario than one in which a zinc deficiency occurs coincidental with drinking during pregnancy.

Although zinc supplementation in relatively well nourished animals has mixed effects in attenuating ARBDs (Fisher, Alcock, Amirian, & Altshuler, 1988; Tanaka et al., 1988), zinc supplementation of diets with an underlying zinc deficiency has the potential for attenuating ARBEs. One such example is a study in which pregnant animals were fed liquid alcohol diets. One group had their diets supplemented with a level of zinc above that recommended for their diets; another's diet had a zinc content below the recommended level. The third group consumed a diet with an amount of zinc normally fed to them. Daily zinc intake for the high-level group was an average 182 micrograms compared to 7 micrograms for the low zinc-supplemented diet. As shown in Figure 13.4, fetuses exposed to the combination of alcohol and a long standing low zinc diet had a higher rate of resorptions and a higher rate of external malformations than those exposed to either alcohol or zinc alone or the combination of alcohol and a high zinc diet (Keppen, Pysher, & Rennert, 1985).

A situation in which alcohol is imposed on an underlying zinc deficiency would seem to reflect the real-life situation vis-à-vis FAS because alcoholism and undernutrition precede pregnancy rather than occur only during that condition. A critically low zinc content in the body combined with a relatively high alcohol exposure may then "provoke" the cellular changes that result in abnormal development. This hypothesis would account for the higher incidence of FAS in women characterized by low socioeconomic status (see Chapter 11) because, as previously noted, foods rich in zinc products are more costly than other foods (Dreosti, 1981). Women of low socioeconomic status tend to have lower dietary zinc intakes (Hambridge et al., 1983) and lower serum zinc levels than more affluent women (Flynn et al., 1981). The corollary to this conclusion is that zinc supplementation should only be effective in reducing ARBDs in animals (and by extension in women) whose daily zinc intake is far below recommended levels.

Embryonic cells are especially vulnerable to free radical stress because they possess fewer active antioxidative defense systems, such as superoxide dismutase, and antioxidants compared with adults (Davis et al., 1990; Dreosti, 1993). Those defense mechanisms may be rendered even more inefficient as a result of poor nutrition.

The CNS is more vulnerable to alcohol than other systems because of its high metabolic rate, which not only demands more oxygenation, but also can be expected to produce more free oxygen radicals in the course of that heightened metabolic state. CNS regions, such as the hippocampus and cerebellum, with their especially high metabolic rates (see earlier), are particularly susceptible to free radical damage because they have low levels of free-radical scavenging enzymes and antioxidants relative to other areas of the brain (LeBel, Odunze, Adams, & Bondy, 1989).

Increased vulnerability of certain cell populations to alcohol may also occur because of the physical structure of their membranes. The CNS, for instance, is especially prone to lipid peroxidation because it has a much higher content of peroxidizable substrates, for example, polyunsaturated fatty acids, than do other organs in the body.

Because cell membranes are a primary site of alcohol's actions and lipid peroxidation, membrane composition may influence alcohol's actions on the cell.

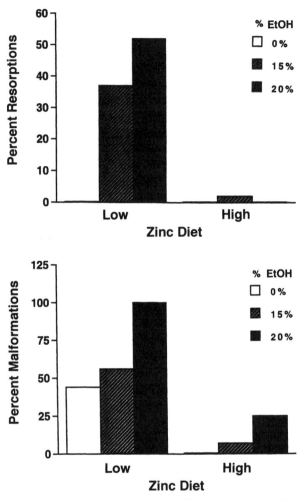

Figure 13.4. Effects of high- and low-zinc diets in combination with prenatal alcohol exposure on resorptions (A) and malformations (B) in mice. (Modified from Keppen et al., 1985, p. 945.)

Since there is a close relationship between the fatty acid content of maternal diets and brain fatty acid composition in offspring (Wainwright, Huang, Mills, Ward, & McCutcheon, 1989; Wainwright et al., 1990), maternal diets high in saturated fats may have the effect of decreasing susceptibility to alcohol's destabilizing effects (Goldstein, 1986).

Although long-term dietary intake of saturated fats may be unhealthy as far as maternal cardiovascular fitness is concerned, epidemiological and experimental studies have suggested that saturated fats can be cytoprotective against alcohol's effects on liver cells (Nanji, Mendenhall, & French, 1989). Dietary saturated fats may also be cytoprotective for fetal development because membranes with a high ratio of saturated to polyunsaturated fatty acids would not only be less susceptible to the "fluidizing" effects of alcohol, they would also be less susceptible to lipid peroxidation (Chautan et al., 1990).

Dietary saturated fat was shown to be a factor in ARBEs by using an animal model in which female rats were fed a standardized laboratory diet or diets high in saturated fats or high in polyunsaturated fats for several weeks prior to pregnancy. After pregnancy, the rats continued to receive these diets along with alcohol.

If mothers had consumed the regular laboratory diet, their offspring exhibited the increased motor activity characteristic of animals prenatally exposed to alcohol. Alcohol-exposed offspring whose mothers had consumed the high-saturated-fat diet, however, were less active than controls, while offspring whose mothers consumed the polyunsaturated fat diet did not differ from their controls (Abel & Reddy, 1997). (For these results, see Figure 13.5.)

The apparently lower incidence/prevalence rates for FAS in England and Italy compared with Germany and the United States (see Chapter 11) could be due in part to culturally or ethnically related dietary preferences. Italy and Great Britain have about 18% lower per capita intakes of polyunsaturated fats (~13.5 g/day) than Germany (26.0 g/day) or the United States (~16.3 g/day) (Liu et al., 1979). Germany, Great Britain, and the United States, on the other hand, have comparable intakes of saturated and monosaturated fatty acids and cholesterol (Liu et al., 1979).

Because the proportion of saturated to unsaturated fats in the diet is higher for Italians and Britons than Americans and Germans (Liu et al., 1979), developing fetuses in Italy and England could also have a higher saturated to unsaturated fatty-acid–cell-membrane ratio, rendering them less susceptible to alcohol-related cell peroxidation.

Other Mechanisms

In proposing that decreased cellular oxygenation and free radical formation initiate cellular events that lead to ARBEs, a number of secondary mechanisms were alluded to. Some of these secondary mechanisms were described in detail; others were mentioned only in passing. (The remainder of this chapter examines some of these latter mechanisms, along with those alluded to in earlier chapters of this book.)

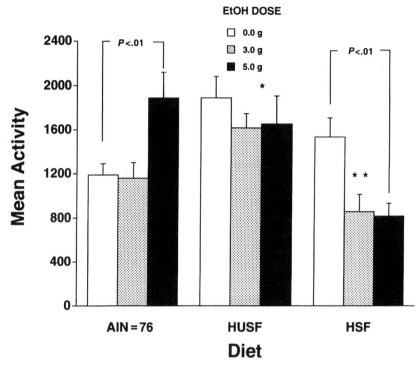

Figure 13.5. Effects of prenatal exposure to alcohol (0, 3.0, or 5 g/kg) and AIN-76 diet, high unsaturated fat (HUSF) diet, and high saturated fat (HSF) diet on ambulation in offspring at 20 days of age (*n* = 10–18/group). Data for males and females have been combined. *Source*: E. L. Abel & P. P. Reddy, Prenatal high saturated fat diet modifies behavioral effects of prenatal alcohol exposure in rats, *Alcohol* (1997), *14* p. 27. Copyright 1997 by Elsevier Science Ltd. Reprinted by permission of the publisher.

Retinoic Acid

Retinoic acid, a metabolite of retinol more commonly known as vitamin A, is a morphogen during embryonic development. As such, retinoic acid is essential for development; deficiencies inhibit embryogenesis, while excesses can lead to birth defects. These effects have been linked to retinoic acid's stimulation of a retinoic-acid gene called homeobox b-1 (Hoxb-1) whose expression occurs early in development (De Luca & Ross, 1996).

Alcohol and retinol are metabolized by the same dehydrogenase enzymes. While ADH metabolizes alcohol to acetaldehyde, it metabolizes *retinol* (which is actually an alcohol) to another aldehyde, *retinal*. Because the same enzyme system is involved, some researchers have hypothesized that one way alcohol produces its teratogenic effects is by preferential metabolism, which results in inhibition of retinoic acid synthesis during embryonic morphogenesis (Duester, 1991; Grummer, Langhough, & Zachman, 1993; Keir, 1991; Pullarkat, 1991).

Alcohol is preferentially metabolized over retinol and other substances for several important reasons, not the least of which is that alcohol is potentially toxic, and, therefore, its detoxification has priority. Because preferential metabolism could produce an imbalance in retinoic acid concentration, and retinoic acid itself can produce some of the same effects as prenatal alcohol exposure, for example, intrauterine growth retardation, CNS anomalies, and limb defects, competitive inhibition of retinoic acid metabolism could be a possible explanation for alcohol's teratogenic effects.

Although the argument for competitive enzyme inhibition was originally based on observations in adult mammalian tissues, such as the liver, a recent study reported a significant inhibition in retinoic acid production in 7.5-day-old mouse embryos exposed to alcohol in vitro (Deltour et al., 1996). No significant inhibition was observed in day 6.5 or day 8.5 embryos, and in day 7.5 embryos, inhibition only occurred with alcohol concentrations of 100 mM (Deltour et al., 1996), a concentration comparable to a blood alcohol level of about 500 mg%.

Although this study provided supporting evidence for the hypothesis that alcohol's teratogenic effects could involve inhibition of retinoic acid, the hypothesis was nevertheless still problematic because there was no way of knowing whether the inhibition was considerable enough to affect subsequent development. (This is the same problem of statistical versus biological significance frequently mentioned in this book.)

The results of a related study that also evaluated alcohol-related inhibition of retinoic acid production in embryos, in fact, suggested that inhibition is unlikely as an explanation. The authors pointed out that the blood alcohol level associated with intoxication is around 33 mM (about 150 mg%), and the average concentration of retinol in human blood is about 2 μM, a ratio of about 16,500:1. When they duplicated this ratio in their animal model, no statistically significant inhibitory effects were observed. Even at a ratio hundreds of times lower, reflecting a blood alcohol level far greater than any one human could tolerate, inhibition was reduced by less than 30%. On the basis of this report, it is unlikely that FAS results from competitive inhibition of retinoic acids during embryonic morphogenesis (Chen, Namkung, & Juchau, 1996). However, the latter study was conducted with 12.5-day-old rat fetuses, whereas the former study indicated inhibition of retinoic acid production on in 7.5-day-old mouse embryos, so differences in age, or species, may make these studies not directly comparable.

Insulin Resistance

Glucose is a critical energy source for embryological and fetal growth and development (Hay, 1979). During the last trimester, it is the fetus's primary fuel source. Any changes in either its availability or metabolism can therefore result in decreased growth and physical anomalies in human and animals (Hunter & Sadler, 1989).

Studies of fetal blood glucose levels associated with in utero alcohol exposure were inconsistent (Falconer, 1990; Lopez-Tejero, Llobera, & Herrera, 1989; Marquis, Leichter, & Lee, 1984; Witek-Janusek, 1986). In large part, these inconsistencies may be because of procedural differences related to sampling time. For instance, because of glucose's importance to the body, changes in glucose availability to cells trigger reactions from the pancreas and peripheral mechanisms to restore homeostasis. Because of the interplay among these various factors, inconsistencies among the studies may be due to sampling before or after homeostatic influences were activated or completed.

For example, there are various "feedback" mechanisms in the body for maintaining glucose levels within relatively narrow limits. In well-fed animals, conditions of hyperglycemia stimulate the pancreas to release insulin. Insulin has the effect of removing glucose from the blood and transporting it to cells until homeostasis is restored. Depending on when sampling is done, hyperglycemia might or might not be found. If pancreatic function were impaired, then the hyperglycemia would remain elevated for a longer time.

The nutritional status of the animal being tested is also important. When animals or humans fast, blood sugar levels are lowered. The ensuing hypoglycemia triggers the release of another of hormone, glucagon, by the pancreas. Glucagon acts to increase blood glucose levels by promoting the release of glucose from the liver by stimulating glycogenolysis in that organ. Because the mother is the sole source of glucose for the developing fetus, fetal glucose levels will in large part depend on her glucose levels and on the placental transport of glucose to the fetus. Sampling time is therefore critical for detecting fetal blood glucose levels following alcohol exposure.

Although this is a very simplistic description of pancreatic control of blood glucose levels, it indicates the potential importance of sampling time, and the condition of the animals being tested, and their nutritional status with respect to resting blood glucose levels.

There is, however, another point that emerges from this brief discussion, namely that fetal disturbances in pancreatic function due to prenatal alcohol exposure could result in impaired glucose homeostasis. Since there are no reports of pancreatic pathology in connection with FAS or in animals prenatally exposed to alcohol, this is an unlikely explanation for either hyper- or hypoglycemia in alcohol-exposed fetuses or offspring after birth, and, therefore, it is an unlikely explanation for alcohol-related birth defects.

The possibility that alcohol affects fetal development by inhibiting glucose transport across the placenta is also unlikely because human placental transport of glucose is not significantly affected in vitro by alcohol even at high concentrations

(500 mg%) (Schenker et al., 1989). In addition, chronic treatment with alcohol in vivo results in only a very minor depression (12%) of glucose transport by the rat placenta (Snyder, Jiang, & Singh, 1986).

A third possibility, and the one for which there is the most experimental support, is that prenatal alcohol exposure results in long-lasting resistance to insulin's actions on cellular glucose transport in the fetus. The implication for the fetus is that despite normal or hyperglycemic conditions brought on by alcohol exposure, the fetus is unable to maximize its cellular glucose content; therefore, it develops in a context functionally tantamount to hypoglycemia. Such a course of development could explain not only why the fetus is growth retarded, but also why it experiences impaired CNS development. Since these conditions persist post-natally, these developments might also explain the child's continued growth retardation. The corollary to this conclusion is that this condition can be reversed by agents that decrease insulin resistance.

Support for this interpretation is not overwhelming, but there is considerable congruent evidence. Children with FAS have normal fasting plasma glucose levels, but some have enhanced glucose responses during glucose tolerance tests; their significantly elevated insulin levels are suggestive of insulin resistance (Castells et al., 1981). Chick embryos exposed to alcohol are likewise refractory to insulin (Sandstrom et al., 1993), as are fetal, newborn, juvenile, and adult rodents prenatally exposed to alcohol (Lopez-Tejero et al., 1989).

Insulin resistance ought to result in decreased fetal growth and development (it would result in decreased uptake of glucose into cells). A significant inhibition of glucose uptake and utilizations by fetal organs resulting from prenatal alcohol exposure has in fact been reported (Singh et al., 1989; Snyder et al., 1992).

Somewhat related to these studies are those examining glucose utilization rates in conjunction with positron emission tomography (PET) in children and its counterpart in animals. These studies have found that basal and activity-related glucose utilization are inhibited in brain areas of children with FAS (Hannigan et al., 1995a; Loock et al., 1993). A comparable study in animals found a 29% decrease in glucose utilization in the neocortex of alcohol-exposed rats (Miller & Dow-Edwards, 1988; Vingan, Dow-Edwards, & Riley, 1986). These measures are believed to reflect brain metabolic activity. Given the possibility that alcohol makes cells refractory to insulin, it is also possible that these areas are less metabolically active because of a decrease in their glucose uptake rather than its utilization.

Under normal conditions, cellular glucose levels are directly related to blood glucose levels. However, if cells are insulin resistant, blood glucose levels could be normal, while cellular levels might contain less glucose than normal. This would account for the lower metabolic activity of brain regions previously mentioned; it could also account for the lower rates of neural transmission elsewhere in the brain, as reflected in the delayed BAEP (see Chapter 9).

Endocrine-Mediated Effects

Hypothalamic-Pituitary-Adrenal (HPA) Axis. Shortly after birth, levels of adrenocorticotropin-releasing-factor in the hypothalamus are elevated in animals prenatally exposed to alcohol. Adrenocorticotropin hormone (ACTH) levels in the pituitary and corticosterone levels in plasma, brain, and adrenal are also increased, while corticosterone-binding globulin (CGB) capacity is diminished (Kim et al., 1996). All of these measures indicate the fetus has experienced heightened HPA activity in conjunction with prenatal alcohol exposure. Because removal of the maternal adrenal cortex abolishes the suppressive effects of prenatal alcohol exposure on birth weight, its immunosuppressive actions (see Chapters 10 and 13), and possibly has other effects as well, one of alcohol's actions on the fetus may be indirectly related to its role as a maternal stressor, or it may act synergistically with other stressors.

Although corticosterone levels in rats return to normal by about the fifth day after birth, the corticosterone and β-endorphin responses to stressors in rats are blunted during the early preweaning period (the first 2 weeks after birth) (Kim et al., 1996). This condition normalizes around weaning in rats (Kim et al., 1996), then it reemerges during adulthood. Although basal plasma corticosterone and beta-endorphin levels are normal in rats, the HPA axis in response to some stressors is exaggerated (Weinberg, 1988), and recovery takes longer (Kim et al., 1996). Although this heightened stress reaction occurs primarily in females (Nelson et al., 1986; Taylor, Branch, Van Zuylen, & Redei, 1986; Weinberg, 1988), under certain conditions, such as prolonged exposure to stressors, males also exhibit increased stress responses (Weinberg, 1992).

The reason for this heightened stress response in animals prenatally exposed to alcohol has not yet been determined. The adrenals themselves are not overly responsive to ACTH, nor is the pituitary overly responsive to its secretagogues (Lee & Rivier, 1994; Taylor, Branch, Van Zuylen, & Redei, 1988). Although it seems likely that this differential responsiveness lies within the central nervous system (Taylor et al., 1988), no such site has yet been identified.

Weinberg and Peterson (1991) have speculated that the hippocampus is probably involved because it is the primary site for glucocorticoid feedback in the brain, and because of the large body of evidence indicating that the hippocampus is one of the areas in the brain most sensitive to alcohol's in utero effects (see Chapter 9). In line with this hypothesis, Weinberg also speculated that this sensitivity might arise from a decrease in the concentration of glucocorticoid receptors in the hippocampus. However, when she tested this hypothesis, there was no evidence to support it because animals prenatally exposed to alcohol did not differ from controls in either specific binding or binding affinity of glucocorticoid receptors (Weinberg & Petersen, 1991; see also, Kim, Yu, Osborn, & Weinberg, 1994).

Other investigators have hypothesized that the basis for this differential stress response lies in the hypothalamus (Taylor et al., 1986), but there is no direct evidence to support this hypothesis. This increased susceptibility to infection has also been associated with the HPA axis (see later).

Altered susceptibility to infection may be related to retarded development of the thymus, as reflected in decreased size or cellularity. Although such decreases were reported in one study of FAS patients (Ammann, Wara, Cowan, Barrett, & Stiehm, 1982) and in animals prenatally exposed to alcohol (Ewald, Huang, & Bray, 1991; Redei, Clark, & McGivern, 1989; Wong et al., 1992), when thymus weight was expressed as a function of body weight in animals, results were very inconsistent, with no changes (Redei et al., 1989), decreases (Redei et al., 1989; Wong et al., 1992) and increases (Redei et al., 1989) being noted.

The most consistently supported association between the increased susceptibility to infection and altered immune responsiveness is the decrease in T-cell lymphocyte responses which occurs in humans and animals (see Chapter 10). Studies by Taylor's group suggested that this decreased proliferation may be specifically related to an altered responsiveness to interleukin-2 (IL-2), rather than to an inhibition of the mitogen-receptor interaction that initiates T-cell activation and production of IL-2 (Weinberg & Jerells, 1991). Natural killer cells (NK), a subtype of lymphocytes different from T cells and B cells, are not significantly affected by prenatal alcohol exposure in animals (Wolcott, Jennings, & Chervenak, 1995).

As alluded to earlier, these changes in immune function in offspring have been related to effects on the HPA axis, which is activated by both alcohol and stress (Kalant, 1990). Prenatal exposure to alcohol or glucocorticoids can cause a decrease in thymus weight (Jerrells & Pruett, 1994). The fact that maternal adrenalectomy abolishes the suppression of lymphocyte proliferation to mitogens in male animals prenatally exposed to alcohol suggests corticosteroids mediate the effects of prenatal alcohol exposure on the immune system (Redei et al., 1993).

Corticosteroids may also mediate the increased susceptibility to infections later in life. In adult humans and animals prenatally exposed to alcohol, basal cortisol and corticosterone levels are not elevated. When challenged by stressors, however, the HPA axis in animals becomes overly stimulated, and it produces significantly more corticosterone than normal. Whether the same increased stimulation occurs in humans is not yet known. If it does, this elevated corticosteroid response to stressors may dampen the immune system, making a person more vulnerable to infection.

Hypothalamic-Pituitary-Thyroid (HPT) Axis. While there is relatively little evidence that alterations in thyroid activity are involved in FAS/ARBEs, this possibility cannot be entirely dismissed yet. Acute and chronic maternal alcohol consumption or infusion in animals during pregnancy suppressed the fetus's response to thyroid-releasing hormones (Rose, Meis, & Castro, 1981) and resulted in decreased plasma thyroxine (T_4) or tridodothyroinine (T_3) levels in mothers and fetuses (Rose et al., 1981). In utero or lactational exposure to alcohol in rats can also result in long-lasting decreases in serum thyroxine or triidodothyroinine levels in rat progeny (Gottesfeld & Silverberg, 1990; Hannigan & Bellisario, 1990) also, the growth of the fetal thyroid in animals is reduced (Yamamoto et al., 1989).

The most interesting evidence linking thyroid hormones and alcohol's in utero effects arises from studies that reported that early postnatal treatment with thyroid hormones attenuated some of the effects of prenatal alcohol exposure in rats (Gottesfeld & Silverberg, 1990; Hannigan, 1993). However, given the absence of any link between hypothyroidism and ARBEs in humans, inferences from these observations are problematic.

Hypothalamic-Pituitary-Gonadal (HPG) Axis.   While there is no clinical or epidemiological evidence of altered testosterone or estrogen activity in FAS, there is considerable evidence of such altered function in animals prenatally exposed to alcohol. One study found that newborn male rats had decreased testicular weights at birth (Kakihana, Butte, & Moore, 1980) and shorter anogenital distances (an effect dependent on androgen levels during sexual differentiation) (Parker, Udani, Gavaler, & Van Thiel, 1984; Rudeen, Kappel, & Lear, 1986), although the latter effect has not been consistently observed (McGivern, 1987). Reports of the persistence of this finding into adulthood have also been inconsistent (Parker et al., 1984).

Structural anomalies in male sex organs associated with prenatal alcohol exposure (see Chapter 8) have been attributed to an attenuation in the testosterone surge that normally occurs prior to birth and shortly afterward (McGivern, Raum, Salido, & Redei, 1988).

Androgenic influences at critical periods of development also influence sexual differentiation in the brain. In the absence of the surge in testosterone or its metabolites, sexual differentiation of many structures in the brain is feminized, regardless of chromosomal factors or external genitalia. For example, male rats whose testosterone levels are markedly reduced by surgical or pharmacological means in a late fetal stage or early neonatal life or those experiencing prenatal stress sometimes exhibit the behavioral characteristics of female rats, including female sexual behavioral patterns (Ward & Ward, 1985).

More than 45 different brain structures exhibit sexual dimorphism (Rudeen, 1992), and several of them have been found to exhibit alcohol-related demasculinization. The sexually dimorphic nucleus of the preoptic area of the hypothalamus is normally larger in volume in males than females, but in male rats prenatally exposed to alcohol, the size differences are considerably diminished (Barron, Tieman, & Riley, 1988; Rudeen et al., 1986).

The corpus callosum is another sexually dimorphic structure for which the normal sexual differentiation in size is reduced following prenatal alcohol exposure (Zimmerberg & Scalzi, 1989). By comparison, the anterior commissure, which is not sexually dimorphic, is not comparably affected (Barron et al., 1988; Zimmerberg & Scalzi, 1989).

Attenuation of masculinizing influences in certain brain structures may underlie the feminimized patterns of sexual behavior in male rats prenatally exposed to alcohol. These animals exhibited lordosis when mounted by other males (Barron et al., 1988; Hard et al., 1984; Rudeen et al., 1986; Ward, Ward, Winn, & Bielawski, 1994), and their own masculine behavior toward females was diminished (Ward et al., 1994; Parker et al., 1984). These males also exhibited other feminized activities, such as maternal behaviors (Hard et al., 1985; McGivern et al., 1984) and altered saccharin preference (McGivern, Clancy, Hill, & Noble, 1984). However, males prenatally exposed to alcohol will still exhibit male copulatory behavior in the presence of females (Hard et al., 1984). Ward et al. (1994) speculated that prenatal alcohol exposure may result in a bisexual orientation because males presented with females will engage in male patterns of sexual behavior but when mounted by other males, exhibit femalelike behavioral patterns.

Although most of the research in this area has been directed at males, some studies have suggested that female sexual function is also influenced by prenatal alcohol exposure. For instance, levels of hypothalamic luteinizing hormone releasing hormone (LHRH) and plasma luteinizing hormone (LH) are decreased in 30- to 40-day-old female rats prenatally exposed to alcohol (Morris, Harms, Petersen, & McArthur, 1989). A delayed onset of menses has been noted in girls of alcoholic mothers (Robe, Robe, & Wilson, 1979), but not in a systematic study. Female rats prenatally exposed to alcohol have been reported to have delayed onset of vaginal opening (Boggan et al., 1979; McGivern, 1991), but onset of vaginal estrus was not delayed (Hard et al., 1984).

Insulin Growth Factor (Somatomedins). Serum insulin growth factor-1 (IGF-I; also called somatomedin C) along with IGF-11 are involved in DNA synthesis, neuronal cytoskeletal protein synthesis, cellular differentiation, and pre- and postnatal growth (see review by LeRoith, Werner, Beitner-Johnson, & Roberts, 1995).

Although levels of these factors were significantly lower in infants with ARBEs compared with nonaffected infants of drinking or abstinent mothers, the decreases did not correlate with birth weight or placenta weights (Halmesmaki et al., 1989a), so their involvement in these and other ARBEs remains to be clarified.

The role of these factors in animal studies also remains to be clarified. IGF-I receptors are present in human and rat placenta (Daughaday et al., 1978). However, IGF-1 does not cross the placenta (Halmesmaki et al., 1989a). Any effects of alcohol on these receptors is therefore problematic with respect to ARBEs.

Effects of alcohol on plasma IGF-1 levels are inconsistent. While IGF-I levels were reduced by over 20% in newborn rats, prenatally exposed to alcohol in two studies (Singh, Srivenugopal, Ehmann, Yuan, & Snyder, 1994), a third study failed to find any significant changes in IGF-1 levels in newborn rats following prenatal alcohol exposure (Mauceri et al., 1993).

Fatty Acid Ethyl Esters (FAEEs)

Although not directly related to normal cell metabolism, oxidative phosphorylation may be compromised by the nonoxidative metabolism of alcohol to toxic fatty acid ethyl esters (FAEEs) (Bearer, Gould, Emerson, Kinnunen, & Cook, 1992). FAEEs are potentially harmful because they bind to mitochondria and can uncouple oxidative phosphorylation, resulting in organ damage (Bora & Lange, 1993); the brain is particularly vulnerable to their effects (Bora & Lange, 1993; Laposata & Lange, 1986).

FAEEs are produced in organs that have little or no ADH activity, such as the brian and placenta (Bearer et al., 1992; Bora & Lange, 1993) production of FAEEs is proportional to alcohol ingestion (Laposata & Lange, 1986). FAEEs have been found in fetal tissues of mice (Bearer et al., 1992), rats (Hungund & Gokhale, 1994), and humans (Bearer et al., 1992) following maternal alcohol administration. The selective nature of alcohol-related organ damage, whereby organs such as the brain and heart may be damaged while the liver or pancreas are unaffected (see Chapter 8, "Liver," "Pancreas"), may thus be related to the production of FAEEs in selective organs.

CHAPTER 14

Conclusions and Implications

A basic argument throughout this book that is alcohol abuse—defined as consumption of five or more drinks per drinking occasion, more than once a week—is responsible for all of the alcohol-related birth effects (ARBEs) currently associated with drinking during pregnancy. Although a single binge at this level during a pregnancy may produce some ARBEs, the more days a woman drinks at this level during her pregnancy, the greater the potential for causing cumulative damage to her unborn child. Consumption of lower levels of alcohol, which currently go by the name of "moderate," "social," or "occasional" drinking, may be found to be damaging in the future, but given all the research done to explore moderate drinking, such a possibility seems unlikely. Rather than exaggerating the dangers of "moderate" drinking, clinicians and researchers who work in this area should recognize that any harm to an unborn child from alcohol exposure is related to acute binge or chronic abusive drinking. Although the number of drinks that make up a binge is certainly arbitrary, it is certain that that number, whatever it may be, will be much closer to five than one.

The fact that ARBEs result from alcohol abuse and not moderate drinking has important implications not only with respect to the terms we use to describe those effects, but also for the strategies we use when we try to prevent them.

Because there is no quantity or health-related risk attached to the "alcohol" in "fetal alcohol syndrome," there is little point in targeting "moderate" drinkers if we are intent on reducing the number of children born with ARBEs, such as FAS. The reason we continue to do so is, in part, due to use of terms like *fetal alcohol syndrome*. Even large numbers of obstetricians have reached the misguided conclusion that as little as one drink a day can lead to FAS (Abel & Krueger, 1998b). This mistake stems in large part from the fact names have revelatory importance—they communicate some fundamental nature about the thing being named. *Alcohol abuse*, undeniably communicates much more about the intrinsic causal nature of FAS than *alcohol*. For that reason, and for the other reasons outlined in Chapter 2, the term *fetal alcohol abuse syndrome* was adopted in this book in lieu of *fetal alcohol syndrome*, and the focus of the discussion was directed at the role of alcohol abuse as the explanation for the syndrome and its related effects.

Labeling the disorder fetal alcohol abuse syndrome does not affect its diagnosis or its impact, but it does undermine the important idea that trivial amounts of alcohol consumption can cause the disorder. Equally important, it implies that alcohol alone is not a sufficient cause of the disorder, we cannot ignore the importance of the mother or her lifestyle in its etiology.

Name changes, especially where health concerns are involved, have to be balanced against the potential negative ramifications attendant on those changes. The argument could be made that as a result of stressing that ARBEs are due to alcohol abuse pregnant women might be lulled into a false complacency concluding that their drinking does not pose a danger to their unborn children as long as it falls short of "abusive drinking," which they would then be free to define anyway they liked. The presumption underlying this argument is that women who are alcohol abusers when they are not pregnant have been restricting their consumption because the message attached to the "alcohol" in FAS has been that any amount of drinking may cause birth defects.

This argument is simply not convincing. An abstainer or a moderate drinker is not suddenly going to begin drinking more because of a name change because, by definition, an abstainer is someone who does not drink, and a "moderate" drinker is someone who does not drink excessively.

A related argument hinges on the idea that alcohol abuse and alcoholism are controllable habits, involving something one chooses or does not choose to do. The implication is that fetal alcohol abuse syndrome is entirely preventable if an alcohol abuser simply wills herself not to drink during pregnancy. But this means that same will power should make alcohol abuse and alcoholism preventable at any time. If the latter argument is vapid, so is the former.

Another obvious question is, are their concerns stemming from a name change for a child who already has "fetal alcohol syndrome"? The answer is that there are none. However, there may be considerable benefits for future children because in focusing limited resources on the real problem instead of becoming entangled in the "wrong problem," we will waste less and do more. By targeting our time and resources where they are needed most, we can focus on the real problem with lasers, not flashlights.

Yet another concern is the possibility that credibility regarding the occurrence of ARBEs and FAS would be fundamentally undermined by any name change. Credibility is always a concern, but a name change does not seem to have deterred the credibility of Down's syndrome, which was once called *mongoloid-*

ism. The fact that German physicians, following Majewski's arguments (Majewski, 1981), have been using the term *alcohol embryopathy* rather than fetal alcohol syndrome has also not affected the credibility of this birth defect. A danger to its credibility was not considered a possibility by, among others, K. Jones, who named the syndrome but later advised dropping the term fetal alcohol effect from the clinical lexicon. Nor did the Institute of Medicine (1996) raise it as an issue in its deliberations over renaming the effects. In fact, the IOM created several new terms of its own, such as *alcohol-related neurodevelopmental disorder* (*ARND*), to distinguish neurodevelopmental problems from the physical anomalies related to alcohol's in utero toxicity. The latter, it suggested, should retain the designation *alcohol-related birth defects* (*ARBDs*), and because it proposed using ARBDs as one of its subcategories, the IOM coined another term, *alcohol-related effects*, to be used as a generic term for effects related to prenatal alcohol exposure that did not fit into any of its categories.

The population most at risk for FAS in the United States lives in America's inner cities and is characterized by abject poverty. FAS has been found in every racial group, but is almost always associated with low socioeconomic status. Although genotype is undoubtedly related to susceptibility to FAS, genotype at the individual, not the population level, is involved. Population studies evaluating racial genotypes for rates of alcohol metabolism or susceptibilities to alcohol abuse may reveal significant group differences, but the relevance of such differences pales when compared with differences related to socioeconomic conditions.

Among other things, low socioeconomic status is associated with poor diet, and poor diet has an effect on the body similar to that associated with smoking. The feature common to both is that poor nutrition and smoking deplete the body of antioxidants, rendering a pregnant woman and her unborn child more susceptible to alcohol's toxicity from free radicals.

As long as it is legal to drink alcohol, alcohol abuse will exist. Few clinicians or biomedical researchers believe that the antidote to this disorder is to "just say no." But these same experts blithely assert that FAS is readily preventable—all that is required is for the alcoholic to stop drinking during pregnancy—as if a disease, which they purport alcoholism to be, can be turned on and off like a spigot. Unless and until simplistic solutions like "just say no" are abandoned, and more attention is focused on the alcohol abuser and the conditions in which she lives, we will not prevent FAS.

If FAS is a distinctive disorder, suggestions offered on behalf of children with FAS need to go beyond platitudes. One such platitude is that people with FAS need supportive, loving, home environments that will allow them to develop their full potential (Giunta & Streissguth, 1988). Is this not true of every child? Likewise, concern over birth control and sex education for adolescents and adults with FAS (Giunta & Streissguth, 1988) should be no different than the concern that ought to be directed at the soaring teen pregnancies that plague the nation? Similarly, comments that "as adolescents, these patients tend to be sexually curious, yet they often lack understanding of socially appropriate sexual behavior" (Giunta & Streissguth, 1988, p. 456) could be applied to the general adolescent population. Whatever the meaning of "appropriate sexual behavior" are teenagers with FAS any different from teenagers without FAS? In the same light, comments that adolescents with FAS "are at higher average risk for sexual victimization due to their impulsive behavior and poor social judgment (Giunta & Streissguth, 1988, p. 456)" are speculation, and again there is no reason to assume that adolescents with FAS are any more at risk for sexual victimization than those without. In fact, given the widespread prevalence of sexual abuse in America, FAS would seem to have no specific relationship to being sexually victimized.

What is required is neither platitudes nor speculation, but a direct effort to determine how people with FAS differ from people with other problems. Until a specific niche is identified wherein children with FAS are shown to be different from mentally retarded children, hyperactive children, or children with learning disorders, any services provided for children with FAS will be the same as those currently available for children with similar problems who do not have FAS, raising the important issue of whether there is any point to labeling children as FAS in the first place. If a child has FAS, and is hyperactive, will the treatment be any different than the treatment offered to hyperactive children who do not have FAS? Studies, such as Coles et al. (1997), that indicate that children with FAS differ from those with attention deficit disorder are an important beginning. If children with FAS do differ, it is important to know how they differ. The "why" is another issue altogether. There is no point in identifying someone as having FAS unless that diagnosis will lead to some specific treatment.

On the other hand, Giunta and Streissguth's (1988) suggestions that teachers at all levels be trained and informed about FAS to help them recognize and understand the problems these children face, and so that they can set realistic performance standards for them are certainly reasonable. But the danger associated with labeling is ever present. If a teacher suspects a child has FAS, that teacher may treat that child differently from others, even if the child does not manifest learning or behavioral problems. Conversely, if a child does manifest learning or behavioral problems, what advantage is it to the child to be labeled FAS if the treatment is the same as that provided for those not labeled as FAS? Early identification of FAS may result in a child's being placed in special education at an earlier age than otherwise, but unless the child exhibits the kinds of learning or behavioral problems that special education is designed to help, it would be injurious to a child with FAS to do so if she or he did not need such help. One should not automatically assume that a child needs to be treated for any particular problem simply because a diagnosis has been made.

One factor that has not received enough attention in the context of ARBEs is the home environment. As noted in Chapter 10, children with FAS are more likely to experience physical and sexual abuse and neglect than those who do not have FAS. Children with FAS are typically raised in "high-risk environments" by mothers who continue to have alcohol-related problems after they give birth, and whose social and monetary resources are pitiful. It is also likely these women live with spouses who are also alcohol abusers. This kind of environment and parenting are well-known factors that contribute to child abuse (Macdonald & Blume, 1986). Growing up in such an environment may make a child excessively fearful or withdrawn and may result in subsequent antisocial behavior. If children prenatally exposed to alcohol are placed in foster care prior to 6 months of age, they may escape the kinds of "psychosocial problems" associated with living in these kinds of chaotic homes (Aronson & Olegard, 1987). FAS needs to be recognized as a condition contributing to child abuse (Giunta & Streissguth, 1988), and unless parents are able to cope with the special needs of children with FAS, there is little reason for optimism.

The home environment may also be one reason why many children with ARBEs are unable to overcome their prenatal insults. In the absence of FAS, for instance, there is little evidence that language development is significantly related to maternal alcohol consumption, even among children with physical anomalies or reduced birth weight attributable to prenatal alcohol exposure. On the other hand, the quality of the caretaking environment is a major factor contributing to language functioning in these children (Greene et al., 1991b).

Platitudes aside, one of the most important sources of help for parents and those with FAS are parent support groups. Parents who have adopted children with FAS need to be aware that they are not "the only ones" encountering the problems they have to deal with on a daily basis in raising children with FAS. By sharing information as to what works and what doesn't work, parents may be able to assist one another in managing and helping children with FAS deal with their problems. At the very least, support groups enable parents to develop reasonable expectations. It is all well and good for parents to be informed of the scientific data regarding children's language and learning skills, but that information should only be used as a guide. The practical everyday experience that parents share with one another is invaluable. Research can give direction, but research in FAS to this point is still in its formative stages and can offer parents little in the way dealing with the everyday problems of raising children with FAS.

References

Aase J. M., Clinical recognition of FAS: Difficulties of detection and diagnosis. *Alcohol Health and Research World 18:*5–9, 1994.

Aase J. M. *Diagnostic Dysmorphology.* New York: Plenum Publishing, 1990.

Aase M. M., Jones K. L., Clarren S. K. Do we need the term "FAE"? *Pediatrics 95:*428–430, 1995.

Abdollah S., Brien J. F. Effect of chronic maternal ethanol administration on glutamate and N-methyl-d-aspartate binding sites in the hippocampus of the near-term fetal guinea pig. *Alcohol 12:*377–382, 1995.

Abel E. L. *Drugs and Behavior.* New York: Wiley, 1974.

Abel E. L. Effects of ethanol on pregnant rats and their offspring. *Psychopharmacology 57:*5–11, 1978.

Abel E. L. Effects of ethanol exposure during different gestation weeks of pregnancy on maternal weight gain and intrauterine growth retardation in the rat. *Neurobehavioral Toxicology 1:*145–151, 1979.

Abel E. L. A critical evaluation of the obstetric use of alcohol in preterm labor. *Drug and Alcohol Dependence 7:*367–378, 1981.

Abel E. L. Characteristics of mothers of fetal alcohol syndrome children. *Neurobehavioral Toxicology and Teratology 4:*3–4, 1982.

Abel E. L. *Marihuana, Tobacco, Alcohol and Reproduction.* Boca Raton, FL: CRC Press, 1983.

Abel E. L. *Fetal Alcohol Syndrome and Fetal Alcohol Effects.* New York: Plenum Press, 1984a.

Abel E. L. Smoking and pregnancy. *Journal of Psychoactive Drugs 16:*327–338, 1984b.

Abel E. L. Alcohol enhancement of marihuana-induced fetotoxicity. *Teratology 31:*35–40, 1985.

Abel E. L. Fetal alcohol syndrome in families. *Neurotoxicology and Teratology 10:*1–2, 1988.

Abel E. L. *Behavioral Teratogenesis and Behavioral Mutagenesis: A Primer in Abnormal Development.* New York: Plenum Press, 1989a.

Abel E. L. Paternal and maternal alcohol consumption: Effects on offspring in two strains of rats. *Alcoholism: Clinical and Experimental Research 13:*533–541, 1989b.

Abel E. L. *Fetal Alcohol Syndrome.* Oradell, NJ: Medical Economics, 1990.

Abel E. L. An update on incidence of FAS: FAS is not an equal opportunity birth defect. *Neurotoxicology and Teratology 17:*437–443, 1995.

Abel E. L. Alcohol-induced changes in blood gases, glucose, and lactate in pregnant and nonpregnant rats. *Alcohol 13:*281–285, 1996a.

Abel E. L. Effects of prenatal alcohol exposure on birth weight in rats: Is there an inverted "U"-shaped function? *Alcohol 13:*99–102, 1996b.

Abel E. L., Dintcheff B. A. Effects of prenatal alcohol exposure on growth and development in rats. *Journal of Pharmacology and Experimental Therapeutics 207:*916–921, 1978.

Abel E. L., Dintcheff B. A. Factors affecting the outcome of maternal alcohol exposure: I. Parity. *Neurobehavioral Toxicology and Teratology 6:*373–377, 1984.

Abel E. L., Dintcheff B. A. Factors affecting the outcome of maternal alcohol exposure: II. Maternal age. *Neurobehavioral Toxicology and Teratology 7:*263–266, 1985.

Abel E. L., Hannigan J. H. "J-shaped" relationship between drinking during pregnancy and birth weight: Reanalysis of prospective epidemiological data. *Alcohol and Alcoholism 30:*345–355, 1995a.

Abel E. L., Hannigan J. H. Maternal risk factors in fetal alcohol syndrome: Provocative and permissive influences. *Neurotoxicology and Teratology 17:*445–462, 1995b.

Abel E. L., Kruger M. L., Hon v. Stroh Brewery Co.: What do we mean by "moderate" and "heavy" drinking. *Alcoholism: Clinical and Experimental Research 19:*1024–1031, 1995.

Abel E. L., Kruger M. L., and Friedl, J. How do physicians define "light," "moderate," and "heavy" drinking? *Alcoholism: Clinical and Experimental Research.* In press, 1998a.

Abel E. L., Kruger M. L. What do physicians know about Fetal Alcohol Syndrome? *Alcoholism: Clinical and Experimental Research,* In press, 1998b.

Abel E. L., Reddy P. P. Prenatal high saturated fat diet modifies behavioral effects of prenatal alcohol exposure in rats. *Alcohol 14:*25–29, 1997.

Abel E. L., Sokol R. J. Incidence of fetal alcohol syndrome and economic impact of FAS-related anomalies. *Drug and Alcohol Dependence 19:*51–70, 1987.

Abel E. L., Sokol R. J. A revised conservative estimate of the incidence of FAS and its economic impact. *Alcoholism: Clinical and Experimental Research 15:*514–524, 1991.

Abel E. L., Berman R. F., Church M. W. Prenatal alcohol exposure attenuates pentylene–tetrazol-induced convulsions in rats. *Alcohol 10:*155–157, 1993.

Abel E. L., Church, M. W., Dintcheff B. A. Prenatal alcohol exposure shortens life span in rats, *Teratology 36:*217–221, 1987.

Abel E. L., Jacobson S., Sherwin B. T. In utero ethanol exposure: Functional and structural brain damage. *Neurobehavioral Toxicology and Teratology 5:*363–366, 1983.

Abel E. L., Martier S., Kruger, M., Ager J., Sokol R. J. Ratings of fetal alcohol syndrome facial features by medical providers and biomedical scientists. *Alcoholism: Clinical and Experimental Research 17:*717–721, 1993.

Adickes E., Shuman R. Fetal alcohol myopathy. *Pediatric Pathology 1:*369–384, 1983.

Adickes E. D., Mollner T. J., Lockwood S. K. Ethanol-induced morphological alterations during growth and maturation of cardiac myocytes. *Alcoholism: Clinical and Experimental Research 14:*827–831, 1990.

Ahluwalia B., Smith D., Adeyiga, O., Akbasak B., Rajguru S. Ethanol decreases progesterone synthesis in human placental cells: Mechanism of ethanol effect. *Alcohol 9:*395–401, 1992.

Alpert J. J., Day N., Dooling E., Hingson R., Oppenheimer E., et al. Maternal alcohol consumption and newborn assessment: Methodology of the Boston City Hospital Prospective Study. *Neurobehavioral Toxicology Teratology 3:*195–201, 1981.

Altura B. M., Altura B. T., Carella A., Chatterjee M., Halevy S., et al. Alcohol produces spasms of human umbilical blood vessels: Relationship to fetal alcohol syndrome (FAS). *European Journal of Pharmacology 86:*311–312, 1983.

Amankwah K. S., Kaufmann, R. C. Ultrastructure of human placenta: Effects of maternal drinking. *Gynecologic and Obstetric Investigation 18:*311–316, 1984.

Amaro H., Fried L. E., Cabral H., Zuckerman B. Violence during pregnancy and substance abuse. *American Journal of Public Health 80:*575–579, 1990.

American Psychiatric Association. *Diagnostic and Statistical Manual of Mental Disorders (4th ed.).* Washington, DC: *Psychiatric Association,* 1994.

Ammann A. J., Wara D. W., Cowan M. J., Barrett D. J., Stiehm E. R. The DiGeorge syndrome and the fetal alcohol syndrome. *American Journal of Disease in Childhood 136:*906–908, 1982.

Andersen A. M. N., Olsen J. Social and public health aspects of alcohol abuse in pregnancy. In Spohr H. L., Steinhausen H. C. (Eds.), *Alcohol, Pregnancy and the Developing Child* (pp. 289–300). Cambridge, UK: Cambridge University Press, 1996.

Andersson S., Halmesmaki E., Koivusalo M., Lapatto R., Ylikorkala O. Placenta alcohol metabolism in chronic alcohol abuse. *Biology of the Neonate 56:*90–93, 1989.

Anokute C. C. Epidemiology of spontaneous abortions: The effects of alcohol consumption and cigarette smoking. *Journal of the National Medical Association 78:*771–775, 1986.

Armstrong B. G., McDonald A. D., Sloan M. Cigarette, alcohol, and coffee consumption and spontaneous abortion. *American Journal of Public Health 82:*85–87, 1992.

Aro T. Maternal diseases, alcohol consumption, and smoking during pregnancy associated with reduction limb defects. *Early Human Development 9:*49–57, 1983.

Aronson M. *Children of alcoholic mothers.* Unpublished M.D. thesis, Departments of Pediatrics and Psychology, University of Göteborg, Göteborg, Sweden, 1984.

Aronson M., Olegard R. Children of alcoholic mothers. *Drug and Alcohol Abuse and Child and Adolescent Pediatrics 14:*57–61, 1987.

Aronson M., Kyllerman M., Sabel K. G., Sandin B., Olegard R. Children of alcoholic mothers: Developmental, perceptual, and behavioral characteristics. *Acta Pediatrica Scandinavica 4:* 27–35, 1985.

Aronson M., Olegard R., Sabel K. G. Dynamics of infant growth and development from birth to 18 months of age in relation to maternal alcohol consumption during pregnancy. In Aronson M. (Ed.), *Children of Alcoholic Mothers.* Sweden: Kompendiet-Lindome, 1984.

Asante K. O., Nelms-Matzke J. Survey of children with chronic handicaps and fetal alcohol syndrome in the Yukon and Northwest B. C. Ottawa. Unpublished report. Canada: Haland Welfare, 1985.

Ashley M. J., Olin J. S., le Riche W. H., Kornaczewski A., Schmidt W., et al. Morbidity in alcoholics: Evidence for accelerated development of physical disease in women. *Archives of Internal Medicine 137:*883–887, 1977.

Assadi F. K., Ziai M. Zinc status of infants with fetal alcohol syndrome. *Pediatric Research 20:* 551–556, 1986.

Astley S. J., Weinberger E., Shaw D. W. W., Richards T. L., Clarren, S. K. Magnetic resonance imaging and spectroscopy in fetal-ethanol-exposed Macaca nemestrina. *Neurotoxicology and Teratology 17:*523–530, 1995.

Aufrere G., LeBourhis B. Effect of alcohol intoxication during pregnancy on foetal and placental weight: Experimental studies. *Alcohol and Alcoholism 22:*401–407, 1987.

Autti-Ramo I., Granstrom M-L. The psychomotor development during the first year of life of infants exposed to intrauterine alcohol of various duration. *Neuropediatrics 22:*59–64, 1991a.

Autti-Ramo I., Granstrom M-L. The effect of intrauterine alcohol exposition in various durations on early cognitive development. *Neuropediatrics 22:*203–210, 1991b.

Autti-Ramo I., Gaily E., Granstrom M-L. Dysmorphic features in offspring of alcoholic mothers. *Archives of Disease in Childhood 67:*712–716, 1992.

Autti-Ramo I., Korkman M., Hilakivi-Clarke L., Lehtonen M., Halmesmaki E., et al. Mental development of 2-year-old children exposed to alcohol in utero. *Journal of Pediatrics 120:*740–746, 1992.

Azouz E. M., Kavianian G., Der Kaloustian V. M. Fetal alcohol syndrome and bilateral tibial exostoses: A case report. *Pediatric Radiology 23:*615–616, 1993.

Baldwin V. J., MacLeod P. M., Benirschke K. Placental findings in alcohol abuse in pregnancy. *Birth Defects 18:*89–94, 1982.

Baran D. T. Alcohol-induced inhibition of fetal 25-(^{3}H)hydroxy-vitamin D and alpha (^{14}C)amino-isobutyric acid accumulation in the pregnant rat. *Endocrinology 111:*1109–1114, 1982.

Barden T. P. Perinatal care. In S. Romney, M. J. Graz, B. Little, E. J. Merrill et al. (Eds.). *Gynecology and Obstetrics*. New York: McGraw-Hill, p. 223, 1975.

Bark N. Fertility and offspring of alcoholic women: An unsuccessful search for the fetal alcohol syndrome. *British Journal of Addiction 74:*43–49, 1979.

Barr H. M., Streissguth A. P., Martin D. C., Herman C. S. Infant size at 8 months of age: Relationship to maternal use of alcohol, nicotine, and caffeine during pregnancy. *Pediatrics 74:*336–341, 1984.

Barrada M. I., Virnig N. L., Edwards L. E., Hakanson E. Y. Maternal intravenous ethanol in the prevention of respiratory distress syndrome. *American Journal of Obstetrics and Gynecology 129:*25–30, 1977.

Barrison I. G., Waterson E. J., Murray-Lyon I. Adverse effects of alcohol in pregnancy. *British Journal of Addiction 80:*11–22, 1985.

Barron S., Tieman S. B., Riley E. P. Effects of prenatal alcohol exposure on the sexually dimorphic nucleus of the preoptic area of the hypothalamus in male and female rats. *Alcoholism: Clinical and Experimental Research 12:*59–64, 1988.

Baruah J. K., Kinder D. Pathological changes in peripheral nerves in experimental fetal alcohol syndrome. *Alcoholism: Clinical and Experimental Research 13:*547–548, 1989.

Bearer C. F., Gould S., Emerson R., Kinnunen P., Cook C. S. Fetal alcohol syndrome and fatty acid ethyl esters. *Pediatric Research 31:*491–495, 1992.

Beattie J. O., Day R. E., Cockburn F., Garg R. A. Alcohol and the fetus in the West of Scotland. *British Medical Journal 287:*17–20, 1983.

Beauchemin R. R., Gartner L. P., Provenza D. V. Alcohol-induced cardiac malformations in the rat. *Anatomischer Anzeiger Jena 155:*17–28, 1984.

Becker M., Warr-Leeper G. A., Leeper H. A. Fetal alcohol syndrome: A description of oral motor, articularity, short-term memory, grammatical, and semantic disabilities. *Journal of Communication Disorders 23:*97–124, 1990.

Becker U., Tonnesen H., Kaas-Claesson N., Gluud C. Menstrual disturbances and fertility in chronic alcoholic women. *Drug and Alcohol Dependence 24:*75–82, 1989.

Beer W. H., Johnson R. F., Guentzel M. N., Lozano J., Henderson G. I., et al. Human placental transport of zinc: Normal characteristics and role of ethanol. *Alcoholism: Clinical and Experimental Research 16:*98–104, 1992.

Bell R., Lumley J. Alcohol consumption, cigarette smoking, and fetal outcome in Victoria, 1985. *Community and Health Studies 13:*484–491, 1989.

Bennett L. A., Ames G. M. (Eds.). *The American Experience with Alcohol*. New York: Plenum Press, 1986.

Bergstrom R. M., Sainion K., Taalas J. The effect of ethanol on the EEG of the guinea pig foetus. *Med Pharmacol Exper 16:*418–452, 1967.

Berkowitz G. S., Holford T. R., Berkowitz R. L. Effects of cigarette smoking, alcohol, coffee, and tea consumption on preterm delivery. *Early Human Development 7:*239–250, 1982.

Berlin, I. *The Hedgehog and the Fox: An Essay on Tolstoy's View of History*. New York: New American Library, 1957.

Berman R. F., Krahl S. E. Neurophysiological correlates of fetal alcohol syndrome. In Abel E. L. (Ed.), *Fetal Alcohol Syndrome: From Mechanism to Prevention* (pp. 69–84). Boca Raton, FL: CRC Press, 1996.

Berman R. F., Beare D. J., Church M. W., Abel E. L. Audiogenic seizure susceptibility and auditory brainstem responses in rats prenatally exposed to alcohol. *Alcoholism: Clinical and Experimental Research 16:*490–498, 1992.

Bielawski D. M., Abel E. L. Acute treatment of paternal alcohol exposure produces malformations in offspring. *Alcohol 14:*397–401, 1997.

Bierich J. R., Majewski F., Michaelis R., Tillner I. Uber das embryo-fetale alkolsyndrom. (On the embryofetal alcohol syndrome.) *European Journal of Pediatrics 121:*155–177, 1976.

Bingol N., Schuster C., Fuchs M., Iosub S., Turner G., et al. The influence of socioeconomic factors on the occurrence of fetal alcohol syndrome. *Advances in Alcoholism and Substance Abuse 6:*105–118, 1987.

Binkiewicz A. M., Robinson M. J., Senior B. Pseudo-Cushing syndrome caused by alcohol in breast milk. *Journal of Pediatrics 6:*956–967, 1978.

Bocking A. D., Carmichael L. J., Abdollah S., Sinervo K. R., Smith G. N., et al. Effects of ethanol on immature ovine fetal breathing movements, fetal prostaglandin E_2, and myometrial activity. *American Journal of Physiology 266:*R1297–R1301, 1994.

Boggan W. O., Monroe B., Turner W. R., Upshurk J., Middaugh L. D. Effect of prenatal ethanol administration on the urogenital system of mice. *Alcoholism: Clinical and Experimental Research 13:*206–208, 1989.

Boggan W. O., Randall C. L., Dodds H. M. Delayed sexual maturation in female $C_{57}BL/6J$ mice prenatally exposed to alcohol. *Research Communications in Pathology Pharmacology 23:*117–125, 1979.

Bolumar F., Rebagliato M., Hernandez-Aguado I., Florey C. du V. Smoking and drinking habits before and during pregnancy in Spanish women. *Journal of Epidemiology and Community Health 48:*36–40, 1994.

Bonati M., Fellin G. Changes in smoking and drinking behavior before and during pregnancy in Italian mothers: Implications for public health intervention. *International Journal of Epidemiology 20:*927–932, 1991.

Bonnemann C., Meinecke P. Holoprosencephaly as a possible embryonic alcohol effect. *American Journal of Medical Genetics 37:*431–432, 1990.

Bonthius D. J., West, J. R. Blood alcohol concentrations and microencephaly: A dose-response study in the neonatal rat. *Teratology 37:*223–231, 1988.

Bora P. S., Lange L. G. Molecular mechanism of ethanol metabolism by human brain to fatty acid ethyl esters. *Alcoholism: Clinical and Experimental Research 17:*28–30, 1993.

Borges G., Lopez-Cervantes M., Medina-Mora M. E., Tapia-Conyer R., Garrido F. Alcohol consumption, low birth weight, and preterm delivery in the national addiction survey (Mexico). *International Journal of Addiction 28:*355–368, 1993.

Boyd T. A., Ernhart C. B., Greene T. H., Sokol R. J., Martier S. Prenatal alcohol exposure and sustained attention in the preschool years. *Neurotoxicology and Teratology 13:*49–55, 1991.

Bray D. L., Anderson P. D. Appraisal of the epidemiology of fetal alcohol syndrome among Canadian native peoples. *Canadian Journal of Public Health 80:*42–45, 1989.

Bresnahan K., Zuckerman B., Cabral H. Psychosocial correlates of drug and heavy alcohol use among pregnant women at risk for drug use. *Obstetrics and Gynecology 80:*976–908, 1992.

Brooke O. G., Anderson H. R., Bland J. M., Peacock J. L., Stewart C. M. Effects on birth weight of smoking, alcohol, caffeine, socioeconomic factors, and psychosocial stress. *British Medical Journal 298:*795–801, 1989.

Brooten D., Peters M. A., Glatts M., Gaffney S. E., Knapp M., et al. A survey of nutrition, caffeine, cigarette and alcohol intake in early pregnancy in an urban clinic population. *Journal of Nurse-Midwifery 32:*85–90, 1987.

Brown N. A., Goulding E. H., Fabro S. Ethanol embryotoxicity: Direct effects on mammalian embryos in vitro. *Science 206:*573–575, 1979.

Brown R. T., Coles C. D., Smith I. E., Platzman K. A., Silverstein J., et al. Effects of prenatal alcohol exposure at school age: II. Attention and behavior. *Neurotoxicology and Teratology 13:*369–376, 1991.

Bruce F. C., Adams M. M., Shulman H. B., Martin M. L. Alcohol use before and during pregnancy. *American Journal of Preventive Medicine 9:*267–273, 1993.

Bruyere H. J., Stith C. E. Strain-dependent effect of ethanol on ventricular sepatal defect frequency in leghorn chick embryos.*Teratology 48:*299–303, 1993.

Bruyere H. J., Stith C. E. Ethyl alcohol reduces cardiac output, stroke volume, and end diastolic volume in the embryonic chick. *Teratology 49:*104–112, 1994.

Buckley J. D., Sather H., Ruccione K., Rogers P. C. J., Hass J. E., et al. A case-control study of risk factors for hepatoblastoma: A report from the children's cancer study group. *Cancer 64:*1169–1176, 1989.

Burd L. I., Martsolf J. T. Fetal alcohol syndrome: Diagnosis and syndromal variability. *Physiological Behavior 46:*39–43, 1989.

Burd L. I., Jones D., Simmons M. A., Makowski E. L., Meschia G., et al. Placental production and fetal utilization of lactate and pyruvate. *Nature 254:*710–711, 1975.

Burd L. I., Shea T. E., Knull H. "Mountain gin": Ingestion of commercial products containing denatured alcohol among Native Americans. *Journal of Studies on Alcohol 48:*388–389, 1987.

Burke J. P., Fenton M. R. The effect of maternal ethanol consumption on aldehyde dehydrogenase activity in neonates. *Research Communications in Psychology, Psychiatriy, and Behavior 3:*169–172, 1978.

Caetano R. Ethnicity and drinking in northern California: A comparison among whites, blacks, and Hispanics. *Alcohol and Alcoholism 19:*31–34, 1984.

Campbell, M. A., Fentel A. G. Terategenicity of acetaldehyde in vitro relevance to the Fetal Alcohol Syndrome. *Life Science 32:*2641–2647, 1987.

Canfield R., Selva I. K. FAS surveillance in a native American population in South Dakota. Unpublished study, 1993.

Cardones F., Brancato R., Venturi E., Bianchi S., Magni R. Corneal endothelial anomalies in the fetal alcohol syndrome. *Archives of Ophthalmology 110:*1128–1131, 1992.

Carmichael-Olson H., Sampson P. D., Barr H., Steissguth A. P., Brookstein F. L. Prenatal exposure to alcohol and school problems in late childhood: A longitudinal prospective study. *Development and Psychopathology 4:*341–359, 1992.

Cartwright M. M., Smith S. M. Stage-dependent effects of ethanol on cranial neural crest cell development: Partial basis for the phenotypic variations observed in fetal alcohol syndrome. *Alcoholism: Clinical and Experimental Research 19:*1454–1462, 1995a.

Cartwright M. M., Smith S. M. Increased cell death and reduced neural crest cell numbers in ethanol-exposed embryos: Partial basis for the fetal alcohol syndrome phenotype. *Alcoholism: Clinical and Experimental Research 19:*378–386, 1995b.

Castells S., Mark E., Abaci F., Schwartz E. Growth retardation in fetal alcohol syndrome. *Developmental Pharmacology and Therapeutics 3:*232–241, 1981.

Castro-Gago M., Novo I., Pena J. Maternal alcohol ingestion and neural tube defects: Observations in four brothers in a family. *Brain Development 9:*321–322, 1987.

Cate, J. C., Hedrick R., Morin R. Fetal alcohol syndrome and lactic acidosis. *Clinical Chemistry 29:*1320, 1983.

Cavallo F., Russo R., Zotti C., Camerlengo A., Ruggenini A. M. Moderate alcohol consumption and spontaneous abortion. *Alcohol and Alcoholism 30:*195–201, 1995.

Centers for Disease Control. Linking multiple data sources in fetal alcohol syndrome surveillance—Alaska. *Morbidity and Mortality Weekly Report 42:*312–314, 1993a.

Centers for Disease Control. Fetal alcohol syndrome–United States, 1979–1992. *Morbidity and Mortality Weekly Report 42:*339–341, 1993b.

Centers for Disease Control. Update: Trends in fetal alcohol syndrome–United States, 1979–1993. *Morbidity and Mortality Weekly Report 44:*249–251, 1995a.

Centers for Disease Control. Use of international classification of diseases coding to identify fetal alcohol syndrome—Indian Health Service Facilities, 1981–1992. *Morbidity and Mortality Weekly Report 44:*253–261, 1995b.

Chautan M., Calaf R., Leonardi J., Charbonnier M., Andre M., et al. Inverse modifications of heart and liver α-tocopherol status by various dietary N-6/N-3 polyunsaturated fatty acid ratios. *Journal of Lipid Research 31:*2201–2208, 1990.

Chen H., Namkung M. J., Jachau M. R. Effects of ethanol on biotransformation of all-trans-retinol and all-trans-retinal to all-trans-retinoic acid in rat conceptual cytosol. *Alcoholism: Clinical and Experimental Research 20:*942–947, 1996.

Chernick V., Childiaeva R., Ioffe S. Effects of maternal alcohol intake and smoking on neonatal electroencephalogram and anthropometric measurements. *American Journal of Obstetrics and Gynecology 146:*41–47, 1983.

Chernoff G. F. The fetal alcohol syndrome in mice: An animal model. *Teratology 15:*223–230, 1977.

Church M. W., Gerkin K. P. Hearing disorders in children with fetal alcohol syndrome: Findings for case reports. *Pediatrics 82:*147–154, 1988.

Church M. W., Holloway J. A. Audiogenic seizure susceptibility in mature rats with fetal alcohol syndrome. *Alcoholism: Clinical and Experimental Research 5:*145, 1981.

Church M. W., Abel E. L., Dintcheff B. A., Gerkin K. P., Gritzke R., et al. Brain-stem and cortical auditory evoked potentials in rats chronically exposed to alcohol in utero. In Johnson R., Pohrbaugh J. W., Parasuraman R. (Eds.), *Current Trends in Event-Related Potential Research* (Vol. 40; pp. 452–460), 1987.

Church M. W., Abel W. L., Dintcheff B. A., Matyjasik C. Maternal age and blood alcohol concentration in the pregnant Long-Evans rat. *Journal of Pharmacology and Experimental Therapeutics 253:*192–199, 1990.

Church M. W., Abel E. L., Kaltenbach J. A., Overbeck G. W. Effects of prenatal alcohol exposure and aging on auditory function in the rat: Preliminary results. *Alcoholism: Clinical and Experimental Research 20:*172–179, 1996.

Church M. W., Eldis F., Blakley B. W., Bawle E. V. Hearing, language, speech, vestibular, and dentofacial disorders in the fetal alcohol syndrome (FAS). *Alcoholism: Clinical and Experimental Research 21:*227–237, 1997.

Church M. W., Gerkin K. P., McPherson E. W. The incidence of sudden infant death syndrome (SIDS) amongst the older siblings of children with fetal alcohol syndrome (FAS). *Alcoholism: Clinical and Experimental Research 1:*93 (Abstract 10), 1986.

Church M. W., Holmes P. A., Overbeck G. W., Tilak J. P., Zajac C. S., Interactive effects of prenatal alcohol and cocaine exposures on postnatal mortality, development, and behavior in the Long-Evans rat. *Neurotoxicology and Teratology 13:*377–386, 1991.

Clarren S. K. Recognition of fetal alcohol syndrome. *Journal of the American Medical Association 45:*2436–2440, 1981.

Clarren S. K. Neuropathology in fetal alcohol syndrome. In West J. R. (Ed.), *Alcohol and Brain Development* (pp. 158–166). New York: Oxford University Press, 1986.

Clarren S. K. Alcohol-related birth defects: The clinical situation as defined over 15 years of experience. In Robinson G. C., Armstrong R. W. (Eds.), *Alcohol and Child/Family Health* (pp. 23–35), Vancouver, BC: University of British Columbia, 1988.

Clarren S. K., Bowden D. M. Fetal alcohol syndrome: A new primate model for binge drinking and its relevance to human ethanol teratogenesis. *Journal of Pediatrics 101:*819–824, 1982.

Clarren S. K., Astley S. J., Bowden D. M. Physical anomalies and development delays in nonhuman primate infants exposed to weekly doses of ethanol during gestation. *Teratology 37:*561–569, 1988.

Clarren S. K., Sampson P. D., Larsen J., Donnell D. J., Barr H. M., et al. Facial effects of fetal alcohol exposure: Assessment by photographs and morphometric analysis. *American Journal of Medical Genetics 26:*651–666, 1987.

Coles C. D. Prenatal alcohol exposure and human development. In Miller M. W. (Ed.), *Development of the Central Nervous System: Effects of Alcohol and Opiates* (pp. 9–36). New York: Wiley-Liss, 1992.

Coles C. D., Brown R. T., Smith I. E., Platzman K. A., Erickson S., et al. Effects of prenatal alcohol exposure at school age: I. Physical and cognitive development. *Neurotoxicology and Teratology 13:*357–367, 1991.

Coles C. D., Platzman K. A., Raskind-Hood C. L., Brown R. T., Falek A., et al. A comparison of children affected by prenatal alcohol exposure and attention deficit hyperactivity disorder (ADHD). *Alcoholism: Clinical and Experimental Research 21:*150–161, 1997.

Coles C. D., Platzman K. A., Smith, I., James M. E., Falek A. Effects of cocaine and alcohol use in pregnancy as neonatal growth and neurobehavioral status. *Neurotoxicology and Teratology 14:*22–33, 1992.

Coles C. D., Smith I. E., Falek A. A neonatal marker for cognitive vulnerability to alcohol's teratogenic effects. *Alcoholism: Clinical and Experimental Research 11:*197, 1987a.

Coles C. D., Smith I. E., Falek A. Prenatal alcohol exposure and infant behavior: Immediate effects and implications for later development. *Advances in Alcoholism and Substance Abuse 6:*87–104, 1987b.

Coles C. D., Smith I. E., Fernoff P. M., Falek A. Neonatal ethanol withdrawal: Characteristics in clinically normal nondysmorphic neonates. *Journal of Pediatrics 105:*445–451, 1984.

Coles C. D., Smith I. E., Fernhoff P. M., Falek A. Neonatal neurobehavioral characteristics as correlates of maternal alcohol use during gestation. *Alcoholism: Clinical and Experimental Research 9:*454–460, 1985a.

Coles C. D., Smith I. E., Lancaster J. A., Falek A. Persistence over the first month of neurobehavioral deficits in infants exposed to alcohol prenatally. *Alcoholism: Clinical and Experimental Research 9:*206, 1985b.

Collingridge G. L., Lester R. A. Excitatory amino acid receptors in the vertebrate central nervous system. *Pharmacological Reviews 40:*143–210, 1989.

Conry J. Neuropsychological deficits in fetal alcohol syndrome and fetal alcohol effects. *Alcoholism Clinical and Experimental Research 14:*650–655, 1990.

Cordero J. F., Floyd R. L., Martin M. L., Davis M., Hymbaugh K. Tracking the prevalence of FAS. *Alcohol Health and Research World 18:*82–85, 1994.

Cornelius M. D., Day N. L., Cornelius J. R., Geva D., Taylor P. M., et al. Drinking patterns and correlates of drinking among pregnant teenagers. *Alcoholism: Clinical and Experimental Research 17:*290–294, 1993.

Cornelius M. D., Richardson G. A., Day N. L., Cornelius J. R., Geva D., et al. A comparison of prenatal drinking in two recent samples of adolescents and adults. *Journal of Studies on Alcohol 55:*412–419, 1994.

Coulter C. L., Leech R. W., Schaefer G. B., Scheithauer B. W., Brumback R. A. Midline cerebral dysgenesis, dysfunction of the hypothalamic-pituitary axis, and fetal alcohol effects. *Archives of Neurology 50:*771–775, 1993.

Counsell A. M., Smale P. N., Geddis D. C. Alcohol consumption by New Zealand women during pregnancy. *New Zealand Medical Journal 107:*278–281, 1994.

Crain L. S., Fitzmaurice N. E., Mondry C. Nail dysplasia and fetal alcohol syndrome. *American Journal of Disease in Childhood 137:*1069–1072, 1983.

Crawford M. A., Doyle W., Leaf A., Laigfield M., Ghebremeskel K., et al. Nutritional and neurodevelopmental disorders. *Nutrition and Health 9:*81–85, 1993.

Criqui M. H., Ringel B. L. Does diet or alcohol explain the French paradox. *Lancet 344:*1719–1723, 1994.

Da Costa Pereira A., Olsen J., Ogston A. Variability of self-reported measures of alcohol consumption: Implications for the association between drinking in pregnancy and birth weight. *J. Epidemiology and Community Health 47:*326–330, 1993.

Dahl-Regis M. M., Jayam-Trought A. Fetal alcohol syndrome and myathenia gravis. *Journal of the National Medical Association 78:*1111–1117, 1986.

Daughaday J. H., Maritz I. K., Trivedi B. A preferential binding site for insulinlike growth factor II in human and rat placental membranes. *Journal of Clinical Endocrinology and Metabolism 46:*649–652, 1978.

Davis P. J., Partridge J. W., Storrs C. N. Alcohol consumption in pregnancy. How much is safe. *Archives of Disease in Childhood 57:*940–943, 1982.

Davis W. L., Crawford L. A., Cooper O. J., Farmer G. R., Thomas D. L., et al. Ethanol induces the generation of reactive free radicals by neural crest cells in vitro. *Journal of Craniofacial Genetics and Developmental Biology 10:*277–293, 1990.

Dawkins M. P., Harper F. D. Alcoholism among women: A comparison of black and white problem drinkers. *International Journal of Addictions 18:*333–349, 1983.

Day N. L., Cornelius M., Goldschmidt L., Richardson G., Robles N., et al. The effect of prenatal tobacco and marijuana use on offspring growth from birth through 3 years of age. *Neurotoxicology and Teratology 14:*407–414, 1992.

Day N. L., Goldsmith L., Robles N., Richardson G., Cornelius M., et al. Prenatal alcohol exposure and offspring growth at 18 months of age: The predictive validity of two measures of drinking. *Alcoholism: Clinical Experimental Research 15:*913–918, 1991.

Day N. L., Jasperse D., Richardson G., Robles N., Sambamoorthi U., et al. Prenatal exposure to alcohol: Effect on infant growth and morphologic characteristics. *Pediatrics 84:*536–541, 1989.

Day N. L., Richardson G. A., Geva D., Robles N., Alcohol, marijuana, and tobacco: Effects of prenatal exposure on offspring growth and morphology at age six. *Alcoholism: Clinical and Experimental Research 18:*786–794, 1994.

Day N. L., Richardson G. A., Geva D., Taylor P., Scher M., et al. The effects of prenatal alcohol use on the growth of children at three years of age. *Alcoholism: Clinical and Experimental Research 15:*67–71, 1991.

Day N. L., Richardson G., Robles N. Effect of prenatal alcohol exposure on growth and morphology of offspring at 8 months of age. *Pediatrics 85:*748–752, 1990.

De Groot H., Littauer A. Hypoxia, reactive oxygen, and cell injury. *Free Radical Biology and Medicine 6:*541–551, 1989.

De Luca L. M., Ross, S. A. Retinoic acid response elements as positive and negative regulators of the expression of the homeobox b-1 genes. *Nutrition Review 54:*61–63, 1996.

Dehaene P. H., Crepin G., Delahousse G., Querleu D., Walbaum R., et al. Aspects epidemiologiques du syndrome d'alcoolisme foetal: 45 observations en 3 ans. [Epidemiological aspects of the foetal alcoholism syndrome: 45 cases.] *Nouvelle Presse Medical 10:*2639–2649, 1981.

Dehaene, P. H., Samaille-Villette C., Samaille P. P., Crepin G., Waldbaum R., et al. Le syndrome d'alcoolisme, foetal dans le nord de la France. *Revere de l'Alcoolisme 23:*145–158, 1977.

Dehaene P. H., Samaille-Villette C., Fordaiger-Fasquelle P., Subtel D., Delahouse G., et al. Diagnostic et prevalence du syndrome d'alcoolisme foetal en maternite. *La Presse Medicale 20:*1002, 1991.

Deltour L., Ang H. L., Duester G. Ethanol inhibition of retinoic acid synthesis as a potential mechanism for fetal alcohol syndrome. *FASEB Journal 10:*1050–1057, 1996.

De Nigris, C., Awabdeh, F., Tomassini, A., and Remotti, G., Alcool e gravidanza (Alcohol and pregnancy). *Annali di Ostetricia Ginlcologia Medicina Perinatale 102:*419–430, 1981.

Dexter J. D., Tumbleson M. E., Decker J. D., Middleton C. C. Fetal alcohol syndrome in Sinclair (s-1) miniature swine. *Alcoholism: Clinical and Experimental Research 4:*146–151, 1980.

Dianzani M. U. Role of free radical-mediated reactions in ethanol-induced liver damage. *Advances in Bioscience, Alcohol Toxicology and Free Radical Mechanisms 71:*35–41, 1988.

Dlugosy L., Bracken M. B. Reproductive effects of caffeine: A review and theoretical analysis. *Epidemiologic Reviews 14:*83–100, 1992.

Dombrowski M., Berry S. M., Johnson M. P., Salai A. A. Birth weight/length ratio, ponderal index, placental weight, and birth weight/placental weight ratio. *Archives of Pediatrics and Adolescent Medicine 148:*508–512, 1994.

Dominguez-Rojas V., de Juanes-Pardo J. R., Astasio-Arbiza P., Ortega-Molina P., Gordillo-Florencio E. Spontaneous abortion in a hospital population: Are tobacco and coffee intake risk factors? *European Journal of Epidemiology 10:*665–668, 1994.

Dorris M. *The Broken Cord*. New York: Harper & Row, 1989.

Dow K. E., Riopelle R. J. Ethanol neurotoxicity: Effects on neurite formation and neurotrophic factor production in vitro. *Science 228:*591–593, 1985.

Dreosti I. E. Zinc deficiency and the fetal alcohol syndrome. *Medical Journal of Australia 1:*3–4, 1981.

Dreosti I. E. Nutritional factors underlying the expression of the fetal alcohol syndrome. *New York Academy of Science 678:*193–204, 1993.

Dreosti I. E., Ballard J., Belling B., Record I. R., Manuel S. J., et al. The effect of ethanol and acetaldehyde on DNA synthesis in growing cells and on fetal development in the rat. *Alcoholism: Clinical and Experimental Research 5:*357–362, 1981.

Druse M. J., Rathbun W. E., McNulty J. A., Nyquist-Battie C. Maternal ethanol consumption: Lack of effect on synaptogenesis in layer I of the motor cortex in 19-day-old rat offspring. *Experimental Neurology 94:*497–508, 1986.

Duester G. A hypothetical mechanism for fetal alcohol syndrome involving ethanol inhibition of retinoic acid synthesis at the alcohol dehydrogenase step. *Alcoholism: Clinical Experimental Research 15:*568–572, 1991.

Dufour M. C., FeCaces M. Epidemiology of the medical consequences of alcohol. *Alcohol Health World 17:*265–271, 1993.

Duimstra C., Johnson D., Kutsch C., Wang B., Zentner M., et al. A fetal alcohol syndrome surveillance pilot project in American Indian communities in the northern Plains. *Public Health Reports 108:*225–229, 1993.

Duncan R. J. S., Woodhouse B. The lack of effect on liver alcohol dehydrogenase in mice of early exposure to alcohol. *Biochemical Pharmacology 27:*2755–2756, 1978.

Dupuis C., Dehaene P., Deroubaix-Tella P., Blanc-Garin A. P., Rey C., et al. Les cardiopathies des enfants nes de mere alcoolique. *Archives des Maladies du Coeur et des Vaisseaux 71:*565–572, 1978.

Edwards C. H., Cole O. J., Oyemade J., Knight E. M., Johnson A. A., et al. Maternal stress and pregnancy outcome in a prenatal clinic population. *Journal of Nutrition 124:*10065–10215, 1994.

Egeland G. M., Perham-Hester K. A., Hook E. B. Use of capture-recapture analyses in fetal alcohol syndrome surveillance in Alaska. *American Journal of Epidemiology 141:*335–341, 1995.

Eguchi Y., Yamamoto M., Arishima K., Shirai M., Wakabayashi K., et al. Histological changes in the placenta induced by maternal alcohol consumption in the rat. *Biology of the Neonate 56:*158–164, 1989.

Ellis F. W., Pick J. R. An animal model of the fetal alcohol syndrome in beagles. *Alcoholism: Clinical and Experimental Research 4:*123–134, 1980.

Ernhart C. B. Clinical correlations between ethanol intake and fetal alcohol syndrome. *Recent Developments in Alcoholism 9:*127–150, 1991.

Ernhart C. B. A critical review of low-level prenatal lead exposure in the human: 1. Effects on the fetus and newborn. *Reproductive Toxicology 6:*9–19, 1992.

Ernhart C. B., Green T., Sokol R. J., Martier S., Boyd T. A., et al. Neonatal diagnosis of fetal alcohol syndrome: Not necessarily a hopeless prognosis. *Alcoholism: Clinical and Experimental Research 19:*1550–1557, 1995.

Ernhart C. B., Morrow-Tlucak M., Sokol R. J., Martier S. Underreporting of alcohol use in pregnancy. *Alcoholism: Clinical and Experimental Research 12:*506–511, 1988.

Ernhart C. B., Sokol R. J., Martier S., Moron P., Nadler D., et al. Alcohol teratogenicity in the human: A detailed assessment of specificity, critical period, and threshold. *American Journal of Obstetrics and Gynecology 33:*156–161, 1987.

Ernhart C. B., Wolf A. W., Linn P. L., Sokol R. J., Kennard M. J., et al. Alcohol-related birth defects: Syndromal anomalies, intrauterine growth retardation, and neonatal behavioral assessment. *Alcoholism: Clinical and Experimental Research 9:*447–453, 1985a.

Ernhart C. B., Wolf A. W., Sokol R. J., Brittenham G. M., Erhard P. Fetal lead exposure: Antenatal factors. *Environmental Research 38:*54–66, 1985b.

Erskine R. L., Ritchie J. W. K. The effects of maternal consumption of alcohol on human umbilical artery blood flow. *American Journal of Obstetrics and Gynecology 154:*318–321, 1986.

Escobar L. F., Bixler D., Padilla L. M. Quantitation of craniofacial anomalies in utero: Fetal alcohol and Crouzon syndromes and thanatophoric dysplasia. *American Journal of Medical Genetics 45:*25–29, 1993.

Espina N., Lima V., Lieber C. S., Garro A. J. In vitro and in vivo inhibitory effect of ethanol and acetaldehyde on methylguanine transferase. *Carcinogenesis 9:*761–766, 1988.

Ewald S. J., Huang C., Bray L. Effect of prenatal alcohol exposure on lymphocyte populations in mice. *Advances in Experimental Medicine and Biology 288:*237–244, 1991.

Falconer J. The effect of maternal ethanol infusion on placental blood flow and fetal glucose metabolism in sheep. *Alcohol and Alcoholism 25:*413–416, 1990.

Faustman E. M., Streissguth A. P., Stevenson L. M., Omenn G. S., Yoshida A. Role of maternal and fetal-alcohol-metabolizing genotypes in fetal alcohol syndrome. *Toxicologist 12:*1562, 1992.

Ferrer I., Galofre E. Dendritic spine anomalies in fetal alcohol syndrome. *Neuropediatrics 18:*161–163, 1987.

Finucane B. T. Difficult intubation associated with the foetal alcohol syndrome. *Canadian Anaesthesia Society Journal 27:*574–575, 1980.

Fisher S. E., Karl P. I. Ethanol-nutrient interaction and the fetus. In Abel E. L. (Ed.), *Fetal Alcohol Syndrome: From Mechanism to Prevention* (pp. 269–284). Boca Raton, FL: CRC Press, 1996.

Fisher S. E., Alcock N. W., Amirian J., Altshuler H. L. Neonatal and maternal hair zinc levels in a nonhuman primate model of the fetal alcohol syndrome. *Alcoholism: Clinical and Experimental Research 12:*417–421, 1988.

Fisher S. E., Atkinson M., Jacobson S., Sehgal P., Burnap J., et al. Selective fetal malnutrition: The effect of in vivo ethanol exposure upon in vitro placental uptake of amino acids in the nonhuman primate. *Pediatric Research 17:*704–707, 1983.

Fisher S. E., Duffy L., Atkinson M. Selective fetal malnutrition: Effect of acute and chronic ethanol exposure upon rat placental Na-K-ATPase activity. *Alcoholism: Clinical and Experimental Research 10:*150–153, 1986.

Fisher S. E., Inselman L. S., Duffy L., Atkinson M., Spencer H., et al. Ethanol and fetal nutrition: Effects of chronic ethanol exposure on rat placental growth and membrane-associated folic acid receptor binding activity. *Journal of Pediatric Gastroenterology and Nutrition 4:*645–649, 1985.

Flynn A., Martier S. S., Sokol R. J., Miller S. I., Golder N. L., et al. Zinc status of pregnant alcoholic women: A determinant of fetal outcome. *Lancet 1:*572–574, 1981.

Fogel B. J., Nitkowsky K. H. M., Gruenwald P. Discordant abnormalities in monozygotic twins. *Journal of Pediatrics 66:*64–72, 1965.

Forrest F., du V. Florey C., Taylor D., McPherson F., Young J. A. Reported social alcohol consumption during pregnancy and infant's development at 18 months. *British Medical Journal 303:*22–26, 1991.

Foster U. G., Baird P. A. Congenital defects of the limbs and alcohol exposure in pregnancy: Data from a population based study. *American Journal of Medical Genetics 44:*782–785, 1992.

Fox S. H., Brown C., Koontz A. M., Kessel S. S. Perceptions of risks of smoking and heavy drinking during pregnancy: 1985 NHIS findings. *Public Health Reports 102:*73–79, 1987.

Francis v. State, 529 So. 2d 670 (Fla. 1988).

Freeza M., di Padova C., Pozzato G., Terpin M., Baroana E., et al. High blood alcohol levels in women. *New England Journal of Medicine 322:*95–99, 1990.

Fricker H. S., Bürgi W., Kaufmann H., Bruppacher R., Kipfer H., et a. Schwangerschaftsverlauf in einem repräsentativen Schweizer Kollektiv (Aarauer Schwangerschafts-und Neugeborenenstudie): II. Genussmittel in der Schwangerschaft. *Schweizerische Medizinische Wochenschrift Journal Suisse de Medecine 115:*381–386, 1985.

Fried P. A., Makin J. E. Neonatal behavioral correlates of prenatal exposure to marihuana cigarettes and alcohol in a low-risk population. *Neurotoxicology and Teratology 9:*1–7, 1987.

Fried P. A., O'Connell C. M. A comparison of the effects of prenatal exposure to tobacco, alcohol, cannabis, and caffeine on birth size and subsequent growth. *Neurotoxicology and Teratology 9:*79–85, 1987.

Fried P. A., Watkinson B. 12- and 24-month neurobehavioural follow-up of children prenatally exposed to marihuana, cigarettes, and alcohol. *Neurotoxicology and Teratology 10:*305–313, 1988.

Fried P. A., Innes K. S., Barnes M. W. Soft drug use prior to and during pregnancy: A comparison of sample over a four-year period. *Drug and Alcohol Dependence 13:*161, 1984.

Fried P. A., Watkinson B., Grant A. Changing patterns of soft drug use prior to and during pregnancy: A prospective study. *Drug and Alcohol Dependence 6:*323–328, 1980.

Friedman J. M. Can maternal alcohol ingestion cause neural tube defects? *Journal of Pediatrics 101:*232–234, 1982.

Fryns J. P., Deroover J., Parloir C., Goffaux P., Lebas E., et al. The foetal alcohol syndrome. *Acta Paediatrica Belgica 30:*117–121, 1977.

Fuchs M., Isoub S., Bingol N., Gromisch D. Palpebral fissure size revisited. *Journal of Pediatrics 96:*77–78, 1980.

Fukunaga T., Sillanaukee P., Eriksson C. J. Occurrence of blood acetaldehyde in women during ethanol intoxication: Preliminary findings. *Alcoholism: Clinical and Experimental Research 17:*1198–1200, 1993.

Gabrielli O., Salvolini U., Coppa G. V., Catassi C., Rossi R., et al. Magnetic resonance imaging in the malformative syndromes with mental retardation. *Pediatric Radiology 21:*16–19, 1990.

Gage J. C., Sulik K. K. Pathogenesis of ethanol-induced hydronephrosis and hydroureter as demonstrated following in vivo exposure of mouse embryos. *Teratology 44:*299–312, 1991.

Garber J. M. Steep corneal curvature in the fetal alcohol syndrome: A fetal alcohol syndrome landmark. *Journal of the American Optometric Association 8:*641–644, 1982.

Garro A. J., McBeth D. L., Lima V., Lieber C. S. Ethanol consumption inhibits fetal DNA methylation in mice: Implications for the fetal alcohol syndrome. *Alcoholism: Clinical and Experimental Research 15:*395–398, 1991.

Ghishan F. K., Patwardhan R., Greene H. L. Fetal alcohol syndrome: Inhibition of placental zinc transport as a potential mechanism for fetal growth retardation in the rat. *Journal of Clinical and Laboratory Medicine 100:*45–52, 1982.

Gibson G. T., Baghurst P. A., Colley D. P. Maternal alcohol, tobacco, and cannabis consumption and the outcome of pregnancy. *Australia and New Zealand Journal of Obstetrics and Gynaecology 23:*15–19, 1983.

Giknis M. L. A., Damjanov I., Rubin E. The differential transplacental effects of ethanol in four mouse strains. *Neurobehavioral Toxicology 2:*235–237, 1980.

Gilliam D. M., Kotch L. E., Dudek B. C., Riley, E. P. Ethanol teratogenesis in selectively bred long-sleep and short-sleep mice: A comparison to inbred $C_{57}BL/6J$ mice. *Alcoholism: Clinical and Experimental Research 13:*667–672, 1989.

Giunta C. T., Streissguth A. P. Patients with fetal alcohol syndrome and their caretakers: Social casework. *Journal of Contemporary Social Work (Sept.):*453–459, 1988.

Glass R. H., Golbus H. S. Habitual abortion. *Fertility and Sterility 29:*257, 1978.

Godel J. C., Pabst H. F., Hodges P. E., Johnson K. E., Froese G. J., et al. Smoking and caffeine and alcohol intake during pregnancy in a northern population: Effects on fetal growth. *Canadian Medical Association Journal 147:*181–188, 1992.

Golden N. L., Sokol R. J., Kuhnert B. R., Bottoms S. Maternal alcohol use and infant development. *Pediatrics 70:*931–934, 1982.

Goldstein D. B. Effect of alcohol on cellular membranes. *Annals of Emergency Medicine 15:*1013–1018, 1986.

Goldstein G., Arulanantham K. Neural tube defect and renal anomalies in a child with fetal alcohol syndrome. *Journal of Pediatrics 93:*636–637, 1978.

Goodlett C. R., Marcussen B. L., West J. R. A single day of alcohol exposure during the brain growth spurt induces brain weight restriction and cerebellar Purkinje cell loss. *Alcohol 7:*107–114, 1990.

Gordon B. H. J., Streeter M. L., Winick M. Prenatal alcohol exposure: Abnormalities in placental growth and fetal amino acid uptake in the rat. *Biology of the Neonate 47:*113–119, 1985.

Gottesfeld Z. Fetal alcohol exposure and functional implications of the neuroimmune-endocrine networks. In Abel E. L. (Ed.), *Fetal Alcohol Syndrome: From Mechanism to Prevention* (pp. 113–144). Boca Raton, FL: CRC Press, 1996.

Gottesfeld Z., Silverberg P. B. Developmental delays associated with prenatal alcohol exposure are reversed by thyroid hormone treatment. *Neuroscience Letters 109:*42–47, 1990.

Gottesfeld Z., Trippe K., Wargovich M. J., Berkowitz A. S. Fetal alcohol exposure and adult tumorigenesis. *Alcohol 9:*465–471, 1992.

Gould S. J., *The Mismeasure of Man.* New York: W. W. Norton, 1989.

Greeley S., Johnson W. T., Schafer D., Johnson P. E. Gestational alcoholism and fetal zinc accretion in Long-Evans rats. *Journal of American College of Nutrition 9:*265–271, 1990.

Greenamyre J. T., Olson J. M. M., Penney J. B., Young A. B. Autoradiographic characterization of N-methyl-d-aspartate, quisqualate-, and kainate-sensitive glutamate binding sites. *Journal of Pharmacology and Experimental Teratology 233:*254–263, 1985.

Greene T., Ernhart C. B., Ager J., Sokol R., Martier S., et al. Prenatal alcohol exposure and cognitive development in the preschool years. *Neurotoxicology and Teratology 13:*57–68, 1991a.

Greene T., Ernhart C. B., Sokol R. J., Martier S., Marler M. R., et al. Prenatal alcohol exposure and preschool physical growth: A longitudinal analysis. *Alcoholism: Clinical and Experimental Research 15:*905–913, 1991b.

Greizerstein H. B., Aldrich L. K. Ethanol and diazepam effects on intrauterine growth of the rat. *Developmental Pharmacology and Therapeutics 6:*409–418, 1983.

Griso J. A., Roman E., Inskip H., Beral V., Donovan J. Alcohol consumption and outcome of pregnancy. *Journal of Epidemiology and Community Health 38:*232–235, 1984.

Grossman D. C., Krieger J. W., Sugarman J. R., Forquera R. A. Health status of urban American Indians and Alaska natives. *Journal of the American Medical Association 271:*845–850, 1994.

Grummer M. A., Langhough R. E., Zachman R. D. Maternal ethanol ingestion effects on fetal rat brain vitamin A as a model for fetal alcohol syndrome. *Alcoholism: Clinical and Experimental Research 17:*592–597, 1993.

Guilmet G. M. Oral linguistic and nonoral-visual styles of attending: Navajo and Caucasian children compared in an urban classroom and on an urban playground. *Human Organization 40:*145–150, 1981.

Gusella J., Fried P. Effects of maternal social drinking and smoking on offspring at 13 months. *Neurobehavioral Toxicology and Teratology 6:*13–17, 1984.

Haddad J., Messer J. Fetal alcoholism syndrome: Report of three siblings. *Neuropediatrics 25:*109–111, 1994.

Hagberg B., Kyllerman M. Epidemiology of mental retardation—A Swedish survey. *Brain and Development 5:*441–449, 1983.

Hakkola J., Pasanem M., Purkunen R., Saarikoski S., Pelkonen O., et al. Expression of xenobiotic-metabolizing cytochrome P_{450} forms in human and adult fetal liver. *Biochemical Pharmacology 48:*59–64, 1994.

Halmesmaki E., Ylikorkala O. A retrospective study on the safety of prenatal ethanol treatment. *Obstetrics and Gynecology 72:*545–549, 1988.

Halmesmaki E., Autti-Ramo I., Granstrom M. L., Heikinheimo M., Raivio K. O., et al. Alpha-fetoprotein, human placental lactogen, and pregnancy-specific beta-1-glycoprotein in pregnant women who drink: Relation to fetal alcohol syndrome. *American Journal of Obstetrics and Gynecology 155*:598–602, 1986.

Halmesmaki E., Raivio K. O., Ylikorkala O. Patterns of alcohol consumption during pregnancy. *Obstetrics and Gynecology 69*:594–599, 1987.

Halmesmaki E., Valimaki M., Karonen S., Ylikorkala O. Low somatomedin C and high-growth-hormone levels in newborns damaged by maternal alcohol abuse. *Obstetrics and Gynecology 74*:366–370, 1989a.

Halmesmaki E., Valimaki M., Rione R., Ylikahri R., Ylikorkala O. Maternal and paternal alcohol consumption and miscarriage. *British Journal of Obstetrics and Gynecology 96*:188–191, 1989b.

Halperin D. S., Assimacopoulos A., LaCourt G., Beguin F., Ferrier P. E. Maternal serum gamma-glutamyl transferase in the prenatal screening of fetal alcohol effects. *Pediatric Research 19*:1086, 1985.

Halvorsen P. R., Gross T. L., Sokol R. J. The effect of heavy maternal alcohol intake on amniotic fluid phospholipids in late pregnancy. *American Journal of Perinatology 2*:173–177, 1985.

Hambridge K. M., Krebs N. F., Jacobs M. A., Xavier A., Guyett L., et al. Zinc nutritional status during pregnancy: A longitudinal study. *American Journal of Clinical Nutrition 37*:429–434, 1983.

Hamilton M. A. *Linguistic abilities of children with fetal alcohol syndrome.* Ann Arbor, MI: University Microfilms International, 1981.

Hay Y. H. Why do chronic alcoholics require more anesthesia? *Anesthesiology 30*:341–342, 1969.

Hannigan J. H. Alcohol exposure and maternal-fetal thyroid function: Impact on biobehavioral maturation. In Zakhari S. (Ed.), *Alcohol and Endocrine System* (pp. 313–336). Bethesda, MD: National Institute on Alcoholism and Alcoholism, 1993.

Hannigan J. H. The effects of prenatal exposure to alcohol plus caffeine in rats: Pregnancy outcome and early offspring development. *Alcoholism: Clinical and Experimental Research 19*:238–246, 1995.

Hannigan J. H., Bellisario R. L. Lower serum thyroxine levels in rats following prenatal exposure to ethanol. *Alcoholism: Clinical and Experimental Research 14*:456–460, 1990.

Hannigan J. H., Abel E. L., Kruger M. L. "Population" characteristics of birth weight in an animal model of alcohol-related developmental effects. *Neurotoxicology and Teratology 15*:97–105, 1993a.

Hannigan J. H., Berman R. F., Zajac C. S. Environmental enrichment and the behavioral effects of prenatal exposure to alcohol in rats. *Neurotoxicology and Teratology 15*:261–266, 1993b.

Hannigan J. H., Martier S. S., Chugani H. T., Sokol R. J. Brain metabolism in children with fetal alcohol syndrome (FAS): A positron emission tomography study. *Alcoholism: Clinical and Experimental Research 19*:53A, 1995a.

Hannigan J. H., Martier S. S., Naber J. M. Independent associations among maternal alcohol consumption and infant thyroxine levels and pregnancy outcome. *Alcoholism: Clinical Experimental Research 19*:135–141, 1995b.

Hanson J. W., Jones K. L., Smith D. W. Fetal alcohol syndrome: Experience with 41 patients. *Journal of the American Medical Association 235*:1458–1460, 1976.

Hanson J. W., Streissguth A. P., Smith D. W. The effect of moderate alcohol consumption during pregnancy on fetal growth and morphogenesis. *Journal of Pediatrics 92*:457–460, 1978.

Hard E., Dahlgren I. L., Engel J., Larsson K., Liljequist S., et al. Developmental of sexual behavior in prenatally ethanol-exposed rats. *Drug and Alcohol Dependence 14*:51–61, 1984.

Hard E., Musi B., Dahlgren I. L., Engel J., Larsson K., et al. Impaired maternal behavior and altered central serotonergic activity in the adult offspring of chronically ethanol treated dams. *Acta Pharmacologica Toxicologica 56*:347–353, 1985.

Harlap S., Shiono P. H. Alcohol, smoking, and incidence of spontaneous abortions in the first and second trimester. *Lancet 2*:173–176, 1980.

Harlap S., Shiono P. H., Ramecharan S. Alcohol and spontaneous abortions. *American Journal of Epidemiology 110:*372, 1979.

Harris S. R., MacKay L. L. J., Osborn J. A. Autistic behaviors in offspring of mothers abusing alcohol and other drugs: A series of case reports. *Alcoholism: Clinical and Experimental Research 19:*660–665, 1995.

Harris S. R., Osborn J. A., Weinberg J., Loock C., Junald K. Effects of prenatal alcohol exposure on neuromotor and cognitive development during early childhood: A series of case reports. *Physical Therapy 73:*608–617, 1993.

Hart R. S., Frame L. T. Toxicological defense mechanisms and how they may affect the nature of dose-response relationships. *Belle Newsletter 5*(1):June, 1996.

Haste F. M., Brooke O. B., Anderson H. R., Bland J. M., Shaw A., et al. Nutrient intakes during pregnancy: Observations on the influence of smoking and social class. *American Journal of Clinical Nutrition 51:*29–36, 1990.

Haughton G., Mohr D., Ellis F. Increased susceptibility to induction of primary Rosa sarcoma in $C_{57}BL/10ScSn$ mice following perinatal exposure to dietary ethanol. *Alcoholism: Clinical and Experimental Research 5:*347 (abstract), 1981.

Havlicek V., Chiliaeva R., Chernick V. EEG frequency spectrum characteristics of sleep states in infants of alcoholic mothers. *Neuropadiatrie 8:*3690–373, 1977.

Hay W. W. Fetal glucose metabolism. *Seminars in Perinatology 3:*157–176, 1979.

Hazlett L. D., Barrett R. P., Berg R. S., Abel E. L. Maternal and paternal alcohol consumption increase offspring susceptibility to Pseudomonas aeruginosa ocular infection. *Ophthalmic Research 21:*381–387, 1989.

Heaton M. B., Swanson D. J., Paiva M., Walker D. W. Ethanol exposure affects trophic factor activity and responsiveness in chick embryo. *Alcohol 9:*161–166, 1992.

Henderson G. I., Schenker S. The effects of maternal alcohol consumption on the viability and visceral development of the newborn rat. *Research Communications in Chemical Pathology and Pharmacology 16:*15–32, 1977.

Henderson G. I., Devi B. G., Perez A., Schenker S. In utero ethanol exposure elicits oxidative stress in the rat fetus. *Alcoholism: Clinical and Experimental Research 19:*714–720, 1995.

Henderson G. I., Hoyumpa A. M. Jr., McClain C., Schenker S. The effects of chronic and acute alcohol administration on fetal development in the rat. *Alcoholism: Clinical and Experimental Research 3:*99–106, 1979.

Henderson G. I., Hoyumpa A. M. Jr., Rothschild M. A., Schenker S. Effect of ethanol and ethanol-induced hypothermia on protein synthesis in pregnant and fetal rats. *Alcoholism: Clinical and Experimental Research 4:*165–177, 1980.

Henderson G. I., Patwardhan R. V., McLeroy S., Schenker S. Inhibition of placental amino acid uptake in rats following acute and chronic ethanol. *Alcoholism: Clinical and Experimental Research 6:*495–505, 1982.

Henderson G. I., Turner D., Patwardhan R. V., Lumeng L., Hoyumpa A. M., et al. Inhibition of placental valine uptake after acute and chronic maternal ethanol consumption. *Journal of Pharmacology and Experimental Therapeutics 216:*465–472, 1981.

Hexter A. C., Harris J. A., Roeper P., Croen L. A., Kruger P., et al. Evaluation of the hospital discharge index and the birth certificate as sources of information on birth defects. *Public Health Reports 105:*296–306, 1990.

Higuchi S., Maramatsu T., Matsushita S., Murayama M., Hayashida M. Polymorphisms of ethanol-oxidizing enzymes in alcoholics with inactive $ALDH_2$. *Human Genetics 97:*431–434, 1996.

Higuchi Y., Matsumoto N. Embryotoxicity of ethanol and acetaldehyde: Direct effects of mouse embryo in vitro. *Congenital Anomalies 24:*9–28, 1984.

Hingson R., Alpert J. J., Day N., Dooling E., Kayne H., et al. Effects of maternal drinking and marijuana use on fetal growth and development. *Pediatrics 70:*539–546, 1982.

Hinzpeter E. N., Renz S., Loser H. Augenveranderungen bei Alkoholembryohopathie (Eye manifestations of alcohol embryopathy). *Klinische Monatsblatter fur Augenheilkunde 200:*33–38, 1992.

Hoff S. F. Synaptogenesis in the hippocampal dentate gyrus: Effects of in utero ethanol exposure. *Brain Research Bulletin 21:*47–54, 1988.

Hoffman H. J., Damas K., Hillman L., Krongrad E. Risk factors for SIDS: Results of the National Institute of Child Health and Human Developments SIDS Cooperative Epidemiological Study. *Annals of the New York Academy of Sciences 533:*13–27, 1988.

Hogue C. J. R., Buehler J. W., Strauss L. T., Smith J. C. Overview of the National Infant Mortality Surveillance (NIMS) project—design, methods, results. *Public Health Reports 102:*126–138, 1987.

Holliday R. The inheritance of epigenetic defects. *Science 238:*163–169, 1987.

Hollstedt C., Dahlgren L., Rydberg U. Alcoholic women in fertile age treated at an alcoholic clinic. *Acta Psychiatric Scandinavica 67:*195–204, 1983a.

Hollstedt C., Dahlgren L., Rydberg U. Outcome of pregnancy in women treated at an alcoholic clinic. *Acta Psychiatrica Scandinavica 67:*236–248, 1983b.

Holzman A. E., Chrousos G. A., Kozma C., Traboulsi E. I. Duane's retraction syndrome in the fetal alcohol syndrome. *American Journal of Ophthalmology 110:*656–566, 1990.

Hooper S. H., Harding R., Deayton J., Thorburn G. D. Role of prostaglandins in the metabolic responses of the fetus to hypoxia. *American Journal of Obstetrics and Gynecology 166:*1568–1575, 1992.

Hungund B. L., Gokhale V. S. Reduction of fatty acid ethyl ester accumulation by ganglioside GM_1 in rat fetus exposed to ethanol. *Biochemical Pharmacology 37:*3001–3004, 1994.

Hunt E., Streissguth A. P., Kerr B., Carmichael-Olson H. Mothers' alcohol consumption during pregnancy: Effects on spatial-visual reasoning in 14-year-old children. *Psychological Sciences 6:*339–342, 1995.

Hunter E. S., Sadler T. W. Fuel-mediated teratogenesis: Biochemical effects of hypoglycemia during neurulation in mouse embryos in vitro. *American Journal of Physiology 257:*E269–E276, 1989.

Hutchings D. E. Prenatal opioid exposure and the problem of causal inference. In Pinkert T. M. (Ed.), *Current Research on the Consequences of Maternal Drug Abuse* (pp. 6–19). Rockville, MD: National Institute on Drug Abuse, 1985.

Hutchings D. E. The puzzle of cocaine's effects following maternal use during pregnancy: Are their reconcilable differences? *Neurotoxicology and Teratology 15:*281–286, 1993.

Hynd G. W., Scott S. A. Propositional and appositional modes of thought and differential cerebral speech lateralization in Navajo Indian and Anglo children. *Child Development 51:*909–911, 1980.

Hynd G. W., Teeter A., Stewart J. Acculturation and the lateralization of speech in the bilingual Native American. *International Journal of Neuroscience 11:*1–7, 1980.

Ihemelandu E. C. Effect of maternal alcohol consumption on pre- and post-natal muscle development of mice. *Growth 45:*35–43, 1984.

Institute of Medicine. *Fetal Alcohol Syndrome.* Washington, DC: National Academy Press, 1996.

Ioffe S., Chernick V. Maternal alcohol ingestion and the incidence of respiratory distress syndrome. *American Journal of Obstetrics and Gynecology 156:*1231–1235, 1987.

Ioffe S., Chernick V. Development of the EEG between 30 and 40 weeks gestation in normal and alcohol-exposed infants. *Developmental Medicine and Child Neurology 30:*797–807, 1988.

Ioffe S., Chernick V. Predition of subsequent motor and mental retardation newborn infants exposed to alcohol in utero by computerized EEG analysis. *Neuropediatrics 21:*11–17, 1990.

Ioffe S., Childiaeva R., Chernick V. Prolonged effects of maternal alcohol ingestion on the neonatal electroencephalogram. *Pediatrics 74:*330–335, 1984.

Iosub S., Fuchs M., Bingol N., Gromisch D. S. Fetal alcohol syndrome revisited. *Pediatrics 68:*475–479, 1981.

Jacobson J. L., Jacobson S. W., Sokol R. J. Effects of prenatal exposure to alcohol, smoking, and illicit drugs on postpartum somatic growth. *Alcoholism: Clinical and Experimental Research 18:*317–323, 1994a.

Jacobson J. L., Jacobson S. W., Sokol R. J. Increased vulnerability to alcohol-related birth defects in the offspring of mothers over 30. *Alcoholism: Clinical and Experimental Research 20:*359–363, 1996.

Jacobson J. L., Jacobson S. W., Sokol R. J., Martier S. S., Ager J. W., et al. Effects of alcohol use, smoking, and illicit drug use on fetal growth in black infants. *Journal of Pediatrics 124:*757–764, 1994b.

Jacobson J. L., Jacobson S. W., Sokol R. J., Martier S. S., Ager J. W., et al. Teratogenic effects of alcohol on infant development. *Alcoholism: Clinical and Experimental Research 17:*174–183, 1993a.

Jacobson S. W., Fein G. G., Jacobson J. L., Schwartz P. M., Dowler J. K. Neonatal correlates of prenatal exposure to smoking, caffeine, and alcohol. *Infant Behavior and Development 7:*253–265, 1984.

Jacobson S. W., Jacobson J. L., Bihun J. T., Chiodo L., Sokol R. J. Effects of prenatal alcohol exposure on poststress cortisol levels in infants. *Alcoholism: Clinical and Experimental Research 17:*456, 1993b.

Jacobson S. W., Jacobson J. L., Frye K. F. Incidence and correlates of breast-feeding in disadvantaged women. *Pediatrics 88:*728–736, 1991a.

Jacobson S. W., Jacobson J. L., Sokol, R. J., Martier S. S., Ager J. W. Prenatal alcohol exposure and infant information-processing ability. *Child Development 64:*1706–1721, 1993c.

Jacobson S. W., Jacobson J. L., Sokol R. J., Martier S. S., Ager J. W., et al. Maternal recall of alcohol, cocaine, and marijuana use during pregnancy. *Neurotoxicology and Teratology 13:*535–540, 1991b.

Jacobson S. W., Rich J., Tovsky N. J. Delayed myelination and lamination in the cerebral cortex of the albino rat as a result of fetal alcohol syndrome. In Galanter M. (Ed.), *Currents in Alcoholism* (pp. 123–133). New York: Grune & Stratton, 1979.

Jaffer Z., Nelson M., Beighton P. Bone fusion in the fetal alcohol syndrome. *Journal of Bone and Joint Surgery 63B:*569–571, 1981.

Janzen L. A., Nanson J. L., Block G. W. Neuropsychological evaluation of preschoolers with fetal alcohol syndrome. *Neurotoxicology and Teratology 17:*273–279, 1995.

Jellinger K., Gross H., Kaltenback E., Grisold W. Holoprosencephaly and agenesis of the corpus callosum: Frequency of associated malformations. *Acta Neuropathologica 55:*1–10, 1981.

Jerrells T. R., Pruett S. B. Immunotoxic effects of ethanol. In Dean J. H., Luster M. I., Munson A. E., Kimber I. (Eds.), *Immunotoxicology and Immunopharmacology* (pp. 323–347). New York: Raven Press, 1994.

Johnson K. G. Fetal alcohol syndrome: Rhinorrhea, persistent otitis media, choanal stenosis, hypoplastic sphenoids and ethmoid. *Rocky Mountain Medical Journal 76:*64–65, 1979.

Johnson S., Knight R., Marmer D. J., Steele R. W. Immune deficiency in fetal alcohol syndrome. *Pediatric Research 15:*908–911, 1981.

Johnston L. D., O'Malley P. M., Bachman J. G. *Drug use, drinking, and smoking: National survey results from high school, college, and young adult populations, 1975–1988* (DHHS Publication No. ADM 89-1638). Washington DC: U.S. Government Printing Office, 1989.

Jones K. L., Smith D. W. Recognition of the fetal alcohol syndrome in early infancy. *Lancet 2:*999–1001, 1973.

Jones K. L., Smith D. W., Streissguth S., Myrianthopoulos N. C. Outcome in offspring of chronic alcoholic women. *Lancet 1:*1076–1078, 1974.

Jones K. L., Smith D. W., Ulleland C. N., Streissguth A. P. Pattern of malformation in offspring of chronic alcoholic mothers. *Lancet 1:*1267–1271, 1973.

Jones P. J. H., Leichter J., Lee M. Uptake of zinc, folate, and analogs of glucose and amino acid by the rat fetus exposed to alcohol in utero. *Nutrition Reports International 24:*75–83, 1981.

Jorgensen M. B., Diemer N. H. Selective neuron loss after cerebral ischemia in the rat: Possible role of transmitter glutamate. *Acta Neurologica Scandinavica 66:*536–546, 1982.

Kahn A. J. Effect of ethanol exposure during embryogenesis and the neonatal period on the incidence of hepatoma in C_3H male mice. *Growth 32:*311–316, 1968.

Kakihana R., Butte J. C., Moore J. A. Endocrine effects of maternal alcoholization: Plasma and brain testosterone, dihydrotestosterone, estradiol, and corticosterone. *Alcoholism: Clinical and Experimental Research 1:*57–61, 1980.

Kalant H. Stress-related effects of ethanol in mammals. *Critical Reviews in Biotechnology 9:*265–272, 1990.

Kaminski M., Franc M., Lebouvier M., Du Mazubrun D., Rumeau-Rouquette C. Moderate alcohol use and pregnancy outcome. *Neurobehavioral Toxicology and Teratology 3:*173–181, 1981.

Kaminski M., Rumeau C., Schwartz D. Alcohol consumption in pregnant women and the outcome of pregnancy. *Alcoholism: Clinical and Experimental Research 2:*155–163, 1978.

Kaminski M., Rumean-Rouqueette C., Schwartz D. Consummation d'alcool chez les femmes enceintes et issue de la grosses. *Revue Epidemiologie Medecine Sociale et Sante Publique 24:* 27–40, 1976.

Kandall S. R., Gaines J. Maternal substance use and subsequent sudden infant death syndrome (SIDS) in offspring. *Neurotoxicology and Teratology 13:*235–240, 1991.

Kaneko W. M., Ehlers C. L., Phillips E. L., Riley E. P. Auditory event-related potentials in fetal alcohol syndrome and Down's syndrome in children. *Alcoholism: Clinical Experimental Research 20:*35–42, 1996.

Kaneko W. M., Riley E. P., Ehlers C. L. Electrophysiological and behavioral findings in rats prenatally exposed to alcohol. *Alcohol 10:*169–178, 1993.

Kapamadzija A., Horvat K. Alkohol u trudnoci (Alcohol in pregnancy). *Medicinski Pregled 44:*41–33, 1991.

Kariniemi V., Rosti J. Maternal smoking and alcohol consumption as determinants of birth weight in an unselected study population. *Journal of Perinatal Medicine 16:*249–252, 1988.

Keir W. J. Inhibition of retinoic acid synthesis and its implications in fetal alcohol syndrome (editorial). *Alcoholism: Clinical and Experimental Research 15:*560–564, 1991.

Kennedy L. A. Changes in the term mouse placenta associated with maternal alcohol consumption and fetal growth deficits. *American Journal of Obstetrics and Gynecology 149:*518–522, 1984.

Kennedy L. A., Sheppard M. S., Bhaumick B., Laverty W. H. Reduced binding of basic somatomedin by mouse placental membranes following maternal alcohol administration. *Developmental Pharmacology and Therapeutics 9:*132–144, 1986.

Keppen L. D., Pysher T., Rennert O. M., Zinc deficiency acts as a coteratogen with alcohol in fetal alcohol syndrome. *Pediatric Research 19:*944–947, 1985.

Kesaniemi Y. A., Sippel H. W. Placental and foetal metabolism of acetaldehyde in rat: I. Contents of ethanol and acetaldehyde in placenta and foetus of the pregnant rat during ethanol oxidation. *Acta Pharmacology Toxicology 37:*43–48, 1975.

Kesby G., Parker G., Barrett E. Personality and coping style as influences on alcohol intake and cigarette smoking during pregnancy. *Medical Journal of Australia 155:*229–223, 1991.

Khera K. S. Maternal toxicity in humans and animals: Effects on fetal development and criteria for detection. *Teratugenesis Carcinogenesis and Mutagenesis 7:*287–295, 1987.

Kim C. K., Osborn J. A., Weinberg J. Stress reactivity in fetal alcohol syndrome. In Abel E. L. (Ed.), *Fetal Alcohol Syndrome: From Mechanism to Prevention* (pp. 215–216). Boca Raton, FL: CRC Press, 1996.

Kim C. K., Weinberg J., Pinel J. P. J. Effects of prenatal ethanol exposure on susceptibility to convulsions and response to the anticonvulsant effects of ethanol in rats. *Alcoholism: Clinical and Experimental Research 15:*337, 1991.

Kim C. K., Yu W., Osborn J., Weinberg J. Prenatal ethanol exposure and glucocorticoid receptors in the hippocampus and hypothalamus. *Alcoholism: Clinical and Experimental Research 18:*470, 1994.

Klein K. L., Scott W. J., Clark K. E., Wilson J. G. Indomethacin-placental transfer, cytotoxicity, and teratology in the rat. *American Journal of Obstetrics and Gynecology 141:*448–452, 1981.

Kleinfeld J., Wescott S. (Eds.), *Fantastic Antoine Succeeds! Experiences in Educating Children with Fetal Alcohol Syndrome.* Anchorage, Alaska: University of Alaska Press, 1993.

Kline J., Shrout P., Stein A., Susser M., Warburton D. Drinking during pregnancy and spontaneous abortion. *Lancet 2:*176–180, 1980.

Kline J., Stein Z., Hutzler M. Cigarettes, alcohol, and marijuana: Varying associations with birth weight. *International Journal of Epidemiology 16:*44–51, 1987.

Knight J. E., Kodituwakku P. W., Orrison W. W., Lewine J. D., Maclin E. L., et al. Magnetic resonance imaging in high-functioning children with fetal alcohol syndrome who exhibit neuropsychological deficits. *Alcoholism: Clinical and Experimental Research 17:*485, 1993.

Knupfer G. The risk of drunkenness (or *Ebrietas resurrecta*). A comparison of frequent intoxication indices and of population subgroups as to problems risks. *British Journal of Addiction 79:*185–196, 1984.

Knupfer G. Drinking for health: The daily light drinker's fiction. *British Journal of Addiction 82:* 547–555, 1987a.

Knupfer G. New directions for survey research in the study of alcoholic beverage consumption. *British Journal of Addiction 82:*583–585, 1987b.

Kodituwakku P. W., Handmaker N. S., Cutler S. K., Weathersby E. K., Handmaker S. D. Specific impairments in self-regulation in children exposed to alcohol prenatally. *Alcoholism: Clinical and Experimental Research 19:*1558–1564, 1995.

Kokotailo P. K., Adger H., Duggan A. K., Repke J., Joffe A. Cigarette, alcohol, and other drug use by school-age pregnant adolescents: Prevalence, detection, and associated risk factors. *Pediatrics 90:*328–334, 1992.

Kokotailo P. K., Langhough R. E., Cox N. S., Davidson S. R., Fleming M. F. Cigarette, alcohol, and other drug use among small city pregnant adolescents. *Journal of Adolescent Health 15:*366–373, 1994.

Kolata G. B. Fetal alcohol advisory debated. *Science 214:*642–645, 1981.

Kotch L. E., Sulik K. K. Experimental fetal alcohol syndrome: Proposed pathogenic basis for a variety of associated facial and brain anomalies. *American Journal of Medical Genetics 44:*168–176, 1992a.

Kotch L. E., Sulik K. K. Patterns of ethanol-induced cell death in the developing nervous system of mice: Neural fold states through the time of anterior neural tube closure. *International Journal of Developmental Neuroscience 10:*273–279, 1992b.

Kotch L. E., Chen S.-Y., Sulik K. K. Ethanol-induced teratogenesis: Free radical damage as a possible mechanism. *Teratology 52:*128–136, 1995.

Kotch L. E., Dehart D. B., Alles A. J., Chernoff N., Sulik K. K. Pathogenesis of ethanol-induced limb reduction defects in mice. *Teratology 46:*323–332, 1992.

Kotkoskie L. A., Norton S. Acute response of the fetal telencephalon to short-term maternal exposure to ethanol in the rat. *Acta Neuropathologica 79:*513–519, 1990.

Kruse J., Lefevre M., Zweig S. Changes in smoking and alcohol consumption during pregnancy: A population-based study in a rural area. *Obstetrics and Gynecology 67:*627–632, 1986.

Kuzma J. S., Kissinger D. G. Patterns of alcohol and cigarette use in pregnancy. *Neurobehavioral Toxicology and Teratology 3:*211–221, 1981.

Kuzma J. W., Sokol R. J. Maternal drinking behavior and decreased intrauterine growth. *Alcoholism: Clinical and Experimental Research 6:*396–402, 1982.

Kyllerman M., Aronson M., Sabel K. G., Karlberg E., Sandin B., et al. Children of alcoholic mothers:

Growth and motor performance compared to matched controls. *Acta Paediatrica Scandinavica 74:*10–26, 1985.

LaDue R. A., Streissguth A. P., Randels S. P. Clinical considerations pertaining to adolescents and adults with fetal alcohol syndrome. In Sonderegger T. B. (Ed.), *Perinatal Substance Abuse* (pp. 104–131). Baltimore, MD: Johns Hopkins University Press, 1992.

Lancaster F., Samorajski T. Prenatal ethanol exposure decreases synaptic density in the molecular layer of the cerebellum. *Alcohol and Alcoholism 1:*477–480, 1987.

Landesman-Dwyer S., Keller L. S., Streissguth A. P. Naturalistic observations of newborns: Effects of maternal alcohol intake. *Alcoholism: Clinical and Experimental Research 2:*171–177, 1978.

Langman, J., Cordell, E. L., Ultrastructural observations on FVaR-induced cell death an subsequent elimination of cell debris. *Teratology 17:*229–269, 1978.

Lapatto R., Raisanen J. A rapid method for the quantification of C, N, and O in biomedical samples by proton-induced gamma-ray-emission analysis applied to human placental samples. *Physics in Medicine and Biology 33:*75–81, 1988.

Laposata E. A., Lange L. G. Presence of nonoxidative ethanol metabolism in human organs commonly damaged by ethanol abuse. *Science 231:*497–499, 1986.

Lorroque B., Kaminski M., Dehaene P., Subtil D., Delfosse M., et al. Moderate prenatal alcohol exposure and psychomotor development at preschool age. *American Journal of Public Health 85:*1654–1661, 1995.

Larroque B., Kaminski M., Lelong N., d'Herbomez M., Dehaene P., et al. Folate status during pregnancy: Relationship with alcohol consumption and other maternal risk factors and pregnancy outcome. *European Journal of Obstetrics, Gynecology, and Reproductive Biology 43:*19–27, 1992.

Larroque B., Kaminski M., Lelong N., Subtil D., Dehaene P. Effects on birth weight of alcohol and caffeine consumption during pregnancy. *American Journal of Epidemiology 137:*941–950, 1993.

Larsson G. Prevention of fetal alcohol effects: An antenatal program for early detection of pregnancies at risk. *Acta Obstetricia et Gynecologica Scandinavica 62:*171–178, 1983.

Larsson G., Bohlin A. B., Tunell R. Prospective study of children exposed to variable amounts of alcohol in utero. *Archives of Disease in Childhood 60:*316–321, 1985.

Larsson G., Ottenblad C., Hagenfeldt L., Larsson A., Forsgren M. Evaluation of serum γ-glutamyl transferase as a screening method for excessive alcohol consumption during pregnancy. *American Journal of Obstetrics and Gynecology 147:*654–657, 1983.

Laukaran V. H., VandenBerg, B. J. The relationship of maternal attitude toward pregnancy outcomes and obstetric complications. *American Journal of Obstetrics and Gynecology 136:*374–479, 1980.

Lazzaroni F., Bonasi S., Magnani M., Calvi A., Repetto E., et al. Moderate maternal drinking and outcome of pregnancy. *European Journal of Epidemiology 9:*599–606, 1993.

LeBel C. P., Odunze I. N., Adams J. D., Bondy S. C. Perturbations in cerebral oxygen radical formation and membrane order following vitamin E deficiency. *Biochemical and Biophysical Research Communications 163:*860–866, 1989.

Ledig M., Tholey G., Kopp P., Mandel P. An experimental study of fetal alcohol syndrome in the rat: Biochemical modifications in brain and liver. *Alcohol and Alcoholism 24:*231–240, 1989.

Lee M., Leichter J. Effect of litter size on the physical growth and motivation of the offspring of rats given alcohol during gestation. *Growth 44:*327–335, 1980.

Lee M., Leichter J. Skeletal development in fetuses of rats consuming alcohol during gestation. *Growth 47:*254–262, 1983.

Lee S., Rivier C. Prenatal alcohol exposure alters the hypothalamic-pituitary-adrenal axis response of offspring to interleukin-1: Possible mechanisms. *Alcoholism Clinical and Experimental Research 18:*470, 1994.

Lee-Chuan C., Cerklewski F. L., Soeldner A. Effect of maternal ethanol ingestion at two dietary levels of zinc on molar composition and dental caries of rat offspring. *Nutrition Research 5:*951–957, 1985.

Lemoine P., Lemoine P. H. Avenir des enfants de mere alcoolique (etudes des 105 cas retrouves a l'age adulte) et quelque constations d'interet prophylactique. *Annales de Pediatrie 39:*226–235, 1992.

Lemoine P., Harousseau H., Borteryu J. P., Menuet J. C. Les enfants de parents alcooliques: Anomalies observées à propos de 127 cas. [The children of alcoholic parents: Anomalies observed in 127 cases.] *Ouest Medicale 21:*476–482, 1968.

LeRoith D., Werner H., Beitner-Johnson D., Roberts C. T. Molecular and cellular aspects of the insulinlike growth factor I receptor. *Endocrine Reviews 16:*143–163, 1995.

Lesure J. F. L'embryo foetopathie alcoolique à l'Ile de la réunion: Un drame social (Embryonic fetal alcohol pathology in Reunion Island: A social drama). *La Revue Pediatrie 24:*265–271, 1988.

Lieber C. S. Alcohol, protein metabolism, and liver injury. *Gastroenterology 79:*373–390, 1980.

Lieber C. S. Alcohol, liver, and nutrition. *Journal of the American College of Nutrition 10:*602–632, 1991.

Lindblad B., Olsson R. Usually high levels of blood alcohol? *Journal of the American Medical Association 236:*1600–1602, 1976.

Lindor E., McCarthy A. M., McRae M. G. Fetal alcohol syndrome: A review and case presentation. *Journal of Gynecological Nursing 9:*222–223, 225–228, 1980.

Lipson A. H., Walsh D. A., Webster W. S. W. Fetal alcohol syndrome: A great pediatric imitator. *Medical Journal of Australia 1:*266–269, 1983.

Little R. E. Moderate alcohol use during pregnancy and decreased infant birth weight. *American Journal of Public Health 67:*1154–1156, 1977.

Little R. E. History of spontaneous abortion and its relation to tobacco and alcohol use in 513 pregnant women. *American Journal of Epidemiology 108:*223, 1978.

Little R. E., Streissguth A. P. Drinking during pregnancy in alcoholic women. *Alcoholism: Clinical and Experimental Research 2:*179–183, 1978.

Little R. E., Weinberg C. R. Risk factors for antepartum and intrapartum stillbirth. *American Journal of Epidemiology 137:*1177–1189, 1993.

Little R. E., Wendt J. K. The effects of maternal drinking in the reproductive period: An epidemiologic review. *Journal of Substance Abuse 3:*187–204, 1991.

Little R. E., Asker R. L., Sampson P. D., Renwick J. H. Fetal growth and moderate drinking in early pregnancy. *American Journal of Epidemiology 123:*270–278, 1986.

Little R. E., Schultz F. A., Mandell W. Drinking during pregnancy. *Journal of Studies on Alcohol 37:*375–379, 1976.

Little R. E., Streissguth A. P., Barr H. M., Herman C. S. Decreased birth weight in infants of alcoholic women who abstained during pregnancy. *Journal of Pediatrics 96:*974–977, 1980.

Liu K., Stamler J., Moss D., Garside D., Persky V., et al. Dietary cholesterol, fat, and fiber, and colon-cancer mortality: Analysis of international data. *Lancet 2:*782–785, 1979.

Lodewijckx E., DeGroof V. Smoking and alcohol consumption by Flemish pregnant women, 1966–1983. *Journal of Biosocial Science 22:*43–47, 1990.

Lohr M. J., Gillmore M. R., Gilchrist L. D., Butler S. S. Factors related to substance use by pregnant, school-age adolescents. *Journal of Adolescent Health 13:*475–482, 1992.

Longo L. D. Environmental pollution and pregnancy: Risks and uncertainties for the fetus and infant. *American Journal of Obstetrics and Gynecology 137:*162–173, 1980.

Loock C. A., Conry J. L., Li D. B. K., Clark C. M. Disregulation of caudate/cortical metabolism in FAS: A case study. *Alcoholism: Clinical and Experimental Research 17:*485, 1993.

Lopez-Tejero D., Ferrer I., Llobera M., Herra E. Effects of prenatal ethanol exposure on physical growth, sensory reflex maturation, and brain development in the rat. *Neuropathology and Applied Neurobiology 12:*251–260, 1986.

Lopez-Tejero D., Llobera M., Herrera E. Permanent abnormal response to a glucose load after prenatal ethanol exposure in rats. *Alcohol 6:*469–473, 1989.

Loser H. *Alkohol-embryopathie und Alkoholeffekte* (Alcohol Embryopathy and Alcohol Effects). Stuttgart, Germany: Gustav Fischer Verlag, 1995.

Loser H., Themann H., Welim W., Dittrich H. Congenital alcoholic cardiomyopathy and cardiac anomalies in three children. *Deutsche Medzinische Wochenschrift 113:*1630–1634, 1988.

Lower J. B., Windsor R. A., Adams, B., Morris J., Reese V. Use of bogus pipeline method to increase accuracy of self-reported alcohol consumption among pregnant women. *Journal of Studies on Alcohol 47:*173–175, 1986.

Lumley J., Correy J. F., Newman N. M., Curran J. T. Cigarette smoking, alcohol consumption, and fetal outcome in Tasmania 1981–1982. *Australian and New Zealand Journal of Obstetrics and Gynaecology 25:*33–40, 1985.

Macdonald D. I., Blume S. A. Children of alcoholics. *American Journal of Diseases in Children 140:*750–754, 1986.

Magarian G. J. Hyperventilation syndromes: Infrequently recognized common expressions of anxiety and stress. *Medicine 81:*219–236, 1982.

Majewski F. Alcohol embryopathy: Some facts and speculations about pathogenesis. *Neurobehavioral Toxicology and Teratology 3:*129–144, 1981.

Majewski F. Alcohol embryopathy: Experience in 200 patients. *Development Brain Dysfunction 6:*248–265, 1993.

Majewski F., Bierich J. R., Loser H., Michaelis R., Leiber B., et al. Zur klinik und pathogenese der alkohol-embryopathie; berich uber 68 falle (Clinical aspects and pathogenesis of alcohol embryopathy: A report of 68 cases). *Munchen Medizinische Wochenschrift 118:*1635–1642, 1976.

Majewski F., Goecke T. Alcohol embryopathy: Studies in Germany. In E. L. Abel (Ed.), *Fetal Alcohol Syndrome* (Vol. 2, pp. 65–88). Boca Raton, FL: CRC Press, 1982.

Majewski F., Fischback H., Pfeiffer J., Bierich J. R. Zur Frage der Interruptiones der alkohkrankken Frauen (A question concerning interruption of pregnancy in alcoholic women). *Deutsche Medizinesche Wochenschrift 103:*895–898, 1978.

Maling H. M. Toxicity of single doses of ethyl alcohol. In Temolieres S. (Ed.), *Alcohol and Derivatives* (Vol. 2, pp. 277–295). Oxford, UK: Pergamon Press, 1970.

Mankes R. M., Battles A. H., LeFebre R., van der Hoeven T., Glick S. D. Preferential alcoholic embryopathy: Effects of liquid diets. *Laboratory Animal Science 42:*561–566, 1992.

Mankes R. F., Hoffman T., LeFebre R., Bates H., Abraham R. Acute embryopathic effects of ethanol in the Long-Evans rat. *Journal of Toxicology and Environmental Health 11:*583–590, 1983.

Manzke H., Spreter von Kruedenstein P. Embryofetales Alkolsyndrome (Embryofetal alcohol syndrome). *Suchtegefahren 25:*157–166, 1979.

Maprurira M. J., Msamati B. C., Banadda B. M. Correlations between weights of newborn babies, placental parameters, and gestational age. *Central African Journal of Medicine 38:*414–420, 1992.

Marbury M. C., Linn S., Monson R. P., Schoenbaum S., Stubblefield P. G., et al. The association of alcohol consumption with outcome of pregnancy. *American Journal of Public Health 73:*1165–1168, 1983.

Marcus J. D. Neurological findings in the Fetal Alcohol Syndrome. *Neuropediatrics 18:*158–160, 1987.

Marquis S. M., Leichter J., Lee M. Plasma amino acids and glucose levels in the rat fetus and dam after chronic maternal alcohol consumption. *Biology of the Neonate 46:*36–43, 1984.

Martin D. C., Martin J. C., Streissguth A. P., Lund C. A. Sucking frequency and amplitude in newborns as a function of maternal drinking and smoking. In Galanter M. (Ed.), *Currents in Alcoholism* (Vol. 5, pp. 359–366). New York: Grune & Stratton, 1979.

Matilainen R., Airaksinen E., Mononen T., Launiala K., Kaarianinen R. A population-based study on the causes of mild and severe mental retardation. *Acta Paediatrica 84:*261–266, 1995.

Mattson S. N., Riley E. Brain anomalies in fetal alcohol syndrome. In Abel E. L. (Ed.), *Fetal Alcohol Syndrome: From Mechanism to Prevention* (pp. 51–68). Boca Raton, FL: CRC Press, 1996.

Mattson S. N., Carlos R., Riley E. P. The behavioral teratogenicity of alcohol is not affected by pretreatment with aspirin. *Alcohol 10:*51–57, 1993.

Mattson S. N., Riley E. P., Jernigan T. L., Ehlers C. L., Delis D. C., et al. Fetal alcohol syndrome: A case report of neuropsychological, MRI, and EEG assessment of two children. *Alcoholism: Clinical and Experimental Research 16:*1001–1003, 1992.

Mattson S. N., Riley E. P., Jernigan T. L., Garcia A., Kaneko W. M., et al. A decrease in the size of the basal ganglia following prenatal alcohol exposure: A preliminary report. *Neurotoxicology and Teratology 16:*283–289, 1994.

Mau G. Moderate alcohol consumption during pregnancy and child development. *European Journal of Pediatrics 133:*233–237, 1980.

Mauceri H. J., Unterman T., Dempsey S., Lee W.-H., Conway S. Effect of ethanol exposure on circulating levels of insulin-like growth factors I and II, and insulinlike growth factor-binding proteins in fetal rats. *Alcoholism: Clinical and Experimental Research 17:*1201–1206, 1993.

May P. A. Fetal alcohol effects among North American Indians: Evidence and implications for society. *Alcohol Health and Research World 15:*239–247, 1991.

May P. A., Hymbaugh K. J., Aase J. M., Samet J. M. Epidemiology of fetal alcohol syndrome among American Indians of the Southwest. *Social Biology 30:*374–387, 1983.

McCaffery P., Drager U. C. High levels of a retinoic-acid-generating dehydrogenase in the meso-telencephalic dopamine system. *Proceedings of the National Academy of Sciences 91:*7772–7776, 1994.

McDonald A. D., Armstrong B. G., Sloan M. Cigarette, alcohol, and coffee consumption and prematurity. *American Journal of Public Health 82:*87–90, 1992.

McDonald J. W., Johnston M. V. Physiological and pathophysiological roles of excitatory amino acids during central nervous system development. *Brain Research Reviews 15:*41–70, 1990.

McGivern R. F. Influence of prenatal exposure to cimetidine and alcohol on selected morphological parameters of sexual differentiation: A preliminary report. *Neurotoxicology and Teratology 9:*223–226, 1987.

McGivern R. F. Effects of prenatal alcohol exposure on male and female gonadal organ weights. *Alcoholism: Clinical and Experimental Research 15:*341, 1991.

McGivern R. F., Clancy A. N., Hill M. A., Noble E. P. Prenatal alcohol exposure alters adult expression of sexually dimorphic behavior in the rat. *Science 224:*896–898, 1984.

McGivern R. F., Raum W. J., Salido E., Redei E. Lack of prenatal testosterone surge in fetal rats exposed to alcohol: Alterations in testicular morphology and physiology. *Alcoholism: Clinical and Experimental Research 12:*243–247, 1988.

McLeod J. D. Spouse concordance for alcohol dependence and heavy drinking: Evidence from a community sample. *Alcoholism: Clinical and Experimental Research 17:*1146–1155, 1993.

McNeill D. L., Fagan E. L., Harris C. H., Shew R. L. Effects of maternal ethanol consumption prior to and during gestation on the spinal cord of the neonatal rat. *Society for Neuroscience Abstract 15:*1024, 1989.

McShane D. A., Plas J. M. The cognitive functioning of American Indian children moving from the WISC to the WISC-R school. *Psychological Review 13:*61–73, 1984.

Mena M., Casanueva V., Fernandez E., Carraso R., Perez H. Fetal alcohol syndrome at schools for mentally handicapped children in Concepcion, Chile. *PAHO Bulletin 20:*157–169, 1986.

Mezzich A. C., Arria A. M., Tarter R. E., Moss H., Van Thiel D. H. Psychiatric comorbidity in alcoholism: Importance of ascertainment source. *Alcoholism: Clinical and Experimental Research 15:*893–898, 1991.

Middaugh L. D., Boggan W. O. Postnatal growth deficits in prenatal ethanol-exposed mice: Characteristics and critical periods. *Alcoholism: Clinical and Experimental Research 15:*919–926, 1991.

Middaugh L. D., Boggan W. O. Perinatal maternal ethanol effects on pregnant mice and on offspring viability and growth. Influences of exposure time and weaning diet. *Alcoholism: Clinical and Experimental Research 19:*1351–1358, 1995.

Miller M., Israel J., Cuttone J. Fetal alcohol syndrome. *Journal of Pediatric Ophthalmology and Strabismus 18:*6–15, 1981.

Miller M. W. Effects of alcohol on the generation and migration of cerebral cortical neurons. *Science 233:*1308–1311, 1986.

Miller M. W., Dow-Edwards D. L. Structural and metabolic alterations in rat cerebral cortex induced by prenatal exposure to ethanol. *Brain Research 474:*316–326, 1988.

Miller M. W., Muller S. J. Structure and histogenesis of the principal sensory nucleus of the trigeminal nerve: Effects of prenatal exposure to ethanol. *Journal of Comparative Neurology 282:*570–580, 1989.

Miller M. W., Potempa G. Numbers of neurons and glia in mature rat somatosensory cortex: Effects of prenatal exposure to ethanol. *Journal of Comparative Neurology 293:*92–102, 1990.

Mills J. L., Graubard B. I. Is moderate drinking during pregnancy associated with an increasing risk for malformation? *Pediatrics 80:*309–314, 1987.

Mills J. L., Graubard B. I., Harley E. E., Rhoads G. G., Berendes H. W. Maternal alcohol consumption and birth weight. *Journal of the American Medical Association 252:*1875–1879, 1984.

Miralles-Flores C., Delgado-Baeza D. Histomorphometic analysis of the epiphyseal growth plate in rats after prenatal alcohol exposure. *Journal of Orthopaedic Research 10:*325–336, 1992.

Morris D. L., Harms P. G., Petersen H. D., McArthur N. H. LHRH and LH in peripubertal female rats following prenatal and/or postnatal ethanol exposure. *Life Sciences 44:*1165–1171, 1989.

Morrow-Tlucuk M., Ernhart C. B. Maternal prenatal substance use and behavior at age 3 years. *Alcoholism: Clinical and Experimental Research 11:*213, 1987.

Morrow-Tlucak M., Ernhart C. B., Sokol R. J., Martier S., Ager J. Underreporting of alcohol use in pregnancy: Relationship to alcohol problem history. *Alcoholism: Clinical and Experimental Research 13:*399–401, 1989.

Morse B. A. Information processing. In Kleinfeld J., Wescott S. (Eds.), *Fantastic Antoine Succeeds!: Experiences in Educating Children with Fetal Alcohol Syndrome* (pp. 223–236). Anchorage, Alaska: University of Alaska Press, 1993.

Morse B. A., Cermak S. Sensory processing in children with FAS. *Alcoholism: Clinical and Experimental Research 18:*503, 1994.

Morse B. A., Weiner L. Rehabilitation approaches for fetal alcohol syndrome. In Spohr H. L., Steinhausen H. C. (Eds.), *Alcohol, Pregnancy, and the Developing Child* (pp. 249–268). Cambridge, UK: Cambridge University Press, 1996.

Morton N. E. The inheritance of human birthweight. *Annals of Human Genetics 20:*123–134, 1955.

Mukherjee S. P., Hodges, G. D. Maternal ethanol exposure induces transient impairment of umbilical circulation and fetal hypoxia in monkeys. *Science 218:*700–702, 1982.

Mulder E. J. H., Kamstra A., O'Brien M. J., Visser G. H. A., Prechte H. F. R. Abnormal fetal behavioral state regulation in a case of high maternal alcohol intake during pregnancy. *Early Human Development 14:*321–326, 1986.

Nanji A. A., Mendenhall C. L., French S. W. Beef fat prevents alcohol liver disease in the rat. *Alcoholism: Clinical and Experimental Research 13:*15–19, 1989.

Nanson J. L. Autism in fetal alcohol syndrome: A report of six cases. *Alcoholism: Clinical and Experimental Research 16:*558–565, 1992.

Nanson J. L., Hiscock M. Attention deficits in children exposed to alcohol prenatally. *Alcoholism: Clinical and Experimental Research 14:*656–661, 1990.

National Institute on Alcohol Abuse and Alcoholism. *Seventh Special Report to the U.S. Congress on Alcohol and Health.* Washington, DC: U.S. Department of Health and Human Services, 1990.

National Institute on Alcohol Abuse and Alcoholism. *Eighth Special Report to the U.S. Congress on Alcohol and Health.* Washington, DC: U.S. Department of Health and Human Services, 1993.

Nelson L. R., Taylor A. N., Kewis J. W., Poland R. E., Redei E., et al. Pituitary-adrenal response to morphine and footshock stress are enhanced following prenatal alcohol exposure. *Alcoholism: Clinical and Experimental Research 10:*397–402, 1986.

Niki E., Minamisawa S., Oikawa M., Komuro E. Membrane damage from lipid oxidation induced by free radicals and cigarette smoke. *Annals of the New York Academy of Science 686:*29–38, 1993.

Nordstrom M.-L., Cnattingius S., Haglund B. Social difference in Swedish infant mortality by cause of death, 1983 to 1986. *American Journal of Public Health 83:*26–30, 1993.

Norkus E. P., Hsu H., Cehelsky M. R. Effect of cigarette smoking on the vitamin C status of pregnant women and their offspring. *Annals of the New York Academy of Science 498:*500–501, 1987.

Nugent J. K., Lester B. M., Greene S. M., Wieczorek-Deering D., O'Mahony P. The effects of maternal alcohol consumption and cigarette smoking during pregnancy on acoustic cry analysis. *Child Development 67:*1806–1815, 1996.

O'Connor M. J., Brill N. J., Sigman M. Alcohol use in primiparous women older than 30 years of age: Relation to infant development. *Pediatrics 78:*444–450, 1986.

O'Connor M. J., Sigman M., Brill N. Disorganization of attachment in relation to maternal alcohol consumption. *Journal of Consulting and Clinical Psychology 55:*831–836, 1987.

O'Gorman S., Bannigan J. The lung in mouse fetal alcohol syndrome. *Teratology 44:*15A, 1991.

O'Shea K. S., Kaufman M. H. Effect of acetaldehyde on the neuroepithelium of early mouse embryos. *Journal of Anatomy 132:*107–118, 1981.

Ogston S. A., Parry G. J. Results—Strategy of analysis and analysis of pregnancy outcome. *International Journal of Epidemiology 21:*S45–S71, 1992.

Olegard R., Sabel K. Effects on the child of alcohol abuse during pregnancy. *Acta Paediatrica Scandinavica 275:*112–121, 1979.

Olegard R., Sabel K. G., Aronsson M., Sandin B., Johansson P. R., et al. Effects on the child of alcohol abuse during pregnancy: Retrospective and prospective studies. *Acta Paediatrica Scandinavica 275:*112–121, 1979.

Olsen J. Effects of moderate alcohol consumption during pregnancy on child development at 18 and 42 months. *Alcoholism: Clinical and Experimental Research 18:*1109–1113, 1994.

Olsen J., Tuntiseranee P. Is moderate alcohol intake in pregnancy associated with the craniofacial features related to the fetal alcohol syndrome? *Scandinavian Journal of Social Medicine 23:*156–161, 1995.

Olsen J., da Costa Pereira A., Olsen S. F. Does maternal tobacco smoking modify the effect of alcohol on fetal growth? *American Journal of Public Health 81:*69–73, 1991.

Olsen J., Rachootin P., Schiodt A. V., Damsbo N. Tobacco use, alcohol consumption, and infertility. *International Journal of Epidemiology 12:*179–184, 1983.

Ouellette E. M., Rosett H. L., Rosman N. P., Weiner L. Adverse effects on offspring of maternal alcohol abuse during pregnancy. *New England Journal of Medicine 297:*528–530, 1977.

Padmanabhan R. Histological and histochemical changes of the placenta in fetal alcohol syndrome due to maternal administration of acute doses of ethanol in the mouse. *Drug and Alcohol Dependence 16:*229–239, 1985.

Padmanabhan R., Wasfi I. A., Craigmyle M. B. L. Effect of pretreatment with aspirin on alcohol-induced neural tube defects in the TO mouse fetuses. *Drug and Alcohol Dependence 36:*175–186, 1994.

Palmer C. Fetal alcohol effects—incidence and understanding in the Cape. *South African Medical Journal 68:*779–780, 1985.

Panes J., Caballeria J., Gyuitart R., Pares A., Soler X., et al. Determinants of ethanol and acetaldehyde metabolism in chronic alcoholics. *Alcoholism: Clinical and Experimental Research 17:*48–53, 1993.

Parazzini F., Bocciolone L., Fedele L., Negri E., La Vecchia C., et al. Risk factors for spontaneous abortion. *International Journal of Epidemiology 20:*157–161, 1991.

Parazzini F., Tozzi L., Chatenoud L., Restelli S., Luchini L., et al. Alcohol and risk of spontaneous abortions. *Human Reproduction 9:*1950–1953, 1994.

Parker S., Udani M., Gavaler J. S., Van Thiel D. H. Adverse effects of alcohol upon the adult sexual behavior of male rats exposed in utero. *Neurobehavioral Toxicology and Teratology 6:*289–293, 1984.

Pasamanick B., Lilienfield A. M. Association of maternal and fetal factors with development of mental deficience: I. Abnormalities in the prenatal and perinatal periods. *Journal of the American Medical Association 159:*155–160, 1955.

Patrick J., Carmichael L., Richardson B., Smith G., Homan J., et al. Effects of multiple-dose maternal ethanol infusion on fetal cardiovascular and brain activity in lambs. *American Journal of Obstetrics and Gynecology 159:*1424–1429, 1988.

Patrick J., Richardson B., Hasen G., Clarke D., Wlodek M., et al. Effects of maternal ethanol infusion on fetal cardiovascular and brain activity in lambs. *American Journal of Obstetrics and Gynecology 151:*859–867, 1985.

Payer L. *Medicine and Culture.* New York: Penguin Books, 1988.

Peacock J. L., Bland M. M., Anderson H. R. Effects on birth weight of alcohol and caffeine consumption in smoking women. *Journal of Epidemiology and Community Health 45:*159–163, 1991.

Peacock J. L., Bland J. M., Anderson H. R. Preterm delivery: Effects of socioeconomic factors, psychological stress, smoking, alcohol, and caffeine. *British Medical Journal 311:*531–535, 1995.

Pennington S. N., Boyd J. W., Kalmus G. W., Wilson R. W. The molecular mechanism of fetal alcohol syndrome (FAS): I. Ethanol-induced growth suppression. *Neurobehavioral Toxicology and Teratology 5:*259–262, 1983.

Persaud T. V. N. Prostaglandins and organogenesis. *Advances in Prostaglandin Thromboxane and Leukotriene Research 4:*139–156, 1978.

Peterson R. G. Consequences associated with nonnarcotic analgesics in the fetus and newborn. *Federation Proceedings 44:*2309–2313, 1985.

Pettigrew A. G., Hutchinson I. Effects of alcohol on functional development of the auditory pathway in the brainstem of infants and chick embryos. In Ciba Foundation (Ed.), *Mechanisms of Alcohol Damage* in utero (pp. 26–42). London, UK: Pitman, 1984.

Pfeiffer J., Majewski F., Fischbach H., Bierich J. R., Volk, B. Alcohol embryo and fetopathy: Neuropathology of 3 children and 3 fetuses. *Journal of Neurological Sciences 41:*125–137, 1979.

Phillips D. E., Krueger S. K. Rydquist J. E. Short- and long-term effects of combined pre- and postnatal ethanol exposure (three trimester equivalency) on the development of myelin and axons in rat optic nerve. *International Journal of Developmental Neuroscience 9:*631–647, 1991.

Phillips D. K., Henderson G. I., Schenker S. Pathogenesis of fetal alcohol syndrome: Overview with emphasis on the possible role of nutrition. *Alcohol Health and Research World 13:*219–227, 1989.

Phillips S. C., Cragg B. G. A change in susceptibility of rat Purkinje cells to damage by alcohol during fetal, neonatal, and adult life. *Neuropathology and Applied Neurobiology 8:*441–454, 1982.

Pierce D. R., Goodlett C. R., West J. R. Differential neuronal loss following early postnatal alcohol exposure. *Teratology 40:*113–126, 1989.

Pierce D. R., West J. R. Differential deficits in regional brain growth induced by postnatal alcohol. *Neurotoxicology and Teratology 9:*129–141, 1987.

Pierog S. P., Chandavasu O., Wexler I. Withdrawal symptoms in infants with fetal alcohol syndrome. *Journal of Pediatrics 90:*630–633, 1977.

Plant M. L. Alcohol consumption during pregnancy: Baseline data from a Scottish prospective study. *British Journal of Addiction 79:*207–214, 1984.

Plant M. L. *Women, Drinking, and Pregnancy.* New York: Tavistock Publications, 1985.

Plant M. L. *Women, Drinking, and Pregnancy* (2nd ed.). London, UK: Tavistock Publications, 1987.

Plant M. L., Plant M. A. Maternal use of alcohol and other drugs during pregnancy and birth abnormalities: Further results from a prospective study. *Alcohol and Alcoholism 23:*229–233, 1988.

Poe A. E. *The Fall of the House of Usher and Other Writings.* London, UK: Penguin Books, 1986.

Polednak A. P. Black-white differences in infant mortality in 38 standard metropolitan statistical areas. *American Journal of Public Health 81:*1480–1482, 1991.

Praeger K. I., Malin H., Graves C., Spiegler D., Richards L., et al. Maternal smoking and drinking behavior before and during pregnancy. In *Health and Prevention Profile* (pp. 19–24). Hyattsville, Maryland: U.S. Department of Health and Human Services, National Center for Health Statistics, 1983.

Praeger K. I., Malin H., Spiegler D., Van Natta P., Placek P. J. Smoking and drinking behavior before and during pregnancy of married mothers of live born infants and stillborn infants. *Public Health Reports 99:*117–127, 1984.

Primatesta P., DelCorno G., Bonazzi M. C., Waters W. E. Alcohol and pregnancy: An international comparison. *Journal of Public Health Medicine 15:*69–76, 1993.

Pryor W. A., Stone K. Oxidants in cigarette smoke: Radicals, hydrogen peroxide, peroxynitrate, and peroxynitrite. *Annals of the New York Academy of Sciences 686:*12–28, 1993.

Pullarkat R. K. Hypothesis: Prenatal alcohol-induced birth defects and retinoic acid. *Alcoholism: Clinical and Experimental Research 15:*565–567, 1991.

Purpura D. P. Dendritic spine "dysgenesis" and mental retardation. *Science 181:*1126–1128, 1974.

Puschel K., Seifert H. Bedeutung des alkohols in der embryofetalperiode und beim neugeborenen. (Significance of alcohol on the embryo, fetus, and newborn.) *Zeitschrift für Rechtsmedizin 83:* 69–76, 1979.

Pyorala E. Trends in alcohol consumption in Spain, Portugal, France, and Italy from the 1950s until the 1980s. *British Journal of Addiction 85:*469–477, 1990.

Randall C. L., Anton R. F. Aspirin reduces alcohol-induced prenatal mortality and malformations in mice. *Alcoholism: Clinical and Experimental Research 8:*513–515, 1984.

Ranganathan S., Davis D. G., Hood R. D. Development toxicity of alcohol in drosophila melanogaster. *Teratology 36:*45–49, 1987.

Rawat A. K. Ribosomal protein synthesis in the fetal and neonatal rat brain as influenced by maternal ethanol consumption. *Research Communications in Chemical Pathology and Pharmacology 12:*723–732, 1975.

Rawat A. K. Derrangement in cardiac protein metabolism in fetal alcohol syndrome. *Research Communications in Chemical Pathology and Pharmacology 25:*365–375, 1979.

Rawat A. K. Nucleic acid and protein synthesis inhibition in developing brain by ethanol in the absence of hypothermia. *Neurobehavioral Toxicology and Teratology 7:*161–166, 1985.

Redei E., Clark W. R., McGivern R. F. Alcohol exposure in utero results in diminished T-cell function and alternations in brain corticotropin-releasing factor and ACTH content. *Alcoholism: Clinical and Experimental Research 13:*439–443, 1989.

Redei E., Halasz I., Li L., Prystowsky B., Aird F. Maternal adrenalectomy alters the immune and endocrine functions of fetal alcohol-exposed male offspring. *Endocrinology 133:*452–460, 1993.

Renau-Piqueras J., Miragali F., Guerri C., Baguena-Cervellera R. Prenatal exposure to alcohol alters the Golgi apparatus of newborn rat hepatocytes: A cytochemical study. *Journal of Histochemistry and Cytochemistry 35:*221–228, 1987.

Renau-Piqueras J., Sancho-Tello M., Cervellera R., Guerri C. Prenatal exposure to ethanol alters the synthesis and glycosylation of proteins in fetal hepatocytes. *Alcoholism: Clinical and Experimental Research 13:*817–823, 1989.

Reynolds J. D., Brien J. F. Effects of acute ethanol exposure on glutamate release in the hippocampus of the fetal and adult guinea pig. *Alcohol 11:*259–267, 1994.

Reynolds J. D., Brien J. F. Ethanol neurobehavioral teratogenesis and the role of L-glutamate in the fetal hippocampus. *Canadian Journal of Physiology and Pharmacology 73:*1209–1223, 1995.

Reynolds J. D., Penning D. H., Dexter F., Atkins B., Hardy J., et al. Ethanol increases uterine blood flow and fetal arterial blood oxygen tension in the near-term pregnant ewe. *Alcohol 13:*251–256, 1996.

Rice P. A., Nesbitt R. E. L. Jr., Cuenca V. G., Zhang W., Gordon G. B., et al. The effect of ethanol on the production of lactate, triglycerides, phospholipids, and free fatty acids in the perfused human placenta. *American Journal of Obstetrics and Gynecology 155:*207–211, 1986.

Richardson B. S., Patrick J. E., Bousquet J., Homan J., Brien J. F. Cerebral metabolism in fetal lamb after maternal infusion of ethanol. *American Journal of Physiology 249:*R505, 1985.

Richardson B. S., Patrick J. E., Homan J., Carmichael L., Brien J. Cerebral oxidative metabolism in fetal sheep with multiple-dose ethanol infusion. *American Journal of Obstetrics and Gynecology 157:*1496–1502, 1987.

Richardson G. A., Day N. L., Goldschmidt L. Prenatal alcohol, marijuana, and tobacco use: Infant mental and motor development. *Neurotoxicology and Teratology 17:*479–487, 1995.

Richardson G. A., Day N. L., Taylor P. The effect of prenatal alcohol, marihuana, and tobacco exposure on neonatal behavior. *Infant Behavioral Development 12:*199–209, 1989.

Riekman G. A., Paedo D. Oral findings of fetal alcohol syndrome patients. *Journal of the Canadian Dental Association 11:*841–842, 1984.

Riikonen R. S. Difference in susceptibility to teratogenic effects of alcohol in discordant twins exposed to alcohol during the second half of gestation. *Pediatric Neurology 11:*332–336, 1994.

Robe L. B., Robe R. S., Wilson A. Maternal heavy drinking related to delayed onset of daughters' menstruation. *Alcoholism: Clinical and Experimental Research 3:*192, 1979.

Robertson W. B., Manning P. J. Elastic tissue in uterine blood vessels. *Journal of Pathology 112:*237–243, 1974.

Robinson G. C., Conry R. F. Maternal age and congenital optic nerve hypoplasia: A possible clue to etiology. *Developmental Medicine and Child Neurology 28:*294–298, 1986.

Robinson G. C., Conry J. L., Conry R. F. Clinical profile and prevalence of fetal alcohol syndrome in an isolated community in British Columbia. *Canadian Medical Association Journal 137:*203–207, 1987.

Rockwood G. A., Riley E. P. Suckling deficits in rat pups exposed to alcohol in utero. *Teratology 33:*145–151, 1986.

Ronen G. M., Andrews W. L. Holoprosencephaly as a possible embryonic effect. *American Journal of Medical Genetics 40:*151–154, 1991.

Root A. W., Reiter E. O., Andriola M., Duckett B. S. Hypothalamic pituitary function in the fetal alcohol syndrome. *Journal of Pediatrics 87:*585–588, 1975.

Rose J. C., Meis P. J., Castro M. I. Alcohol and fetal endocrine function. *Neurobehavioral Toxicology and Teratology 3:*105–109, 1981.

Rosett H. L. A clinical perspective of the fetal alcohol syndrome (editorial). *Alcoholism: Clinical and Experimental Research 4:*119–122, 1980.

Rosett H. L., Weiner L. *Alcohol and the Fetus.* New York: Oxford University Press, 1984.

Rosett H. L., Ouellette E. M., Weiner L., Owens E. Therapy of heavy drinking during pregnancy. *Obstetrics and Gynecology 51:*41–46, 1978.

Rosett H. L., Snyder P., Sander L. W., Lee A., Cook P., et al. Effects of maternal drinking on neonate state regulation. *Developmental Medicine and Child Neurology 21:*464–473, 1979.

Rosett H. L., Weiner L., Edelin K. Strategies for prevention of fetal alcohol effects. *Obstetrics and Gynecology 57:*1–7, 1981.

Rosett H. L., Weiner L., Lee A., Zuckerman B., Dooling E., et al. Patterns of alcohol consumption and fetal development. *Obstetrics and Gynecology 61:*539–546, 1983.

Rosett H. L., Weiner L. Zuckerman B., McKinlay S., Edelin E. C. Reduction of alcohol consumption during pregnancy with benefits to the newborn. *Alcoholism: Clinical and Experimental Research 4:*178–184, 1980.

Rossig C., Wasser S. T., Oppermann P. Audiologic manifestations in fetal alcohol syndrome assessed by brainstem auditory-evoked potentials. *Neuropediatrics 25:*245–249, 1994.

Rostand A., Kaminski M., Lelong N., Dehaene P., Delestret I., et al. Alcohol use in pregnancy, craniofacial features, and fetal growth. *Journal of Epidemiology and Community Health 44:*302–306, 1990.

Rubin D. H., Krasilnikoff P. A., Leventhall J. M., Berget A., Weile B. Cigarette Smoking and alcohol consumption during pregnancy by Danish women and their spouses—a potential source of fetal morbidity. *American Journal of Drug and Alcohol Abuse 14:*405–417, 1988.

Rudeen P. K. Effects of fetal ethanol exposure on androgen-sensitive neural differentiation. In Miller M. W. (Ed.), *Development of the Central Nervous System: Effects of Alcohol and Opiates* (pp. 169–188). New York: Wiley-Liss, 1992.

Rudeen P. K., Kappel C. A., Lear K. Postnatal or in utero ethanol exposure reduction of the volume of the sexually dimorphic nucleus of the preoptic area in male rats. *Drug and Alcohol Dependence 18:*247–252, 1986.

Russell M. Intrauterine growth in infants born to women with alcohol-related psychiatric diagnosis. *Alcoholism: Clinical and Experimental Research 1:*225–231, 1977.

Russell M. Clinical implications of recent research on the fetal alcohol syndrome. *Bulletin of the New York Academy of Medicine 67:*207–222, 1991.

Russell M., Bigler L. R. Screening for alcohol-related problems in an outpatient obstetric-gynecologic clinic. *American Journal of Obstetrics and Gynecology 34:*4–12, 1979.

Russell M., Skinner J. B. Early measures of maternal alcohol use as predictors of adverse pregnancy outcomes. *Alcoholism: Clinical and Experimental Research 12:*824–830, 1988.

Russell M., Cowan R., Czarnecki D. Prenatal alcohol exposure and early childhood development. *Alcoholism 11:*225, 1987.

Russell M., Czarneci D. M., Cowan R., McPherson E., Mudar P. J. Measures of maternal alcohol use as predictors of development in early childhood. *Alcoholism: Clinical and Experimental Research 15:*991–1000, 1991.

Salaspuro M. Nutrient intake and nutritional status in alcoholics. *Alcohol and Alcoholism 28:*85–88, 1993.

Sameroff A. J., Seifer R., Baldwin A., Baldwin C. Stability of intelligence from preschool to adolescence: The influence of social and family risk factors. *Child Development 64:*80–97, 1993.

Sampson P. D., Brookstein F. L., Barr H. M., Streissguth A. P. Prenatal alcohol exposure, birthweight, and measures of child size from birth to age 14 years. *American Journal of Public Health 84:*1421–1428, 1994.

SAMHSA (Substance Abuse and Mental Health Service Administration). *National Household Survey on Drug Abuse.* U.S. Department of Health and Human Services, Rockville, MD, 1996.

Samson H. H., Grant K. A. Ethanol-induced microcephaly in neonatal rats: Relation to dose. *Alcoholism: Clinical and Experimental Research 8:*201–203, 1984.

Samson H. H., Waterman D. L., Woods S. C. Effect of acute maternal ethanol exposure upon fetal development in the rat. *Physiological Psychology 7:*311–315, 1979.

Sanchez J., Casas M., Rama R. Effect of chronic ethanol administration on iron metabolism in the rat. *European Journal of Haematology 4:*321–325, 1988.

Sanchis R., Guerri C. Alcohol-metabolizing enzymes in placenta an fetal liver: Effect of chronic ethanol intake. *Alcoholism: Clinical and Experimental Research 10:*39–44, 1986.

Sanchis R., Sancho-Tello M., Chirivella M., Guerri C. The role of maternal alcohol damage on ethanol teratogenicity in the rat. *Teratology 36:*199–208, 1987.

Sanchis R., Sancho-Tello M., Guerri C. The effects of chronic alcohol consumption on pregnant rats and their offspring. *Alcohol and Alcoholism 21:*295–305, 1986.

Sancho-Tello M., Renau-Piqueras J., Baguena-Cervellera R., Guerri C. A biochemical and stereological study of neonatal rat hepatocyte subpopulations. *Virchows Archive Cell Pathology, B54:*170–181, 1987.

Sander L. W., Snyder P. A., Rosett H. L., Lee A., Gould J. B., et al. Effects of alcohol intake during pregnancy on newborn state regulation: A progress report. *Alcoholism: Clinical and Experimental Research 1:*233–234, 1977.

Sandor G. G. S., Smith D. F., Macleod P. M. Cardiac malformations in the fetal alcohol syndrome. *Journal of Pediatrics 98:*771–773, 1981.

Sandstrom L. P., Sandstrom P. A., Pennington S. N. Ethanol-induced insulin resistance suppresses the expression of embryonic ornithine decarboxylase activity. *Alcohol 10:*303–310, 1993.

Sardesai V. M. Biochemical and nutritional aspects of eicosanoids. *Journal of Nutritional Biochemistry 3:*562–579, 1992.

Savage D. D., Reyes E. Prenatal exposure to ethanol retards the development of kindling in adult rats. *Experimental Neurology 89:*583–591, 1985.

Savage D. D., Queen S. A., Sanchez C. F., Paxton L. L., Mahoney J. C., et al. Prenatal ethanol exposure during the last third of gestation in rat reduces hippocampal NMDA agonist-binding site density in 45-day-old offspring. *Alcohol 9:*37–41, 1991.

Savoy-Moore R. T., Dombrowski M. P., Cheng A., Abel E. L., Sokol R. J. Low-dose alcohol contracts the human umbilical artery in vitro. *Alcoholism: Clinical and Experimental Research 13:*40–42, 1989.

Saxen I. Epidemiology of cleft lip and palate. *British Journal of Prevention and Social Medicine 29:*103–110, 1975.

Saywitz S. E., Caparulo B. K., Hodgsen E. S. Developmental language disability as a consequence of perinatal exposure to ethanol. *Pediatrics 68:*850–855, 1981.

Scarpellini F., Sbracia M., Scarpellini L. Psychological stress and lipoperoxidation in miscarriage. *Annals of the New York Academy of Sciences 709:*210–213, 1994.

Schenker S., Dicke J. M., Johnson R. F., Hays S. E., Henderson G. I. Effect of ethanol on human placental transport of model amino acids and glucose. *Alcoholism: Clinical and Experimental Research 13:*112–119, 1989.

Scher M. S., Richardson G. A., Coble P. A., Day N. L., Stoffer D. S. The effects of prenatal alcohol and marijuana exposure: Disturbances in neonatal sleep cycling and arousal. *Pediatric Research 24:*101–105, 1988.

Scholtes G. Liver function and liver diseases during pregnancy. *Journal of Perinatal Medicine 7:* 55–68, 1979.

Schuller H. M., Jorquera R., Reichert A., Castonguay, A. Transplacental induction of pancreas tumors in hamsters by ethanol and tobacco-specific nitrosamine 4-(methylnitrosamino-)-1-(3-pyridyl)-1-butanone. *Cancer Research 53:*2498–2501, 1993.

Schwartz L. M. The role of cell death genes during development. *Bioessays 13:*389–395, 1991.

Schweitzer J. B., Sulzer-Azaroff B. Self-control in boys with attention deficit hyperactivity disorder: Effects of added stimulation and time. *Journal of Child Psychology Psychiatry 36:*671–686, 1995.

Scott W. J. Jr., Fradkin R. The effects of prenatal ethanol in cynomolgus monkeys Macaca fascicularis. *Teratology 29:*49–56, 1984.

Seidenberg J., Majewski F. On the frequency of alcohol embryopathy in the different phases of maternal alcoholism. *Suchtgefahren 24:*63–75, 1978.

Serdula M., Williamson D. F., Kendrick J. S., Anda R. F., Byers T. Trends in alcohol consumption by pregnant women 1985 throughout 1988. *Journal of the American Medical Association 265:*876–879, 1991.

Sever L. E. Looking for causes of neural tube defects: Where does the environment fit in? *Environmental Health Perspectives 103:*165–171, 1995.

Shanske A. L., Kazi R. Prevalence of the fetal alcohol syndrome in a developmental clinic population. *American Journal of Human Genetics 32:*128A (Abstract), 1980.

Shaywitz S. E., Cohen D. J., Shaywitz B. A. Behavior and learning difficulties in children of normal intelligence born to alcoholic mothers. *Journal of Pediatrics 96:*978–982, 1980.

Shiono P. H., Klebanoff M. A., Rhoads G. G. Smoking and drinking during pregnancy: Their effects on preterm birth. *Journal of the American Medical Association 225:*82–84, 1986.

Shurygin G. I. Ob osobennostiiakh psikhicheskogo razvitiia detei ot materei, stradaiuschikh khronicheskim alkogolizmom. (Characteristics of the mental development of children of alcoholic mothers.) *Pediatriia* (Moscow) *11:*71–73, 1974.

Sinervo K. R., Smith G. N., Bocking A. D., Patrick J., Brien J. F. Effect of ethanol on the release of prostaglandins from ovine fetal brain stem during gestation. *Alcoholism: Clinical and Experimental Research 16:*443–448, 1992.

Singh S. P., Snyder A. K., Pullen G. L. Maternal alcohol ingestion inhibits fetal glucose uptake and growth. *Neurotoxicology and Teratology 11:*215–219, 1989.

Singh S. P., Srivenugopal K. S., Ehmann S., Yuan X., Synder A. K. Insulinlike growth factors (IGF-I and IGF-II), IGF binding proteins, and IGF gene expression in the offspring of ethanol-fed rats. *Journal of Laboratory and Clinical Medicine 124:*183–192, 1994.

Siebert J. R., Astley S. J., Clarren S. K. Holoprosencephaly in a fetal macaque (Macaca nemestrina) following weekly exposure to ethanol. *Teratology 44:*29–36, 1991.

Skog O. Public health consequences of the J-curve hypothesis of alcohol problems. *Addiction 91:*325–337, 1996.

Skosyrea A. M. Effect of ethyl alcohol on the development of embryos at the organogenesis stage. *Akusherstvo I Ginekologiia (Moscow) 4:*15–18, 1973.

Smith I. E., Coles C. D., Lancaster J., Fernhoff P. M., Falek A., The effects of volume and duration of prenatal ethanol exposure on neonatal physical and behavioral development. *Neurobehavioral Toxicology and Teratology 8:*375–381, 1986.

Snyder S. K., Jiang F., Singh S. P. Effects of ethanol on glucose utilization by cultured mammalian embryos. *Alcoholism: Clinical and Experimental Research 16:*466–470, 1992.

Snyder S. K., Singh S. P., Pullen G. L. Ethanol-induced intrauterine growth retardation: Correlation with placental glucose transfer. *Alcoholism: Clinical and Experimental Research 10:*167–170, 1986.

Sokol R. J. Alcohol and spontaneous abortion. *Lancet 2:*1079, 1980.

Sokol R. J., Ager J., Martier S., Debanne S., Ernhart C., et al. Significant determinants of susceptibility to alcohol teratogenicity. *Annals of the New York Academy of Sciences 477:*87–102, 1986.

Sokol R. J., Chik L., Martier S. S., Salari V. Morphometry of the neonatal fetal alcohol syndrome face from "snapshots." *Alcohol and Alcoholism 1:*531–534, 1991.

Sokol R. J., Martier S. S., Ager J. W., Jacobson S., Jacobson J. Fetal alcohol syndrome (FAS): New definition, new prospective sample, same etiology. *Alcoholism: Clinical and Experimental Research 17:*260, 1993.

Sokol R. J., Miller S. I., Reed G. Alcohol abuse during pregnancy: An epidemiologic study. *Alcoholism: Clinical and Experimental Research 4:*135–145, 1980.

Sokol R. J., Smith M., Ernhart C. B., Baumann R., Martier S. S., et al. A genetic basis for alcohol-related birth defects (ARBD)? *Alcoholism: Clinical and Experimental Research 13:*343A, 1989.

Song B. J., Gelboin H. V., Park S. S., Yang C. S., Gonzalez F. J. Complementary DNA and protein sequences of ethanol-inducible rat and human cytochrome P-450s: Transcriptional and post-transcriptional regulation of the rat enzyme. *Journal of Biological Chemistry 261:*16689–16697, 1986.

Sorette M. P., Maggio C. A., Starpoli A., Boissevain A., Greenwood M. R. C. Maternal ethanol intake affects rat organ development despite adequate nutrition. *Neurobehavioral Toxicology 2:*181–188, 1980.

Southall D. P., Alexander J. R., Stebbens V. A., Taylor V. G., Janczynski N. E. Cardiorespiratory patterns in siblings of babies with sudden infant death syndrome. *Archives of Disease in Childhood 62:*721–726, 1987.

Sowell E. R., Mattson S. N., Riley E. P., Jernigan T. L. Abnormal development of the cerebellar vermis in children prenatally exposed to alcohol: Size reductions in lobules I–V. *Alcoholism: Clinical and Experimental Research 20:*31–34, 1996.

Sparks J. W., Cetin I. Intrauterine growth and nutrition. In Polin R. A., Fox W. W. (Eds.), *Fetal and Neonatal Physiology* (pp. 179–197). Philadelphia, Pennsylvania: Saunders, 1992.

Sparks S. Speech and language in fetal alcohol syndrome. *Journal of the American Speech and Hearing Association 26:*27–31, 1984.

Spatz L. Introduction. In Spatz L., Bloom A. D. (Eds.), *Biological Consequences of Oxidative Stress* (pp. 3–22). New York: Oxford University Press, 1992.

Spohr H. L. Discussion. In Pratt O. E., Doshik R., Range of alcohol-induced damage in the developing central nervous system. In Ciba Foundation, Mechanisms of Alcohol Damage In Utero, Pittman, London, p. 153, 1984.

Spohr H. L. Fetal alcohol syndrome in adolescence: Long-term perspective of children diagnosed in infancy. In Spohr H. L., Steinhausen H. C. (Eds.), *Alcohol, Pregnancy, and the Developing Child* (pp. 207–226). Cambridge, UK: Cambridge University Press, 1996.

Spohr H. L., Steinhausen H. Follow-up studies of children with fetal alcohol syndrome. *Neuropediatrics 18:*13–17, 1987.

Spohr H. L., Willms J., Steinhausen H. C. Prenatal exposure and long-term developmental consequences. *Lancet 341:*907–910, 1993.

Spohr H. L., Willms J., Steinhausen H. C. The fetal alcohol syndrome in adolescence. *Acta Paediatrica 404:*19–26, 1994.

Streenathan R. N., Singh S., Padmanabhan R. Implication of the placenta in acetaldehyde-induced intrauterine growth retardation. *Drug and Alcohol Dependence 13:*199–204, 1984.

Starshak R. J., Wells R. G., Sty J. R., Gregg D. C. *Diagnostic Imaging of Infants and Children.* Gaithersburg, MD: Aspen Publishing, 1992.

Steinhausen H. C., Spohr H. Fetal alcohol syndrome. *Advances in Clinical Child Psychology 9:*217–243, 1986.

Steinhausen H. C., Godel D., Nestler V. Psychopathology in the offspring of alcoholic patients. *Journal of the American Academy of Child Psychiatry 23:*465–471, 1984.

Steinhausen H. C., Nestler V., Spohr H. L. Development and psychopathology of children with the fetal alcohol syndrome. *Developmental and Behavioral Pediatrics 3:*49–54, 1982.

Stephens C. J. Alcohol consumption during pregnancy among Southern city women. *Drug and Alcohol Dependence 16:*19–29, 1985.

Stock D. L., Streissguth A. P., Martin D. C. Neonatal sucking as an outcome variable: comparison of quantitative and clinical assessments. *Early Human Development 10:*273–278, 1985.

Stockwell T. R., Lang E., Lewis P. N. Is wine the drink of moderation? *Medical Journal of Australia 162:*578–581, 1995.

Stoffer D. S., Scher M. S., Richardson G. A. A Walsh-Fourier analysis of the effects of moderate maternal alcohol consumption on neonatal sleep-state cycling. *Journal of American Statistical Association 83:*954–963, 1988.

Stoltenburg-Didinger G., Spohr H. L. Fetal alcohol syndrome and mental retardation: Spine distribution of pyramidal cells in pregnant alcohol-exposed rat cerebral cortex: A Golgi study. *Developmental Brain Research 11:*119–123, 1983.

Streissguth A. P. Fetal alcohol syndrome: Early and long-term consequences. In Harris L. (Ed.), *Problems of Drug Dependence 1991: Proceedings of the 53rd Annual Scientific Meeting* (pp. 129–130). Rockville, Maryland: U.S. Department of Health and Human Services, 1992.

Streissguth A. P. Fetal alcohol syndrome: Understanding the problem, understanding the solution; what Indian communities can do. *American Indian Cultural Research Journal 18:*45–83, 1994.

Streissguth A. P., Dehaene P. Fetal alcohol syndrome in twins of alcoholic mothers: Concordance of diagnosis and IQ. *American Journal of Medical Genetics 47:*857–861, 1993.

Streissguth A. P., Giunta C. T. Mental health and health needs of infants and preschool children with fetal alcohol syndrome. *International Journal of Family Psychiatry 9:*29–47, 1988.

Streissguth A. P., Martin J. C. Prenatal effects of alcohol abuse in humans and laboratory animals. In Kissin B., Begleiter H. (Eds.), *The Pathogenesis of Alcoholism* (Vol. 7, pp. 539–589). New York: Plenum Publishing, 1983.

Streissguth A. P., Randels S. Long-term effects of fetal alcohol syndrome. In Robinson G. C., Armstrong R. W. (Eds.), *Alcohol and Child/Family Health* (pp. 135–150). Vancouver, British Columbia: University of British Columbia, 1988.

Streissguth A. P., Aase J. M., Clarren S. K., Randels S. P., LaDue R. A., et al. Fetal alcohol syndrome in adolescents and adults. *Journal of American Medical Association 265:*1961–1967, 1991.

Streissguth A. P., Barr H. M., Carmichael Olson H., Sampson P. D., Brookstein F. L., et al. Drinking during pregnancy decreases word attack and arithmetic scores on standardized tests: Adolescent data from a population-based prospective study. *Alcoholism: Clinical and Experimental Research 18:*248–254, 1994a.

Streissguth A. P., Barr H. M., Martin D. C. Maternal alcohol use and neonatal habituation assessed with the Brazelton Scale. *Child Development 54:*1109–1118, 1983a.

Streissguth A. P., Barr H. M., Martin D. C., Herman C. S. Effects of maternal alcohol, nicotine, and caffeine use during pregnancy on infant mental and motor development at 8 months. *Alcoholism: Clinical and Experimental Research 4:*152–164, 1980.

Streissguth A. P., Barr H. M., Sampson P. D. Moderate prenatal alcohol exposure: Effects on child IQ and learning problems at age 7½ years. *Alcoholism: Clinical and Experimental Research 14:* 461–476, 1990.

Streissguth A. P., Barr H. M., Sampson P. D., Brookstein, F. L. Prenatal alcohol and offspring development: The first fourteen years. *Drug Alcohol Dependence 36:*89–99, 1994b.

Streissguth A. P., Barr H. M., Sampson P. D., Brookstein F. L., Darby B. L. Neurobehavioral effects of prenatal alcohol: Part I. Research strategy. *Neurotoxicology Teratology 11:*461– 479, 1989a.

Streissguth A. P., Barr H. M., Scott M., Feldman J., Mirsky A. F. Maternal drinking during pregnancy: Attention and short-term memory in 14-year-old offspring—a longitudinal prospective study. *Alcoholism: Clinical and Experimental Research 18:*202–218, 1994c.

Streissguth A. P., Brookstein F. L., Sampson P. D., Barr H. M. The Enduring Effects of Prenatal Alcohol Exposure on Child Development, Birth Through 7 Years: A Partial Least Squares Solution. Ann Arbor, Michigan: University of Michigan Press, 1993.

Streissguth A. P., Brookstein F. L., Sampson P. D., Barr H. M. Neurobehavioral effects of prenatal alcohol: Part III. PLS analyses of neuropsychologic tests. *Neurotoxicological Teratology 11:*493–507, 1989b.

Streissguth A. P., Clarren S. K., Jones K. L. Natural history of the fetal alcohol syndrome: A ten-year follow-up of eleven patients. *Lancet 2:*85–91, 1985.

Streissguth A. P., Darby B. L., Barr H. M., Smith J. R., Martin D. C. Comparison of drinking and smoking patterns during pregnancy over a six-year interval. *American Journal of Obstetrics and Gynecology 145:*716–724, 1983b.

Streissguth A. P., Herman C. S., Smith D. W. Intelligence, behavior, and dysmorphogenesis in the fetal alcohol syndrome: A report on 20 patients. *Journal of Pediatrics 92:*363–367, 1978a.

Streissguth A. P., Herman C. S., Smith D. W. Stability of intelligence in the fetal alcohol syndrome: A preliminary report. *Alcoholism: Clinical and Experimental Research 2:*165–170, 1978b.

Streissguth A. P., LaDue R. A., Randelsk S. P. Indian adolescents and adults with fetal alcohol syndrome: Findings and recommendations. *IHS Primary Care Provider 12:*89–91, 1987.

Streissguth A. P., Martin D. C., Buffington V. E. Identifying heavy drinkers: A comparison of eight alcohol scores obtained on the sample. In Sexias F. A. (Ed.), *Currents in Alcoholism* (pp. 395–420). New York: Grune & Stratton, 1977.

Streissguth A. P., Martin D. C., Martin J. C., Barr H. M. The Seattle longitudinal prospective study on alcohol and pregnancy. *Neurobehavioral Toxicology and Teratology 3:*223–233, 1981.

Streissguth A. P., Sampson P. D., Carmichael-Olson H., Brookstein F. L., Barr H. M., et al. Maternal drinking during pregnancy: Attention and short-term memory in 14-year-old offspring—a longitudinal prospective study. *Alcoholism: Clinical and Experimental Research 18:*202–218, 1994d.

Stromland K. Ocular abnormalities in the fetal alcohol syndrome. *Acta Ophthalmologica 171:*63, 1985.

Stromland K. Contribution of ocular examination to the diagnosis of foetal alcohol syndrome in mentally retarded children. *Journal of Mental Deficiency Research 34:*429–435, 1990.

Stuckey E., Berry C. L. The effects of high-dose sporadic (binge) alcohol intake in mice. *Journal of Pathology 142:*175–180, 1984.

Sulaiman N. D., Florey C. du V., Taylor D. J., Ogston S. A. Alcohol consumption in Dundee primigravidas and its effects on outcome of pregnancy. *British Medical Journal 296:*1500–1503, 1988.

Sulik K. K., Cook C. S., Webster W. S. Teratogens and craniofacial malformations: Relationship to cell death. *Development 103:*213–232, 1988.

Sulik K. K., Johnston M. C. Sequence of developmental alterations following acute ethanol exposure in mice: Craniofacial features of the fetal alcohol syndrome. *American Journal of Anatomy 166:*257–262, 1983.

Sulik K. K., Johnston M. C., Webb M. A. Fetal alcohol syndrome embryogenesis in a mouse model. *Science 214:*936–938, 1981.

Sullivan P. F., Wells J. E., Bushnell J. A. Adoption as a risk factor for mental disorders. *Acta Psychiatrica Scandinavica 92:*119–124, 1995.

Sullivan W. C. A note on the influence of maternal inebriety on the offspring. *Journal of Mental Science 45:*489–503, 1899.

Tanaka H., Arima H., Ishizuka H., Suzuki N., Takashima H. Fetal alcohol syndrome in Japan. *Japanese Medical Journal 2897:*27–30, 1979.

Tanaka H., Iwasaki S., Nakazawa K., Inomata K. Fetal alcohol syndrome in rats: Conditions for improvements of ethanol effects on fetal cerebral development with supplementary agents. *Biology of the Neonate 54:*320, 1988.

Taylor A. N., Branch B. J., Van Zuylen J. E., Redei E. Prenatal ethanol exposure alters ACTH stress response in adult rats. *Alcoholism: Clinical and Experimental Research 10:*120, 1986.

Taylor A. N., Branch B. J., Van Zuylen J. E., Redei E. Maternal alcohol consumption and stress responsiveness in offspring. *Advances in Experimental Medicine and Biology 245:*311–347, 1988.

Taylor C. L., Jones K. L., Jones M. C., Kaplan G. W. Incidence of renal anomalies in children prenatally exposed to ethanol. *Pediatrics 94:*209–212, 1994.

Tennes K., Blackard C. Maternal alcohol consumption, birth weight, and minor physical anomalies. *American Journal of Obstetrics and Gynecology 138:*774–780, 1980.

Thanassi N. M., Rokowski R. J., Sheehy J., Hart B., Absher M., et al. Non-selective decrease of collagen synthesis by cultured fetal lung fibroblasts after non-lethal doses of ethanol. *Biochemical Pharmacology 29:*2417–2424, 1980.

Thomas I. T., Hintz R. J., Frias J. L. New methods for quantitative and qualitative facial studies: An overview. *Journal of Craniofacial Genetics and Developmental Biology 9:*107–111, 1989.

Thomasson H. R., Crabb D. W., Edenberg H. J., Li T.-K. Alcohol and aldehyde dehydrogenase polymorphisms and alcoholism. *Behavior Genetics 23:*131–136, 1993.

Tillner I., Majewski F. Furrows and derman ridges of the hand in patients with alcohol embrhyopathy. *Human Genetics 42:*307–314, 1978.

Tolo K. A., Little R. E. Occasional binges by moderate drinkers: Implications for birth outcomes. *Epidemiology 4:*415–420, 1993.

Tritt S. H., Tio D. L., Brammer G. L., Taylor A. N. Adrenalectomy but not adrenal demodulation during pregnancy prevents the growth-retarding effects of fetal alcohol exposure. *Alcoholism: Clinical and Experimental Research 17:*1281–1289, 1993.

Ulleland C. N. The offspring of alcoholic mothers. *Annals of the New York Academy of Sciences 197:*167–169, 1972.

Ulug S., Riley E. P. The effects of methylphenidate on open-field behavior in rats exposed to alcohol prenatally. *Neurobehavioral Toxicology 5:*35–39, 1983.

University of Michigan Alcohol Research Center. *Drink/Drive Calculator.* Ann Arbor, Michigan: Author, n.d.

Urfer F. N., Fouron J. C., Bard H., DeMuylder X. Low levels of blood alcohol and fetal myocardial function. *Obstetrics and Gynecology 63:*401–404, 1984.

U.S. Department of Commerce, Bureau of Census. *Statistical Abstract of the United States, 1993.* Washington, DC: U.S. Government Printing Office, 1993.

U.S. Department of Health and Human Services, Centers for Disease Control and Prevention. Advance report of final natality statistics, 1990. *Monthly Vital Statistics Report 41:*1–51, 1993.

VandenBerg B. J. Epidemiologic observations of prematurity: Effects of tobacco, coffee, and alcohol. In Reed D. M., Stanley F. J. (Eds.), *The Epidemiology of Prematurity* (pp. 157–176). Baltimore, Maryland: Urban & Schwarzenberg, 1977.

Van Dyke D. C., Mackay L., Ziaylek E. N. Management of severe feeding dysfunction in children with fetal alcohol syndrome. *Clinical Pediatrics 21:*336–339, 1982.

Veghelyi P. V., Osztovics M. The alcohol syndromes: The intrarecombinegic effect of acetaldehyde. *Experientia 34:*195–196, 1978.

Verkerk P. H., van Noord-Zaadstra F., Florey du V. C., de Jonge G. A., Verloove-Vanhorick S. P. The effect of moderate maternal alcohol consumption on birth weight and gestational age in a low risk population. *Early Human Development 32:*121–129, 1993.

Vingan R. D., Dow-Edwards D. L., Riley E. P. Cerebral metabolic alterations in rats following prenatal alcohol exposure: A deoxyglucose study. *Alcoholism: Clinical and Experimental Research 10:*22–26, 1986.

Virji S. K. The relationship between alcohol consumption during pregnancy and infant birth weight. *Acta Obstetrica et Gynecologica Scandinavica 70:*303–308, 1991.

Vitez M., Czeizel E. Az iszakos-alkoholista nok termekenysege (On Fetal alcohol syndrome). *Alkohologia 13:*79–83, 1982.

Vitez M., Koranyi G., Gonczy E., Rudas T., Czeizel A. A semiquantitative score system for epidemiological studies of fetal alcohol syndrome. *American Journal of Epidemiology 119:*301–308, 1984.

Vorhees C. V., Rauch S., Hitzermaun R. Effects of short-term prenatal alcohol exposure on neuronal membrane order in rats. *Developmental Brain Research 38:*161–166, 1988.

Wainwright P. E., Huang Y. S., Mills D. E., Ward G. R., McCutcheon D. Interactive effects of prenatal ethanol and n-3 fatty acid supplementation on brain development in mice. *Lipids 24:*989–997, 1989.

Wainwright P. E., Huang Y. S., Simmons V., Mills D. E., Ward R. P., et al. Effects of prenatal ethanol and long chain n-3 fatty acid supplementation on development in mice: 2. Fatty acid composition of brain membrane phospholipds. *Alcoholism: Clinical and Experimental Research 14:*413–420, 1990.

Wainwright P. E., Ward G. R., Blom K. Combined effects of moderate ethanol consumption and low protein diet during gestation on brain development in BALB/c mice. *Experimental Neurology 90:*422–433, 1985.

Walker D. W., Lee N., Heaton M. B., King M. A., Hunter B. E. Chronic ethanol consumption reduces the neurotrophic activity in rat hippocampus. *Neuroscience Letters 147:*77–80, 1992.

Walpole I. R., Aubrick S., Pontré J., Lawrence C. Low to moderate alcohol use before and during pregnancy and neurobehavioral outcome in the newborn infant. *Developmental Medicine and Child Neurology 33:*875–883, 1991.

Walpole I. R., Hoclig A. Fetal alcohol syndrome: Implications to family and society in Australia. *Australian Paediatric Journal 16:*101–105, 1980.

Walpole I. R., Zubrick S., Pontré J. Confounding variables in studying the effects of maternal alcohol consumption before and during pregnancy. *Journal of Epidemiology and Community Health 43:*153–161, 1989.

Walpole I. R., Zubrick S., Pontré J. Is there a fetal effect with low to moderate alcohol use before or during pregnancy? *Journal of Epidemiology and Community Health 44:*297–301, 1990.

Ward I. L., Ward O. B. Sexual behavior differentiation: Effects of prenatal manipulation in rats. In Adler N. A., Pfaff D., Goy R. W. (Eds.), *Handbook of Behavioral Neurobiology* (pp. 77–98). New York: Plenum Press, 1985.

Ward I. L., Ward O. B., Winn R. J., Bielawski D. Male and female sexual behavior potential of male rats prenatally exposed to the influence of alcohol, stress, or both factors. *Behavioral Neuroscience 108:*1188–1195, 1994.

Ward R. E. Facial morphology as determined by anthropometry: Keeping it simple. *Journal of Craniofacial Genetics and Developmental Biology 9:*45–60, 1989.

Warren R. C., Hahn R. A., Bristow L., Yu E. S. H. The use of race and ethnicity in public health surveillance. *Public Health Reports 109:*1–6, 1994.

Washington State Council on Crime and Delinquency. *Fetal Alcohol Syndrome and Effects: Implications for Criminal and Juvenile Justice.* Seattle, Washington, 1991.

Waterson E. J., Murray-Lyon I. M. Drinking and smoking patterns amongst women attending an antenatal clinical: II. Drinking pregnancy. *Alcohol and Alcoholism 24:*163–173, 1989.

Watzl B., Lopez M., Shahbozian M., Chen G., Columbo L. L., et al. Diet and ethanol modulate immune responses in young $C_{57}Bl/6J$ mice. *Alcoholism: Clinical and Experimental Research 17:*623–630, 1993

Webb S., Hochberg M. S., Sher M. R. Fetal alcohol syndrome—report of case. *Journal of the American Dental Association 116:*196–198, 1988.

Webster W. S., Germain M. A., Lipson A., Walsh D. Alcohol and congenital heart defects: An experimental study in mice. *Cardiovascular Research 18:*335–338, 1984.

Webster W. S., Walsh D. A., McEwèn S. E., Lipson A. H. Some teratogenic properties of ethanol and acetaldehyde in $C_{57}Bl/6J$ mice: Implications for the study of the fetal alcohol syndrome. *Teratology 27:*231–243, 1983.

Wegman M. E. Annual summary of vital statistics—1986. *Pediatrics 80:*817–827, 1987.

Weinberg J. Hyperresponsiveness to stress: Differential effects of prenatal ethanol on males and females. *Alcoholism: Clinical and Experimental Research 12:*647–652, 1988.

Weinberg J. Nutritional issues in perinatal alcohol exposure. *Neurobehavioral Toxicology and Teratology 6:*261–269, 1984.

Weinberg J. Prenatal ethanol effects: Sex differences in offspring stress responsiveness. *Alcohol 9:*219–223, 1992.

Weinberg J., Jerrells T. Suppression of immune responsiveness: Sex differences in prenatal ethanol effects. *Alcoholism: Clinical and Experimental Research 15:*525–531, 1991.

Weinberg J., Petersen T. D. Effects of prenatal ethanol exposure on glucocorticoid receptors in rat hippocampus. *Alcoholism: Clinical and Experimental Research 15:*711–716, 1991.

Weiner L., Rosett H. L., Edelin K. C., Alpert J. J., Zuckerman B. Alcohol consumption by pregnant women. *Obstetrics and Gynecology 61:*6–12, 1983.

Weiner S. G., Shoemaker W. J., Koda L. Y., Bloom F. E. Interaction of ethanol and nutrition during gestation: Influences on maternal and offspring development in the rat. *Journal of Pharmacology and Experimental Therapeutics 216:*572–579, 1981.

Werler M. M., Lammer E. J., Rosenberg L., Mitchell A. A. Maternal alcohol use in relation to selected birth defects. *American Journal of Epidemiology 134:*691–698, 1991.

West J. R., Goodlett C. R., Bonthius D. J., Hamre K. M., Marcussen B. L. Cell population depletion associated with fetal alcohol brain damage: Mechanisms of BAC-dependent cell loss. *Alcoholism Clinical and Experimental Research 14:*813–818, 1990.

West J. R., Hamre K. M., Cassell M. D. Effects of ethanol exposure during the third trimester equivalent on neuron number in rat hippocampus and dentate gyrus. *Alcoholism: Clinical and Experimental Research 10:*190–197, 1986.

West J. R., Hamre K. M., Pierce D. R. Delay in brain growth induced by alcohol in artificially reared rat pups. *Alcohol 1:*213–222, 1984.

West J. R., Hodges C. A., Black A. C. Prenatal exposure to ethanol alters the organization of hippocampal mossy fibers in rat. *Science 211:*957–959, 1981.

West J. R., Kelly S. J., Pierce D. R. Severity of alcohol-induced deficits in rats during the third trimester equivalent is determined by the pattern of exposure. *Alcohol and Alcoholism 1:*461–465, 1987.

Williams D. R., Lavizzu-Mourey R., Warren R. C. The concept of race and health status in America. *Public Health Reports 109:*26–41, 1994.

Wilsnack S. C., Klassen A. D., Wilsnack R. W. Drinking and reproductive dysfunction among women in a 1981 national survey. *Alcoholism: Clinical and Experimental Research 8:*451–458, 1984.

Windham G. C., Fenster L., Swan S. H. Moderate maternal and paternal alcohol consumption and the risk of spontaneous abortion. *Epidemiology 3:*364–370, 1992.

Wisniewski K., Dambska M., Sher J. H., Qazi Q. A clinical neuropathological study of the fetal alcohol syndrome. *Neuropediatrics 14:*197–201, 1983.

Witek-Janusek L. Maternal ethanol ingestion: Effect on maternal and neonatal glucose balance. *American Journal of Physiology 251:*178–184, 1986.

Woessner J. F. Age-related changes in the human uterus and its connective tissue framework. *Journal of Gerontology 18:*220–226, 1963.

Wolcott R. M., Jennings S. R., Chervenak R. In utero exposure to ethanol affects postnatal development of T- and B-lymphocytes, but not natural killer cells. *Alcoholism: Clinical and Experimental Research 19:*170–176, 1995.

Wong C. M. K., Chiapelli F., Chang M. P., Norman D. C., Cooper E. L., et al. Prenatal exposure to alcohol enhances thymocyte mitogenic responses postnatally. *International Journal of Immunopharmacology 14:*303–309, 1992.

Wood R. E. Fetal alcohol syndrome: Its implications for dentistry. *Journal of the American Dental Association 95:*596–599, 1977.

Woodrich D. L. *Attention Deficit Hyperactivity Disorder: What Every Parent Wants to Know.* Baltimore, Maryland: P. H. Brookes Publishing, 1994.

Wooten M. W., Ewald, S. J. Alcohols synergize with NGF to induce early differentiation of PC_{12} cells. *Brain Research 550:*333–339, 1991.

Wright J. T., Waterson E. J., Barrison I. G., Toplis P. J., Lewis I. G., et al. Alcohol consumption, pregnancy, and low birth weight. *Lancet 1:*663–665, 1983.

Wunderlich S. M., Baliga B. S., Munro H. N. Rat placental protein synthesis and peptide hormone secretion in relation to malnutrition protein deficiency or alcohol administration. *Journal of Nutrition 109:*1534–1541, 1979.

Wynter J. M., Walsh D. A., Webster W. S., McEwen S. E., Lipson A. H. Teratogenesis after acute alcohol exposure in cultured rat embryos. *Teratogenesis Carcinogenesis and Mutagenesis 3:*421–428, 1983.

Yamamoto M., Toguchi M., Arishima K., Eguchi Y., Leichter J., et al. Effect of maternal alcohol consumption on fetal thyroid in the rat. *Proceedings of the Society for Experimental Biology and Medicine 191:*382–386, 1989.

Yazdani M., Fonteriat F., Gottschalk S. B., Kanemaw Y., Joseph F., et al. Relationship of prenatal caffeine exposure and zinc supplementation on fetal rat brain growth. *Developmental Pharmacology and Therapeutics 18:*108–115, 1992.

Yazdani M., Joseph F., Grant S., Hartman A. D., Nakamoto T. Various levels of maternal caffeine ingestion during gestation affects biochemical parameters of fetal rat brain differently. *Developmental Pharmacology and Therapeutics 14:*52–61, 1991.

Yirmiya R., Pilati M. L., Chiappelli F., Taylor A. N. Fetal alcohol exposure attenuates lipopolysaccharide-induced fever in rats. *Alcoholism: Clinical and Experimental Research 17:*906–910, 1993.

Yla-Outinen A., Tuimala R. The effect of moderate alcohol consumption during pregnancy in the birth weight and early outcome of the infant. *Upsala Journal of Medical Science 89:*16, 1984.

Zagorul'ko A. K., Fisik E. E., Tikus E. N. Effect of alcohol poisoning during pregnancy on the lung surfactant system of newborn rats. *Biulleten Eksperimentalnui Biologie i meditsinz 110:*142–144, 1990; UDC *616:*1031–1034, 1991.

Zeeman-Polderman M. Drinking behavior of various population segments in western countries: Differences and trends. *Alcohol Digest 13:*1–3, 1994.

Zelson C. Acute management of neonatal addiction. *Addiction Disease 2:*159–168, 1975.

Zidenberg-Cherr S., Benak P. A., Hurley L. S., Keen C. L. Altered mineral metabolism: A mechanism underlying the fetal alcohol syndrome. *Drug and Nutrient Interactions 5:*257–274, 1988.

Zigler E., Cascione R. Mental retardation: An overview. In Gollin E. G. (Ed.), *Malformations of Development* (pp. 69–94). New York: Academic Press, 1984.

Zimmerberg B., Scalzi L. V. Commissural size in neonatal rats: Effects of sex and prenatal alcohol exposure. *International Journal of Developmental Neuroscience 7:*81–86, 1989.

Zimmerberg B., Carson E. A., Kaplan L. J., Zuniga J. A., True R. C. Role of noradrenergic innervation of brown adipose tissue in thermoregulatory deficits following prenatal alcohol exposure. *Alcoholism: Clinical and Experimental Research 17:*418–422, 1993.

Zuckerman B. S., Bauchner H., Parker S., Cabral H. Maternal depressive symptoms during pregnancy and newborn irritability. *Developments in Behavioral Pediatrics 11:*190–194, 1990.

Zuckerman B. S., Frank D., Hingson R., Amaro H., Levenson S. M., et al. Effects of maternal marijuana and cocaine use on fetal growth. *New England Journal of Medicine 320:*762–768, 1989.

Zuckerman B. S., Hingson R. Alcohol consumption during pregnancy: A critical review. *Developmental Medicine and Child Neurology 28:*649–661, 1986.

Index